W0050652

THE HEART IN HYPERTENSION

II

DEVELOPMENTS IN CARDIOVASCULAR MEDICINE

Volume 98

The Heart in Hypertension

A Tribute to Robert Tarazi (1925–1986)

edited by

M.E. Safar

Department of Internal Medicine and Hypertension Research Center, Broussais Hospital, Paris, France

and

F. Fouad-Tarazi

Cleveland Clinic Foundation, Cleveland, Ohio, USA

KLUWER ACADEMIC PUBLISHERS

DORDRECHT / BOSTON / LONDON

Library of Congress Cataloging-in-Publication Data

The Heart in Hypertension: a tribute to Robert Tarazi (1925–1986)/
edited by M.E. Safar, F. Fouad-Tarazi.
    p.   cm. – (Developments in cardiovascular medicine; v. 98)
Includes bibliographies.
1. Hypertension – Congresses. 2. Hemodynamics – Congresses.
3. Heart – Pathophysiology – Congresses. 4. Tarazi, Robert C. – Congresses.
I. Tarazi, Robert C. II. Safar, Michel. III. Fouad-Tarazi, F. IV. Series.
[DNLM: 1. Cardiac Output. 2. Coronary Circulation. 3. Heart – physiopathology.
4. Heart Enlargement – drug therapy. 5. Hypertension – complications.
W1 DE997VME / WG 340 H4362] RC685.H8H43 1989
616.1'32 – dc19
DNLM/DLC
for Library of Congress   89-2460

ISBN-13: 978-94-010-6913-7   e-ISBN-13: 978-94-009-0941-0
DOI: 10.1007/ 978-94-009-0941-0

Published by Kluwer Academic Publishers,
P.O. Box 17, 3300 AA Dordrecht, The Netherlands

Kluwer Academic Publishers incorporates
the publishing programmes of
D. Reidel, Martinus Nijhoff, Dr W. Junk and MTP Press.

Sold and distributed in the U.S.A. and Canada
by Kluwer Academic Publishers,
101 Philip Drive, Norwell, MA 02061, U.S.A.

In all other countries, sold and distributed
by Kluwer Academic Publishers Group,
P.O. Box 322, 3300 AH Dordrecht, The Netherlands.

printed on acid free paper

All rights reserved

© 1989 by Kluwer Academic Publishers
Softcover reprint of the hardcover 1st edition 1989

No part of the material protected by this copyright notice may be reproduced or utilized in any
form or by any means, electronic or mechanical, including photocopying, recording or by any
information storage and retrieval system, without written permission from the copyright owner.

Robert C. Tarazi was one of the pioneers of the hemodynamics of Hypertension. He was fond of clinical research and knew the inherent dificulties of this speciality. However, as the great French novelist Albert Camus, he could say on clinical research:

'Quand j'habitais ma ville natale, je patientais toujours dans l'hiver parce que je savais qu'en une nuit, une seule nuit froide et pure de février, les amandiers de la vallée des Consuls se couvriraient de fleurs blanches.'

(L'Eté/Les Amandiers, Essais,
Edition 'Bibliothèque de la Pleïade',
Paris, Gallimard, 1965, p. 836)

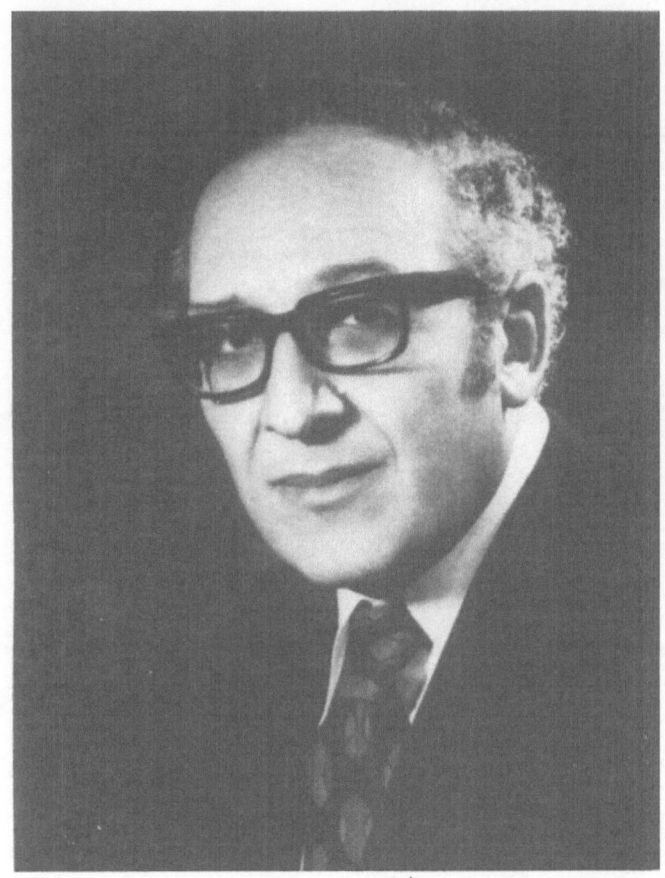

ROBERT CONSTANTIN TARAZI, M.B., B.Ch., M.D. (1925–1986)

Robert Tarazi was born in Cairo in 1925. Following his medical training at Cairo University Hospital, he became head of the Cardiovascular Laboratory at Cairo University Faculty of Medicine in 1960.

From his initial affiliation with the Cleveland Clinic in 1965, he became a member of staff and finally Chairman of the Department of Clinical Science in 1978. From 1974–78 he was also Associate Professor of Medicine at the Case Western Reserve University, School of Medicine in Cleveland, Ohio. Throughout his career, Robert Tarazi received high international acclaim for his work and many publications in the field of cardiovascular research and specifically that pertaining to the heart and hypertension.

Table of contents

CONCLUSION

List of contributors

Agabiti-Rosei, E., Clinical Medica Generale e Terapia Medica, Università degli Studi di Brescia, 25100 Brescia, Italy

Alicandri, C.L., Clinical Medica Generale e Terapia Medica, Università degli Studi di Brescia, 25100 Brescia, Italy

Ayobe, M.H., Physiology Department, Faculty of Medicine, Ain Shams University, Abassia Cairo, Egypt

Birkenhäger, W.H., Erasmus University, Rotterdam, The Netherlands

Bravo, E.L., Cleveland Clinic Foundation, 9500 Euclid Avenue, Cleveland, OH 44195 5071, USA

Bumpus, F.M., Cleveland Clinic Foundation, 9500 Euclid Avenue, Cleveland, OH 44195 5071, USA

Carlier, P.G., Laboratoire de Biochemie Générale et Comparée, Université de L'Etat à Liège, 17 Place Delcour, B-4000 Liège, Belgium

Chaignon, M., Service de Néphrologie, Hôpital Foch, 40 rue Worth, 92151 Suresnes, France

Chobanian, A.V., Cardiovascular Institute, Boston University School of Medicine, Boston, MA 02118, USA

Cody, J., Division of Cardiology, The Ohio State University Hospitals, Columbus, OH 43210, USA

Conway, J., Department of Cardiovascular Medicine, John Radcliffe Hospital, Headington, Oxford, UK

Cuche, J.L., U 228 et Laboratoire de Pharmacologie, Faculté Broussais – Hôtel-Dieu, 2 rue de l'Ecole de Médecine, Paris VI, France

Dustan, H.P., Birmingham VA Medical Center, 700 South 19th Street, Birmingham, AL 35233, USA

Egan, B.M., Division of Hypertension, Department of Internal Medicine, Medical College of Wisconsin, Milwaukee, WI 53226, USA

Estafanous, F.G., Cleveland Clinic Foundation, 9500 Euclid Avenue, Cleveland, OH 44195-5071, USA

Ferrari, A.U., Centro di Fisiologia Clinica e Ipertensione dell'Università di Milano, Via Francesco Sforza 35, 20122 Milano, Italy

Fouad-Tarazi, F.M., Cleveland Clinic Foundation, 9500 Euclid Avenue, Cleveland, OH 44195-5071, USA

Frohlich, E.D., Alton Ochsner Medical Foundation, 1516 Jefferson Highway, New Orleans, LA 70121, USA

Gifford, R.W., Department of Hypertension and Nephrology, The Cleveland Clinic Foundation, 9500 Euclid Avenue, Cleveland, OH 44195-5071, USA

Guazzi, M.D., Istituto di Cardiologia, Via Bonfadini 214, 20138 Milano, Italy

Guédon, J., Service de Néphrologie, Hôpital Foch, 40 rue Worth, 92151 Suresnes, France

Hoffman, J.I.E., Cardiovascular Research Institute, University of California, San Francisco, CA 94143-0130, USA

Ibrahim, M.M., 1, Cardiac Department, Cairo University, Cairo, Egypt

Julius, S., Division of Hypertension, Department of Internal Medicine, The University of Michigan Medical Center, Ann Arbor, Michigan, USA

Korner, P.I., Baker Medical Research Institute, Commercial Road, Prahran, Vic. 3181, Australia

Liard, J.F., Department of Physiology, The Medical College of Wisconsin, 8701 Watertown Plank Road, Milwaukee, WI 53226, USA

London, G.M., Service d'Hémodialyse, Hôpital F.H. Manhès, 8 Grande Rue, 91000 Fleury-Mérogis, France

Lund-Johansen, P., Section of Cardiology, Medical Department, Haukeland Sykehus, 5021 Bergen, Norway

Magrini, F., Centro di Fisiologia Clinica e Ipertensione dell'Università di Milano, Via Francesco Sforza 35, 20122 Milano, Italy

Mancia, G., Centro di Fisiologia Clinica e Ipertensione dell'Università di Milano, Via Francesco Sforza 35, 20122 Milano, Italy

Muiesan, G., Clinical Medica Generale e Terapia Medica, Università degli Studi di Brescia, 25100 Brescia, Italy

Omvik, P., Section of Cardiology, Medical Department, Haukeland Sykehus, 5021 Bergen, Norway

Onoyama, K., 2nd Department of Internal Medicine, Faculty of Medicine, Kyushu University, Maidashi 3, Higashi-Ku, Fukuoka City, 812 Japan

Pedrinelli, R., Hypertension Unit, Clinica Medica, University of Pisa, 56100 Pisa, Italy

Pfeffer, A., Harvard Medical School, Brigham and Women's Hospital, Boston, MA 02118, USA

Reisin, E., Alton Ochsner Medical Foundation, 1516 Jefferson Highway, New Orleans, LA 70121, USA

Rorive, G.L., Laboratoire de Biochemie Générale et Comparée, Université de L'Etat à Liège, 17 Place Delcour, B-4000 Liège, Belgium

Safar, M.E., Service de Médecine 1 et Centre de Recherche de l'Hypertension Arterielle, Hôpital Broussais, 96 rue Didot, 75014 Paris, France

Sen, S., Department of Heart and Hypertension Research, Cleveland Clinic Foundation, 9500 Euclid Avenue, Cleveland, OH 44195-5071, USA

Smelten, N.S., Laboratoire de Biochemie Générale et Comparée, Université de L'Etat à Liège, 17 Place Delcour, B-4000 Liège, Belgium

Weiss, Y.A., Service de Médecine Interne, Centre Hospitalier de Meaux, 6 rue St Fiacre, 77104 Paris, France

Wicker, P., Cleveland Clinic Foundation, 9500 Euclid Avenue, Cleveland, OH 44195-5071, USA

Zanchetti, A., Centro di Fisiologia Clinica e Ipertensione dell'Università di Milano, Via Francesco Sforza 35, 20122 Milano, Italy

INTRODUCTION

A tribute to Robert C. Tarazi, M.D. (1925–1986)

Dr. Robert C. Tarazi was a dedicated clinician, scientist and scholar. My close association with Bob for two decades gave many opportunities to share his great ability to apply the results of basic hypertension research on a clinical problem. His vast experience in cardiology allowed him to establish more firmly the role of the heart in hypertensive disease. He possessed the skill of understanding the physiology of the heart and the vascular system, had vast pleasure in working in this field and was most happy when investigating the adaptive mechanisms controlling the cardiovascular system in health and in disease. In 1969, he introduced the idea of the importance of hypertension in altering the diastolic function of the left ventricle. Later on, in 1980, he revived this idea when non-invasive radioneuclide indices of diastolic function became available. The changes in the left ventricle in hypertension occupied a great deal of his scientific worries not only in terms of their effects on cardiac function but also in terms of their influence on the peripheral vasculature. He stated that 'the heart is not only a sufferer of hypertension but also it may induce hypertension'. This interest did not stop at the descriptive level of what occurs in relation to the diseased heart but Dr. Tarazi aimed at reversing these changes. His studies with Dr. Sen in the rat model were extended to man and opened the field for a new aspect of research in hypertension. Still unsatisfied, he went further to explore the alterations at the cellular level and to relate changes in the heart to those of the coronary circulation. It was his central conviction that 'the heart is not a knob in the cardiovascular tree' but a central organ with important hemodynamic, neural and endocrine mechanisms. He tapped in the field of atrial natriuretic factor, but time did not allow him to satisfy his curious mind. A consolation may be derived from his previous extensive work in the field of blood volume and extracellular fluid volume as well as in relation to diuretic and sodium handling in hypertension.

These are just a few of the achievements of Dr. Tarazi. Much more has been related to his compassion to his patients, his concern regarding treatment of hypertension and the importance of controlling high blood pressure as well as blood pressure dysregulation in autonomic insufficiency.

F.M. BUMPUS
Cleveland, Ohio

2. The multifaceted aspects of cardiac involvement in hypertension

HARRIET P. DUSTAN

Comparing Freis' 1960 review of the hemodynamics of hypertension [1] with our current knowledge concerning the heart in hypertension bears dramatic testimony to the advances in understanding that have come since then – understanding to which Dr. Robert Tarazi with his indefatigable energy and insatiable curiosity contributed significantly.

In the late 1940's, as the investigation of hypertension became serious business, the heart was viewed by some as 'just a nubbin in the cardiovascular system'. After all, cardiac hypertrophy occurred often and cardiac failure was the most common cause of death in that pre-drug era. The finding that the heart pumped blood normally in the absence of failure [2] meant that it worked well and that cardiac hypertrophy was merely a response to arteriolar constriction. Thus, it is not surprising that when Freis reviewed the hemodynamics of hypertension only five of the twenty-three pages of text were devoted to the heart itself, the rest dealing with the blood vessels and control of vascular resistance. How different it is today: the heart is no longer viewed as just a pump but as an organ that has its own unique responses to raised vascular resistance, as not only a victim of hypertension but perhaps also a culprit in the process, as an endocrine organ and as the site of the most commonly fatal complication of hypertension – coronary heart disease.

Thus, cardiac involvement in hypertension is truly multifaceted. What we recognize now as the role of the heart in hypertension is likely just a fraction of its participation. This brief introduction will discuss some of those facets that we know and which will be dealt with in the various contributions that comprise this dedicatory volume. They will focus on the contributions of Tarazi and his colleagues.

M.E. Safar & F. Fouad-Tarazi (eds.), The heart in hypertension.
© *1989 Kluwer Academic Publishers, Dordrecht –*

The heart as a pump

Cardiac output

Pressure/flow relationships in hypertension. The heart is a very special 'nubbin' in the cardiovascular system because it supplies the energy for the circulation of the blood. The early investigations of its pump function in hypertension indicated that the compensated heart pumped the blood normally and the hemodynamic fault was elevated vascular resistance [2]. However, within fifteen years came a series of reports that some hypertensive patients had modestly elevated cardiac output [3, 4] and it eventually became obvious that the hemodynamics of hypertension is one of considerable heterogeneity: that cardiac output can be normal, decreased or increased and vascular resistance, although characteristically increased, is sometimes normal and occasionally slightly decreased [5–7]. These studies have been of inestimable value in that they clearly showed both the heart and the blood vessels – veins as well as arteries – as participating in the hypertensive process. The discussions of cardiac output presented in this volume will exemplify this heterogeneity.

Cardiogenic hypertension. The findings of an elevated cardiac output in some hypertensive patients naturally raised the question whether increased flow is a primary cause of hypertension. From animal studies there was much to support this possibility. Ledingham and Guyton had both proposed increased cardiac output, secondary to fluid retention, as the causative factor in raising vascular resistance through the mechanism of autoregulation [8, 9] and Borst and Borst de Geus had implicated a similar mechanism in man [10].

As attractive as this possibility is there is considerable evidence against it. Tarazi and I reviewed that evidence several years ago and found that the following information did not support increased flow as a causal factor in hypertension, at least not in man and rarely in experimental models [11]. Relevant to this conclusion is that propranolol, given intravenously to patients with elevated cardiac output, reduced flow sharply but arterial pressure did not change because peripheral resistance rose [12]. These patients were treated with propranolol on a long term basis; finally by one year output was near control values and resistance had fallen but not to normal levels. These data provided no insight into mechanisms for the relative vasodilation with long term therapy. Perhaps the chronically decreased flow and perfusion pressure could have allowed vascular remodelling with a resultant decrease in wall/lumen ratio; in that sense, then, the original hypertension could have been a cardiogenic type with vascular thickening a defense against increased flow. However, this would be a long term mechanism and in studies of brief duration there is no evidence that elevated cardiac output causes hypertension.

Hemodynamic studies of the initiation and maintenance of various experimental hypertension have shown a marked heterogeneity in the responses of cardiac output and peripheral resistance to pressorstimuli. A few examples will suffice. Metyrapone-induced hypertension in dogs is characterized by three hemodynamic patterns: (1) an early rise in cardiac output and pressure followed by an increase in peripheral resistance and normalization of output – the autoregulatory model, (2) persistent elevation of output and pressure without any increase in resistance, and (3) an increased resistance as the cause of hypertension without a change in output [13]. Similar results were found in DOCA-salt hypertensive pigs [14]. Both of these being endocrine hypertensions, it is useful to review information from other experimental hypertensions. Left stellate ganglion stimulation in dogs produces hypertension [15]. In the early phase cardiac output rises along with the arterial pressure but within one day, flow is normalized and hypertension is maintained by an elevated vascular resistance. Finally, hypertension in the young SHR is associated with an increased cardiac output but later flow normalizes and the persistent hypertension reflects an increased resistance. If the early phase of increased output is prevented by in utero and subsequent exposure to propranolol, the hypertension is not prevented [16].

In summary, it seems reasonable to conclude that an elevated cardiac output is not a general mechanism for hypertension. It seems more reasonable to conclude that cardiovascular responses to primary pressor factors are individualized and whether the heart or the peripheral circulation responds predominantly is dependent on factors we do not now know.

Cardiac hypertrophy

Adaptations to pressure overload. When Freis wrote his review he cited three possible mechanisms whereby the left ventricle adapts to the increased afterload of hypertension: (1) increased residual volume producing an increased fibre length, (2) increased intrinsic 'contractility' (the parentheses are his) independent of fibre length, and (3) hypertrophy. Only for hypertrophy did he find any supporting evidence. We know a lot more now. It is true that the heart responds to increased pressure by left ventricular hypertrophy (LVH). This hypertrophy is an adaptive mechanism that functions to reduce ventricular wall stress and is brought about by an increase in myocardial cell size [17]. However in the process, collagen synthesis also increases so that the ventricular mass has the potential of being a less efficient organ than its size would suggest [18]. Another problem with hypertrophy concerns an adequate oxygen supply; not only can subendocardial perfusion be reduced in hypertrophied hearts but also hypertension accelerates coronary atherosclerosis that by itself reduces blood flow and oxygen availability.

Echocardiography has added greatly to knowledge concerning the occurrence of cardiac hypertrophy [19]. In the Muscatine study, school children age 9 to 18 were stratified into low, middle and high quintiles of blood pressure [20]. Those with the highest pressures had significantly greater LV mass than the other two groups. It will be important to obtain sequential measurements as these young people age to assess the relationships of arterial pressure and body size to LV mass with aging. Apparently, LVH is not an inevitable consequence of hypertension. Devereux et al. reported that in four studies of mild to moderate essential hypertension and in normotensives, LV mass corrected for body size was greater than $120 \, g/m^2$ in 23 to 48 percent of hypertensives and 0 to 10 percent of normotensives [21]. Although arterial pressure is an important determinant of heart size it is not the only one as Frohlich and Tarazi pointed out some years ago [22]. Additional factors that have been considered are activities of the sympathetic nervous system and renin-angiotensin system.

Another question that will be addressed in this volume, that was a burning one for Tarazi, was whether the regression of LVH is possible and salutary [18]. The work of the Cleveland Clinic group clearly showed that LVH in experimental models of hypertension is variably affected by antihypertensive drug therapy in spite of equivalent reductions of arterial pressure [18]. Generally speaking, the same conclusions can be drawn from studies in man [23]. These studies indicate that there are factors in addition to pressure overload that play a role in hypertrophy. So regression of LVH is possible but is it salutary? Part of the answer is 'yes' because it was shown that LVH regression was not associated with deterioration of pump function [23]. However, it is a hard question to approach because decreased pressure is necessary for regression. Of particular interest, of course, is whether such hearts are able to function well at higher pressure levels such as those that can be expected to recur after drug therapy is discontinued.

Systolic function/dysfunction. For a long time the hypertrophied heart functions well. Frohlich and colleagues have shed considerable light on the functional progress of systolic function in hypertension [24]. They found that hypertensives with normal size hearts had normal or slightly elevated cardiac output and often had slightly increased mean rates of left ventricular ejection. Patients with left atrial abnormalities, indicating some cardiac involvement, had normal cardiac output, slightly decreased rates of left ventricular ejection and a significant increase in the tension time index. The most severely affected patients were those with the highest pressures and ECG and chest X-ray evidence of cardiac involvement. They had decreased cardiac index, still further decrease in left ventricular ejection rate and stroke index and an increased tension time index. Thus, there is evidence for systolic hyperfunction in the early phases of hypertension and systolic dysfunction as hypertension becomes more severe.

Diastolic dysfunction. It seems clear, now, that the earliest cardiac dysfunction in hypertensive heart disease occurs during diastole. Although it had been known for many years that the electrocardiogram could show evidence of atrial abnormality as one of the earliest signs of cardiac dysfunction, it has been the wide application of echocardiography that has clearly delineated these abnormalities [25]. When the heart begins to hypertrophy compliance decreases. Clinically this is expressed as a fourth heart sound and, later, by ECG evidences of left atrial abnormality. Echocardiographic studies have shown a number of abnormalities related to this decreased compliance. There is prolonged isovolumic relaxation time, slow filling of the ventricle and impaired left atrial emptying index. The isovolumic relaxation time was found to correlate significantly with left ventricular mass index in hypertensive patients but only at a correlation coefficient of 0.59. It did not correlate with systolic or diastolic arterial pressure. These findings raise the question whether there is something other than hypertrophy that changes the diastolic compliance of the left ventricle, independent of arterial pressure, leading to diastolic dysfunction in hypertension.

The heart as a source of pressor reflexes

Pressor events in man

It is almost axiomatic that angina can be preceded by an increase in arterial pressure and that myocardial infarction may be accompanied by transient hypertension. It has been thought that the hypertension may be an integral part of the onset of ischemia but a recent study involving both automated blood pressure recordings and Holter monitoring of the electrocardiogram found that painless ischemia was not accompanied by rises in pressure [26].

Blood pressure may rise following operations on the heart [11]. Replacement of the aortic valve may be followed by transient hypertension which can contribute to graft failure [11]. Also, hypertension is well recognized to occur frequently in the early hours following an aortic-coronary arterial bypass graft. This can easily be controlled by intravenous sodium nitroprusside or stellate ganglion infiltration. It clearly seems to be associated with activation of pressor reflexes from the heart.

Pressor events in animals

The heart as the site of powerful pressor reflexes has been defined much better in animals than man. Hypertension can be triggered by distention of coronary vessels, myocardial ischemia and stimulation of chemoreceptors [27–29]. Of particular interest is the hypertensive chemoreflex which can be produced by the injection of seratonin into the left coronary artery of the dog. This is intriguing because of its possible participation in man in the hypertension of angina or myocardial infarction.

The heart as an endocrine organ

Evidence has been rapidly accumulating that the heart plays a role in sodium excretion and blood pressure control through secretion into the circulation of natriuretic peptides. The question comes whether these natriuretic peptides are important in hypertension. Cantin and Genest report that levels of atrial natriuretic factor (ANF) are increased at some time in all forms of experimental hypertension and that infusion of ANF can reduce arterial pressure [30]. However, a causal role for a deficiency of ANF in these hypertensions has not been identified. ANF is not increased in essential hypertension but it has pointed out by Genest that they are inappropriately normal because hypertensive patients tend to have a slightly increased atrial pressure which should increase the levels [31].

In short we recognize the heart as an endocrine organ because it produces a hormone. It is not known how important that hormone is in hypertension or what relationship it has to the multifaceted aspects of cardiac involvement in hypertension.

A tribute

This volume is a tribute to Dr. Robert Tarazi – a tribute from his friends. His research career was relatively brief (about 20 years) but in that short time he had a greater influence on one aspect of hypertension research than most of us do in a full career. Those who knew him will be pleased to see his contributions detailed. Those who did not know him will be amazed that one person in such a short time could have had such an impact on a subject as important as the heart in hypertension.

References

1. Freis ED (1960): Hemodynamics of hypertension. *Physiol Rev* 40: 27–54.
2. Frohlich ED, Brod J, Hoobler SW, Ledingham JM (1968): Hemodynamics, pp. 350–370 in: Page IH, McCubbin JW (eds), *Renal Hypertension*. Chicago: Year Book Medical Publishers.
3. Widimsky J, Fejfarova MH, Fejfar Z (1957): Changes of cardiac output in hypertensive disease. *Cardiologia* 31: 381–389.
4. Eich RJ, Peters RJ, Cuddy RP, Smulyan HI, Lyons RH (1962): Hemodynamics in labile hypertension. *Am Heart J* 63: 188–195.
5. Frohlich ED, Tarazi RC, Dustan HP (1969): Re-examination of the hemodynamics of hypertension. *Am J Med Sci* 257: 9–23.
6. Tarazi RC, Ibrahim MM, Dustan HP, Ferrario CM (1974): Cardiac factors in hypertension. *Circ Res* 34: 1213–1221.
7. Dustan HP (1986): Pathophysiology of hypertension, pp. 1038–1048 in: Hurst JW, Rackley CE, Schlant RC, Sonnenblick EH, Wallace AG, Wenger NK, Logue RB (eds), *The Heart*, 6th edition. New York: McGraw-Hill.
8. Ledingham JM, Cohen RD (1963): The role of the heart in the pathogenesis of renal hypertension. *Lancet* 1963/2: 979–981.
9. Guyton AC, Granger HJ, Coleman TG (1971): Autoregulation of the total systemic circulation and its relation to control of cardiac output and arterial pressure. *Circ Res* 28 (Suppl I): 93–97.
10. Borst JGG, Borst de Geus A (1963): Hypertension explained by Starling's theory of circulatory homeostasis. *The Lancet* 1963/1: 677–682.
11. Dustan HP, Tarazi RC (1978): Cardiogenic hypertension. *Ann Rev Med* 29: 485–493.
12. Tarazi RC, Dustan HP (1972): Beta adrenergic blockade in hypertension: Practical and theoretical implications of long-term hemodynamic variations. *Am J Cardiol* 29: 633–640.
13. Bravo EL, Tarazi RC, Dustan HP (1977): Multifactorial analysis of chronic hypertension induced by electrolyte-active steroids in trained, unanesthetized dogs. *Circ Res* 40 (Suppl I): 140–145.
14. Terris J, Bereck K, Cohen J, et al. (1976): Deoxycorticosterone hypertension in the pig. *Clin Sci Med* 51: 303s–305s.
15. Liard JF, Tarazi RC, Ferrario CM, Manger WM (1975): Hemodynamic and humoral characteristics of hypertension induced by prolonged stellate stimulation in conscious dogs. *Circ Res* 36: 455–464.
16. Pfeffer MA, Frohlich ED, Pfeffer JM, Weiss AK (1974): Pathophysiological implications of the increased cardiac output of young spontaneously hypertensive rats. *Circ Res* 34 (Suppl I): 235–244.
17. Frohlich ED (1983): The heart in hypertension, pp. 791–810 in: Genest J, Kuchel O, Hamet P, Cantin M (eds), *Hypertension,* 2nd edition. New York: McGraw-Hill.
18. Tarazi RC, Fouad FM (1985): Reversal of cardiac hypertrophy by medical treatment. *Ann Rev Med* 36: 407–414.
19. Liebson PR, Devereux RB, Horan MJ (1987): Hypertension research: Echocardiography in the measurement of left ventricular wall mass. *Hypertension* 9 (Suppl II).
20. Schieken RM (1987): Measurement of left ventricular wall mass in pediatric populations. *Hypertension* 9: II 47–52.
21. Devereux RB, Pickering TG, Alderman MH, Chien S, Border JS, Laragh JH (1987): Left ventricular hypertrophy in hypertension prevalence and relationship to pathophysiologic variables. *Hypertension* 9: II 53–60.
22. Frohlich ED, Tarazi RC (1979): Is arterial pressure the sole factor responsible for hypertensive cardiac hypertrophy? *Am J Cardiol* 44: 959–963.

23. Fouad-Tarazi FM, Liebson PR (1987): Echocardiographic studies of regression of left ventricular hypertrophy in hypertension. *Hypertension* 9: II 65–68.
24. Frohlich ED, Tarazi RC, Dustan HP (1971): Clinical-physiological correlations in the development of hypertensive heart disease. *Circulation* 44: 446–455.
25. Smith VE, White WB, Karimeddini MK (1987): Echocardiographic assessment of left ventricular diastolic performance in hypertensive subjects correlation with changes in left ventricular mass. *Hypertension* 9: II 81–84.
26. Crawford MH, Vittitoe J, O'Rourke RA (1987): Ambulatory blood pressure recordings during silent ischemia (abstract). *Circulation* 76: IV–79.
27. Brown AM (1967): Excitation of afferent cardiac sympathetic nerve fibres during myocardial ischaemia. *J Physiol (London)* 190: 35–53.
28. Malliani A, Brown AM (1970): Reflexes arising from coronary receptors. *Brain Res* 24: 352–355.
29. James TN, Isobe JH, Urthaler F (1975): Analyses of components in a cardiogenic hypertensive chemoreflex. *Circulation* 52: 179–192.
30. Cantin M, Genest J (1987): The heart as an endocrine gland. *Hypertension* 10: I 118–121.
31. Genest J (1988): Atrial natriuretic factor and hypertension. *Am J Med Sci* 295: 299–304.

PART ONE

Cardiac output level and systemic hemodynamics

3. Cardiac output in hypertension
Basic concepts and experimental studies

JEAN-FRANÇOIS LIARD

1. Cardiac output and blood pressure control

Simple hydrodynamic considerations indicate that the systemic blood flow from the aorta back to the heart is driven by the difference of total fluid energy between aorta and right atrium (RA), which for all practical purpose is equal to the gradient between mean arterial pressure and right atrial pressure, MAP – RAP. This flow can thus be calculated as MAP – RAP/TPR, where TPR is the total peripheral resistance. Systemic blood flow is equal to cardiac output (CO), and since RAP is small and does not change markedly under most conditions, the usual expression of these relations becomes: MAP = CO × TPR. Thus, mean arterial pressure is determined by cardiac output and peripheral resistance.

Although this relation is very useful, the analogy with Ohm's law cannot be carried too far because of the nature of the power generator in the cardiovascular system, namely the cardiac pump. In a simple electrical circuit, an increase in resistance reduces current proportionately. In the circulation without reflexes, increasing peripheral resistance predominantly increases arterial pressure without decreasing flow. This is in large part because the heart generates more power when exposed to an increased load, through both heterometric and homeometric autoregulation. Therefore, systemic flow can be maintained despite increased TPR, and arterial pressure increases. An increased power also results from increasing the filling pressure of the heart (preload). Since the power generated by the heart is dependent upon the characteristics of the circuit, flows and pressures resulting from changes in this circuit cannot be predicted simply.

Another limitation of the relation MAP = CO × TPR is the danger of thinking of TPR as a global index of arteriolar diameter, when TPR is an operational description including viscosity factors as well as inhomogeneous

M.E. Safar & F. Fouad-Tarazi (eds.), The heart in hypertension.
© *1989 Kluwer Academic Publishers, Dordrecht –*

regional vascular beds in which the diameter, length, and number of the constituting vessels play a variable role. There are many instances when vascular resistance in one bed increases while TPR is decreasing, and vice-versa. Increased vascular tone and decreased density of the vessels in a tissue represent two completely different ways of increasing vascular resistance. Even in a single vessel, the control of its diameter encompasses a large number of phenomena including structural components, events at the vascular smooth muscle cell membrane, as well as the complex neuro-humoral control systems known to modify vascular tone. All these mechanisms are unlikely to play a similar role throughout the body, and TPR certainly does not represent the state of vasoconstriction of each and every single arteriole.

Finally, hypertension may be more than an increase in mean arterial pressure. Systolic pressure is a better predictor than mean pressure of some of the harmful consequences of hypertension, and alterations of pulsatile phenomena may have substantial effects beyond those of a simple increase in the mean level of the pressure. Thus, aortic compliance could play a role independent of total peripheral resistance.

Despite these reservations, a chronic increase of mean arterial pressure must be accounted for, hemodynamically, by an increase of peripheral resistance or of cardiac output. Since cardiac output is normal in most, if not all, forms of established hypertension, the basic abnormality is obviously an increased total peripheral resistance. However, this does not imply any knowledge of the mechanisms involved.

As pointed out by Harris [1], high arterial blood pressure appeared in phylogeny with warm blood and a greatly increased oxygen uptake. Reptiles, amphibia and fishes have mean arterial pressures below 40 mmHg. Harris suggested that in order to maintain oxygen uptake, cardiac output had to increase. Peripheral resistance changed little, and the increased cardiac output appears to account for the increased arterial pressure of warm blooded animals. These observations and conjectures emphasize the potential role of cardiac output in setting the chronic level of arterial pressure. However, it is important to recognize that in any individual, whether normotensive or hypertensive, arterial pressure is tightly controlled. This suggests that mechanisms have evolved after the transition to warm-blooded animals, or that preexisting control mechanisms must have reset, in order to maintain pressure constant at the new elevated level.

Indeed, a number of very efficient short-term and long-term control mechanisms regulate blood pressure. A disturbance that alters arterial pressure triggers compensatory changes of cardiac output and/or total peripheral resistance. Conversely, if the set point of a powerful blood pressure controller is changed in such a way that arterial pressure must increase, cardiac output and/or peripheral resistance will increase, and it does not really matter which mechanism is called upon. Thus, cardiac output is a variable manipulated to achieve pressure control, but it can also be a determinant of mean arterial pressure.

Before discussing the significance of cardiac output in hypertension, it is important to recall some aspects of its regulation. From the graphical analysis of cardiac output regulation described by Guyton et al. [2], it can be determined that the steady-state value of cardiac output (equilibrium point) can change as a result of (1) an alteration of mean circulatory pressure, (2) an alteration in the resistance to venous return, and (3) an alteration in the cardiac output curve. These three major factors can change in various combinations that describe most of the conditions associated with an alteration of cardiac output. Changes in mean circulatory pressure reflect essentially modifications of venous tone or changes in blood volume, whereas changes in the resistance to venous return are brought about by factors that modify vascular resistance. An alteration in the cardiac output curve reflects modifications of the effectiveness of the heart as a pump or alterations of extracardiac pressures.

The cause of an increase in systemic flow has major implications for its possible importance in the development of increased arterial pressure. Increases in cardiac output triggered by peripheral resistance changes and due to an increased slope of the venous return curve are, for example, those associated with opening an arterio-venous fistula, with increasing tissue metabolism, as in exercise, or with a decrease in blood viscosity, as in anemia. They do not increase blood pressure, because the increase in cardiac output is essentially flowing through areas of reduced resistance. Thus, the presence of chronically elevated cardiac output without the development of high blood pressure under these or similar conditions cannot be used as an argument against the significance of cardiac output changes in other situations. On the contrary, cardiac output changes due to an increase of mean circulatory pressure can raise arterial pressure, as can alterations in the cardiac output curve.

Ferrario and Page [3] have emphasized the methodological problems associated with cardiac output measurements. They pointed out that the variability of cardiac output under control conditions is larger than that of arterial pressure (31% vs. 14%). This presumably reflects in part the fact that cardiac output is manipulated to control arterial pressure. The implication of this variability is that moderate increases of cardiac output are difficult to interpret, in particular in the absence of long-term measurements.

2. Cardiac output in experimental hypertension

Although chronic hypertension is characterized by normal systemic blood flow and increased peripheral resistance, several clinical forms exhibit a phase of increased cardiac output. This is usually the case in borderline essential hypertension, and it is also observed in renovascular and mineralocorticoid hypertension [4]. These observations have led to the question of the significance of an increased cardiac output for the development of the hypertension. Experimental studies have been designed to examine this question, and we will review hemodynamic patterns that have been described in various models of hypertension. Because of space limitations, only canine models will be discussed. However, we believe that the conclusions that can be drawn from these models apply to other models as well.

Coleman and Guyton [5] carefully described what has become a classical account of the hemodynamic changes in volume-expanded hypertension. Continuous infusion of isotonic saline after surgical reduction of renal mass produced hypertension, with a transient increase in cardiac output. Total peripheral resistance was initially depressed, then increased. This sequence of events appeared to be triggered by blood volume expansion and increased venous return. Although the time course and magnitude of hemodynamic changes differed somewhat in subsequent studies using the same model, the basic sequence observed was the same [6–8].

In renovascular hypertension, the picture is not as uniform. In the 1-kidney, 1-clip hypertension model, Conway [9] measured unchanged cardiac output 4 and 15 days after renal artery constriction and unilateral nephrectomy while arterial pressure increased. Bianchi et al. [10] found an increase of cardiac output between 3 and 7 days after renal artery constriction in conscious dogs. Ferrario [11] observed that cardiac output rose within 48 hours after renal artery constriction and remained significantly elevated for several weeks. Rise in peripheral resistance lagged behind the increase in cardiac output and became progressively the predominant cause of hypertension. Ferrario et al. [12] had previously reported similar hemodynamic changes in dogs with one kidney wrapped in cellophane and the other intact. Anderson et al. [13] found in dogs that renal artery stenosis of varying degrees increased arterial pressure without changing cardiac output over a 3 day period. In sodium-depleted dogs, renal artery constriction still induced hypertension, but cardiac output fell transiently [14].

In the 2-kidney, 1-clip hypertension model, Bianchi et al. [15] reported a slight, non-significant increase in cardiac output. Maxwell et al. [16] found a rapid increase in cardiac output, between 2 hours and 3 days post constriction. Greenberg et al. [17] reported an increase in flow in the descending aorta from day 2 to 12 after renal artery constriction while arterial pressure increased progressively and remained elevated. Preventing the increase in flow with vena cava constriction did not prevent the blood pressure increase.

In mineralocorticoid hypertension, using metyrapone, Bravo et al. [18]

found wide variations in cardiac output and reported that the rise in pressure was not uniformly associated with an increase in cardiac output. Nor did prevention of cardiac output increase by beta-blockade prevent the development of hypertension. In DOCA hypertension, Conway and Hatton [19] described a variable increase in cardiac output. Beta-adrenergic blockade reduced cardiac output, but did not affect the development of hypertension. Pan and Young [20] studied aldosterone induced hypertension in dogs and showed that arterial pressure increased without an increase in cardiac output. Mean circulatory pressure increased significantly. Kageyama and Bravo [21] studied DOCA-salt hypertension and found that cardiac output tended to increase, but not significantly, whether the dogs received a normal or an increased calcium intake. However, in these dogs fed a high calcium diet, the increase in arterial pressure was reduced and total peripheral resistance tended to decrease.

In dogs on high sodium intake receiving angiotensin II infusions, hypertension develops with a decrease in cardiac output despite an increase in mean circulatory pressure [22].

In summary, cardiac output is frequently elevated in the early stages of various forms of canine experimental hypertension, but this is not always the case. Furthermore, even when cardiac output is increased, pharmacological or mechanical interference with this increase does not prevent the development of hypertension. Although common, an increase in cardiac output may therefore not be a necessary component in many forms of experimental hypertension, and its existence may merely coincide with blood pressure elevation. In this respect, an interesting observation was made by Ganguli et al. in Dahl hypertensive rats [23]. The 'R' rats, when exposed to a high salt intake, increase their cardiac output as the 'S' rats, but their blood pressure does not increase because total peripheral resistance declines. On the other hand, the S rats develop increased blood pressure because their TPR does not fall.

This and other similar observations explain the diverging views about the hemodynamic significance of an increased cardiac output early in hypertension. One view is that the early hemodynamic changes in hypertension are not really relevant to the development of increased vascular resistance, which would be accounted for by alternative mechanisms, such as circulating factors which modify vascular smooth muscle function or changes in sympathetic nervous system activity. On the other hand, it is conceivable that a cardiac output increase, when present, triggers peripheral resistance changes. Mechanisms which could transform an increase of cardiac output into a high total peripheral resistance are generally considered autoregulatory responses. The pressure increase resulting from the increase in cardiac output would trigger peripheral responses similar to those seen in the well documented acute autoregulation of various peripheral tissues. Indeed, in these tissues, resistance increases very rapidly when perfusion pressure increases, through myogenic mechanisms, metabolic mechanisms and/or factors intrinsic to the vessel wall (such as the release of endothelium derived substances, prostanoids, angiotensin, etc.). These rapid responses could account for a substantial change in total peripheral resistance [24]. However, such changes may be completely masked by the neuroendocrine control of the circulation. Indeed, as an increase in cardiac output tends to increase arterial pressure, baroreceptor and other reflexes buffer this increase by lowering vascular resistance. At the same time, the circulating levels of various vasoconstrictor hormones (angiotensin, vasopressin) decline. With time, these neuroendocrine factors adapt, which would unmask the resistance changes due to autoregulatory responses. Furthermore, functional vascular changes appear to alter vascular smooth muscle responsiveness to oxygen [25] and lead to functional rarefaction. Finally, long-term structural autoregulatory responses, including vascular wall thickness changes and true anatomical vessel rarefaction, may account for further increase in vascular resistance in prolonged volume-expanded hypertensions. The possibility that perfusion of tissues in excess of their needs could be an important factor in these responses has been particularly advocated by Coleman et al. [26].

There is evidence for the participation of functional and structural autoregulatory components in the resistance changes of various forms of hypertension. In the development of renal hypertension in rats, protecting the hindquarters from the increased arterial pressure clearly blunted the vascular resistance increase [27], which strongly suggested that an autoregulatory component was acting as a vasoconstrictor mechanism in this vascular bed. In another study of the very early stages of renal hypertension in rats, Meininger et al. reported that protection of the superior mesenteric vascular bed from the elevated pressure also markedly blunted the increase in mesenteric resistance [28]. These findings suggest that pressure-dependent, local autoregulatory mechanisms account for a portion of the increased resistance of this model of hypertension. In more chronic situations, structural changes in the vasculature clearly contribute to the hemodynamic characteristics of all kinds of hypertension [29].

Since the distribution of cardiac output may not be homogeneous following volume expansion, we studied regional blood flows in salt-loading hypertension in renal mass reduced dogs. We found that most of the increase of cardiac output measured within 24 hours after the start of the isotonic saline infusion was diverted to skeletal muscle vascular bed [8]. The vast majority of other vascular beds did not appear to ever experience overperfusion, which provides no support for the idea that perfusion in excess of metabolic needs contributes to the development of high resistance in these beds. The analysis of total peripheral resistance changes during hemodynamic transients is obviously complicated by the inhomogeneous nature of the resistance changes in various individual beds. It is unlikely that generalized overperfusion is a necessary step in the development of increased resistance in volume-expanded hypertension. However, we showed in a later study that the baroreceptor reflex was responsible for the transient vasodilatation seen in skeletal muscle, which accounted for the buffering effect of the reflex in the early phases of the volume expansion [30]. In the absence of the baroreceptor reflex, significant overperfusion of several vascular beds took place (skin, bone, splanchnic area) after 1 day of infusion, which might have contributed to the development of increased resistance in the later stages.

Coarctation of the aorta has been claimed to support the concept of the all important nature of local mechanisms in the control of regional blood flows. It has indeed been reported that flow to various tissues is the same whether the perfusion pressure is increased (proximal to the coarctation) or not (distal). However, it appears from recent measurements made in coarctation of the aorta that regional blood flows are not maintained at a tightly controlled value. In dogs, several vascular beds perfused at the reduced pressure distal to the coarctation, and which never experienced an increased blood flow nor an increased perfusion pressure, showed decreased blood flows one month after coarctation [31]. In rats [32], blood flows in the lower part of the body were found to be increased above control values. Although the results in rats differ from those in dogs, both indicate that regional blood flows can be significantly different from control and are therefore not tightly controlled.

3. Cardiogenic hypertension

As indicated before, several models of hypertension are accompanied by an initial increase in cardiac output, but the significance of this increase is not clear since other mechanisms could account for the development of hypertension in most of these models, including the presence of inhibitors of sodium-potassium ATPase in volume expanded forms of hypertension, or alterations of the sympathetic control of the circulation. Bob Tarazi, in the early 70's, was interested in finding out whether increasing cardiac output by changing the cardiac function curve (that is by increasing cardiac contractility) would provide a model in which increased systemic blood flow could exist independently of blood volume expansion and other complicating factors. He therefore initiated experiments with stellate ganglion stimulation in dogs. When I joined the Cleveland Clinic, we tested the hypothesis that prolonged electrical stimulation of cardiac sympathetic innervation might produce sustained hypertension in conscious dogs [33]. Indeed, we found a moderate degree of hypertension that was maintained as long as the stimulation lasted. During the first hours of stimulation, cardiac output was increased, but later on it decreased back to control as calculated peripheral resistance increased progressively. Circulating catecholamines and plasma renin activity could not account for the development of hypertension, and there was no evidence of body fluid volume expansion. Thus, the results were compatible with the idea that a primary increase in cardiac output could lead to hypertension characterized, at a late stage, by increased periperal resistance. However, since the stellate ganglion was not decentralized, we could not exclude the possibility that stimulation of afferent fibers from the heart contributed to the development of the high blood pressure.

I then attempted to enhance myocardial contractility more selectively by chronic infusion of dobutamine through a catheter implanted in the left coronary artery of conscious dogs [34]. Hypertension developed and was maintained for the duration of the infusion. Cardiac output increased during the first few days, then decreased back toward control as peripheral resistance increased progressively. Since intravenous infusion of the drug at the same dose did not increase arterial pressure [35], systemic effects of dobutamine could not explain the development of hypertension upon intracoronary administration. Thus, blood pressure increased in the absence of volume retention and in face of decreased plasma renin activity, presumably as a result of an increase in cardiac output. Preventing the cardiac output increase with propranolol eliminated any increase in arterial pressure [35].

Several criticisms have been raised to these experiments. First, increasing the pumping capability of he heart should not increase cardiac output substantially if one judges from heart-lung bypass experiments [36]. However, the mechanism of the increase in cardiac output upon stimulation of ventricular contractility in intact animals is in part to transfer blood volume from the lungs to the periphery [37]. Thus, it is theoretically possible to increase cardiac output with an isolated increase in cardiac contractility. A second theoretical objection has been that the renal volume-pressure controller would prevent a sustained increase in arterial pressure by excreting increased amount of sodium and water until blood pressure came all the way back to its control value [36]. We and others [38, 39] have argued that the renal mechanism does not have an infinite gain in the control of blood pressure because it partially adapts to a change in pressure. It is well established that when arterial pressure increases, sodium and water are excreted in increasing amounts, which tends to lower arterial pressure. However, this increased urinary excretion also decreases the total amount of sodium in the body as well as body fluid volumes. This in turn modifies the renal function curve and decreases its slope, as a result of several mechanisms such as increased plasma protein concentration, decreased renal interstitial fluid pressure and increased concentration of sodium retaining hormones. The result of this change in the renal function curve is that the new equilibrium point may be different from the original control value, allowing blood pressure to increase some without any primary renal abnormality.

We therefore believe that cardiogenic hypertension may indeed develop as a result of a primary increase in myocardial contractility causing cardiac output to increase. Obviously, this does not mean that other forms of experimental hypertension necessarily share a common mechanism with cardiogenic hypertension.

4. Conclusions

Mean arterial pressure is maintained within a narrow range, indicating that it is controlled by powerful mechanisms. If hypertension is viewed as the result of an alteration in the set point of the main blood pressure controller(s) [36], then the changes in cardiac output and total peripheral resistance that account hemodynamically for the increase in pressure are not really critical. Blood flow through many organs and tissues tends to be maintained close to a 'normal' value under resting conditions, although this control is not nearly as tight as that of blood pressure. Since cardiac output is the sum of all peripheral blood flows, it also tends to remain constant. Thus, if arterial pressure must go up because of an alteration of its controller's set point, the steady state is likely to be characterized by an increased peripheral resistance.

It is also conceivable that some forms of hypertension do not result from an alteration of the pressure controller(s), but from a primary disturbance of the effectors of that control, such as vascular geometry and amount of energy imparted to the blood by the cardiac pump. In this instance, the main pressure controllers are thought to adapt partially to the increased pressure and to become reset at a new operating point secondarily. Possible examples of such hypertensions have been presented in Part Three.

Acknowledgements

Supported by Grant NIH HL 29587.

References

1. Harris P (1983): Evolution and the cardiac patient, 3: Origins of blood pressure. *Cardiovasc Res* 17: 373–378.
2. Guyton AC, Jones CE, Coleman TG (1973): *Circulatory Physiology, II: Cardiac Output and Its Regulation.* Philadelphia: WB Saunders.
3. Ferrario CM, Page IH (1978): Current views concerning cardiac output in the genesis of experimental hypertension. *Circ Res* 43: 821–831.
4. Dustan HP, Tarazi RC (1978): Cardiogenic hypertension. *Ann Rev Med* 29: 485–493.
5. Coleman TG, Guyton AC (1969): Hypertension caused by salt loading in the dog, III: Onset transients of cardiac output and other circulatory variables. *Circ Res* 25: 153–160.
6. Cowley AW, Guyton AC (1975): Baroreceptor reflex effects on transient and steady-state hemodynamics of salt-loading hypertension in dogs. *Circ Res* 36: 536–546.
7. Manning RD, Coleman TG, Guyton AC, Norman RA, McCaa RE (1979): Essential role of mean circulatory filling pressure in salt-induced hypertension. *J Physiol* 236: R40–R47.
8. Liard JF (1981): Regional blood flows in salt loading hypertension in the dog. *Am J Physiol* 240: H261–H267.
9. Conway J (1968): Changes in sodium balance and hemodynamics during development of experimental renal hypertension in dogs. *Circ Res* 22: 763–767.
10. Bianchi G, Tenconi LT, Lucca R (1970): Effect in the conscious dog of constriction of the renal artery to a sole remaining kidney on haemodynamics, sodium balance, body fluid volumes, plasma renin concentration and pressor reponsiveness to angiotensin. *Clin Sci* 38: 741–766.
11. Ferrario CM (1974): Contribution of cardiac output and peripheral resistance to experimental renal hypertension. *Am J Physiol* 226: 711–717.
12. Ferrario CM, Page IH, McCubbin JW (1970): Increased cardiac output as a contributory factor in experimental renal hypertension in dogs. *Circ Res* 27: 799–810.
13. Anderson WP, Korner PI, Angus JA, Johnston CI (1981): Contribution of stenosis resistance to the rise in total peripheral resistance during experimental renal hypertension in conscious dogs. *Clin Sci* 61: 663–670.
14. Stephens GA, Davis JO, Freeman RH, DeForrest JM, Early DM (1979): Hemodynamic, fluid, and electrolyte changes in sodium-depleted, one-kidney, renal hypertensive dogs. *Circ Res* 44: 316–321.
15. Bianchi G, Baldoli E, Lucca R, Barbin P (1972): Pathogenesis of arterial hypertension after the constriction of the renal artery leaving the opposite kidney intact both in the anaesthetized and in the conscious dog. *Clin Sci* 42: 651–664.
16. Maxwell MH, Lupu AN, Viskoper RJ, Aravena LA, Waks UA (1977): Mechanisms of hypertension during the acute and intermediate phases of the one-clip, two-kidney model in the dog. *Circ Res* 40 (Suppl I): I:24–28.
17. Greenberg S, McGowan C, Gaida M (1982): Effect of an increased cardiac output on vascular responses to vasoactive agents in two-kidney, one-clip Goldblatt hypertension. *Clin Exp Hypertens* 4: 1287–1302.
18. Bravo EL, Tarazi RC, Dustan HP (1977): Multifactorial analysis of chronic hypertension induced by electrolyte-active steroids in trained, unanesthetized dogs. *Circ Res* 40 (Suppl I): I: 140–145.
19. Conway J, Hatton R (1978): Development of deoxycorticosterone acetate hypertension in the dog. *Circ Res* 43 (Suppl I): I: 82–86.
20. Pan YJ, Young DB (1982): Experimental aldosterone hypertension in the dog. *Hypertension* 4: 279–287.
21. Kageyama Y, Bravo EL (1987): Neurohumoral and hemodynamic responses to dietary

calcium supplementation in deoxycorticosterone-salt hypertensive dogs. *Hypertension* 9 (Suppl III): III: 166–170.

22. Young DB, Murray RH, Bengis RG, Markov AK (1980): Experimental angiotensin II hypertension. *Am J Physiol* 239: H391–H398.

23. Ganguli M, Tobian L, Iwai J (1979): Cardiac output and peripheral resistance in strains of rats sensitive and resistant to NaCl hypertension. *Hypertension* 1: 3–7.

24. Cowley AW, Barber WJ, Lombard JH, Osborn JL, Liard JF (1986): Relationship between body fluid volumes and arterial pressure. *Fed Proc* 45: 2864–2870.

25. Lombard JH, Cowley Jr AW, Smits GJ, Mazzeo AJ, Stekiel WJ (1985): Microcirculatory changes in rats in the early stages of reduced renal mass (RRM) hypertension. *Microvasc Res* 29: 236.

26. Coleman TG, Samar RE, Murphy WR (1979): Autoregulation versus other vasoconstrictors in hypertension: A critical review. *Hypertension* 1: 324–330.

27. Meininger GA, Lubrano VM, Granger HJ (1984): Hemodynamic and microvascular responses in the hindquarters during the development of renal hypertension in rats: Evidence for the involvement of an autoregulatory component. *Circ Res* 55: 609–622.

28. Meininger GA, Routh LK, Granger HJ (1985): Autoregulation and vasoconstriction in the intestine during acute renal hypertension. *Hypertension* 7: 364–373.

29. Folkow B (1982): Physiological aspects of primary hypertension. *Physiol Rev* 62: 347–504.

30. Liard JF, Silenzio R (1982): Baroreceptor reflex influence on peripheral circulations in salt-loading hypertension in dogs. *Hypertension* 4: 597–603.

31. Liard JF, Spadone JC (1985): Regional circulations in experimental coarctation of the aorta in conscious dogs. *J Hypertens* 3: 281–291.

32. Stanek KA, Coleman TG, Murphy WR (1987): Overall hemodynamic pattern in coarctation of the abdominal aorta in conscious rats. *Hypertension* 9: 611–618.

33. Liard JF, Tarazi RC, Ferrario CM, Manger WM (1975): Hemodynamic and humoral characteristics of hypertension induced by prolonged stellate ganglion stimulation in conscious dogs. *Circ Res* 36: 455–464.

34. Liard JF (1978): Hypertension induced by prolonged intracoronary infusion of dobutamine in conscious dogs. *Clin Sci Mol Med* 54: 153–160.

35. Liard JF (1980): Cardiogenic hypertension: experimental evidence from a comparison between intravenous and intracoronary administration of dobutamine in conscious dogs. *Clin Sci* 58: 271–277.

36. Guyton AC (1980): *Circulatory Physiology, III: Arterial Pressure and Hypertension*. Philadelphia: W.B. Saunders.

37. Liard JF, Tarazi RC, Ferrario CM (1976): Hemodynamic effects of stellate ganglion stimulation in conscious dogs, pp. 151–160 in: Julius S, Esler MD (eds), *The Nervous System in Arterial Hypertension*. Springfield: C.C. Thomas.

38. Liard JF (1979): Cardiogenic hypertension, pp. 317–355 in: Guyton AC, Young DB (eds), *Cardiovascular Physiology*, Vol. 3. Baltimore: University Park Press (International Review of Physiology 18).

39. Omvik P, Tarazi RC, Bravo EL (1980): Regulation of sodium balance in hypertension. *Hypertension* 2: 515–523.

4. Haemodynamic development

F. MAGRINI

1. Genesis of arterial blood pressure

Pulsatile arterial pressure is generated by the first heart beat. Prior to this, although circulation of blood can be demonstrated in the 16 somite embryo, no pulsatile pressure can be recorded [1].

When the ambryo has 20–21 somites clearcut pulsatile waves rapidly make their appearance, and this is thought to reflect the change in the character of the ventricular contraction waves from peristaltoid to synchronous and rhythmic. The simultaneous elaboration of endocardial masses provides a wave-like mechanism which encourages direct fluid movement within what is essentially a gel-like medium [2].

The kinetic force of the stream stresses the surrounding fluid and gel-like medium in such a way as to develop vascular cavities and channels. The formation of a more elastic cellular line of demarcation between the moving fluid and stressed extravascular gel is encouraged by the movement of the pulsatile fluid stream [3].

The growing heart is likewise exposed to these dynamically fluctuating and responds by expanding its cavity; due to the limited capacity of the musculature to withstand and support peak stress there is also a slow rise in the internal pressure.

To what extent the resistance to flow presented by the gel-like medium governs the size and geometry of the developing ventricular cavity remains unknown, and likewise experimental data to determine whether the heart plays an active role in generating its own afterload are lacking [3].

The fact that ventricular pumping activity precedes temporally the structural development of vascular channels has been cited as evidence that pulsatile pressure is generated by the intermittent impact of the pulsatile flow on the gel-like medium, which constitutes a resistance to flow [4].

M.E. Safar & F. Fouad-Tarazi (eds.), The heart in hypertension.
© *1989 Kluwer Academic Publishers, Dordrecht –*

Whatever the initiating factor in the genesis of pulsatile pressure it is clear that from the 20 somite stage onwards it is governed by the interaction of cardiac output and vascular resistance, and during intra-uterine growth a linear relationship has been demonstrated between the increasing systolic pressure, which rises gradually, and the elaboration of the embryonic vasculature [1].

It is obvious that at birth the cardiovascular and respiratory systems undergo enormous modification [4], but a discussion of these changes is beyond the scope of this chapter.

2. Cardiovascular dynamics during infancy

Profound differences exist between the dynamics of the circulation at maturity and that in the early phases of extrauterine life in terrestrial mammals [5–9], namely:

a) Mean arterial blood pressure (MAP) is 45–50% lower than that found in adults. This infantile hypotension is the result of an extremely low total peripheral resistance (TPR), about one third of the adult value.

b) Cardiac output per unit of body weight (CO/W) is 40–50% higher than that of the adult, attributable to the significantly higher heart rate (HR) (55–60%) and significantly lower stroke output (SV/W) (35–40%) characteristic of the infantile cardiovascular system.

c) Plasma volume per unit of body weight (PV/W) and central venous pressure (CVP) exceed adult values by 25–30% and 35–40% respectively.

Thus a series of haemodynamic features – low resistance, high venous pressure, augmented plasma volume and high CO – distinguish the adult and infantile profiles and it is generally accepted that these characteristics serve to facilitate capillary ultrafiltration [10].

Furthermore, it is probable that the high oxygen consumption and the greater metabolic needs of the tissues and organs during growth [11] represent a stimulus to the cardiovascular system to maintain adequate tissue perfusion and may, as such, also be considered as factors which determine the haemodynamic profile of infancy [12, 13].

The mechanisms underlying the lower TPR of immature animals remain unclear. Incomplete development of the muscle of the arterial wall, high capillary density, and the influence of nervous, humoral and metabolic factors upon the precapillary sphincter tone, have all been considered as possible determinants of the reduced resistance to flow [14–17].

It has been suggested that the elevated CVP characterizing the infantile haemodynamic profile may reflect poorer compliance of the systemic venous

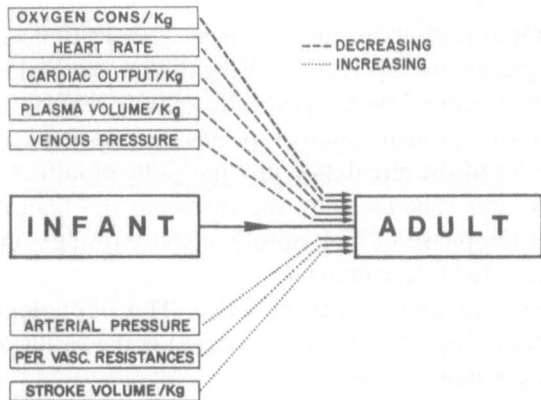

Fig. 1. Haemodynamic remodelling during growth: direction of changes of basic circulatory variables.

system in the early phases of extrauterine life compared to the greater adult compliance with lower CVP [7].

However, the existence of elevated plasma and extracellular fluid volumes suggest that the CVP may result from the interaction of numerous factors, namely: relatively well developed veins with thick walls [18] but reduced compliance, expansion of body fluids [19], and elevated heart rate with low compliance of the right ventricle [20], which in the fetus is thicker walled than the left ventricle [21, 22] thereby reducing its distensibility during diastole.

Nonetheless, it is obvious that the most significant haemodynamic consequence of the elevated HR is a significantly higher cardiac output compared to the adult. Data on the mechanisms responsible for the physiological tachycardia of infancy are inconclusive. Hypotheses suggested include an imbalance in youths between the sympathetic and parasympathetic effects on the heart [23, 24], the presence of hypersensitivity to the cardiac receptors [25], and the possible reflex stimulation of the left ventricle by the low afterload [7].

Thus, analysis of the haemodynamic profile in infancy has shown that the cardiovascular system at this age is characterized by a regime of high flow, low resistance and probably of low venous compliance. The design of the circulation is thus well suited to the need to meet the high oxygen demand which hallmarks the growth process.

3. Heamodynamic changes during development

Body growth is defined as an increase in body weight determined by the augmentation of cell numbers which comprise the organism and associated with profound modifications in the chemical composition and biochemical activity of the organism itself [11, 26]. During this process, which in terrestrial mammals is of the 'definite' type [3] (mitotic activity ceases with the arrest of bone growth and with the acquisition of species specific definitive body dimensions) the dynamics of the circulation are markedly modified.

Figure 1 represents schematically the direction of change of circulatory parameters from the phase of high mitotic activity (infancy) to the phase of mitotic arrest (maturity). In summary:

a) *MAP increases to double its initial value.* This physiological increase in blood pressure (the pressure maturation curve) is the result of a progressive increase in TPR per unit of body weight.

b) *The CO/V diminishes by 45–50%.* Despite the net reduction in CO, the MAP increases by 90–95% indicating that the effect of the increased TPR dominates over the effect of the reduction of systemic blood flow on the blood pressue. The fall in CO is a consequence of a progressive fall in HR; but due to the accompanying 30–35% increase in stroke output, CO/W is maintained.

c) *There is a reduction in CVP and PV/W.* The mechanism(s) underlying the progressive reduction in body fluids with growth have not yet been elucidated.

Longitudinal studies during maturation of the dynamics of body fluids and especially of their distribution within the intra- and extra-vascular compartments will need to be conducted, given their critical importance in the natural history of the circulation and in determining adult blood pressure values [7].

Clearly the distribution of intravascular volume both between the central and peripheral vascular beds and between the arterial and venous circulation will be influenced by structural changes in both the pulmonary vasculature [27, 28] and the peripheral arteries [14] and veins [18] known to occur during development from infancy to adulthood. Indeed, the concept that the cardiovascular sstem may be divided into capacitance and resistance compartments, although valid in the adult circulation, is invalid in the infantile circulation, so that the structural and haemodynamic differences between the capacitance and resistance vessels are also probably acquired during extrauterine development [7].

Thus, it is likely that the reduction in CVP during growth is the result of complex interactions between the development of peripheral venous capacitance, reduction in plasma volume, redistribution of circulating volume between the pulmonary and peripheral circulations and the lowering of the HR.

In essence, therefore, the maturation of mammals is accompanied by haemodynamic 'remodelling' from a regime of high flow with low pressure in infancy to the adult regime of lower blood flow with elevated blood pressure. There is a parallel reduction in total body water, and a redistribution of circulating volume consequent upon the development of the capacitance and resistance vessel compartments.

4. The sequence of events leading to the adult circulatory regime

During growth all haemodynamic parameters are modified progressively and simultaneously.

Figure 2 represents the sequence of events (based upon the varying rates of change) which determines the formation of the stable circulatory regime found in adulthood [7].

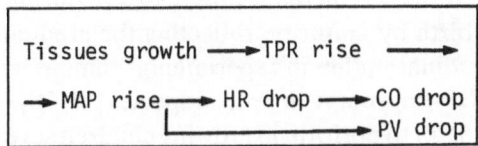

Fig. 2. Haemodynamic remodelling during growth. The process of body maturation offers a completely physiological and 'time-metabolic dependent' model for the localization of circulatory feedback mechanisms.

The rate of increase of body weight (BW), taken as an index of body growth, represents the most rapid event and is followed in a cascade fashion by the increase in TPR, increase in MAP and decrease in HR and CO/W.

A high degree of correlation was found between the increase in BW and TPR and MAP, and between the increase in MAP and decrease in HR CO/W and PV/W [7].

This sequence suggests that numerous circulatory feedback mechanisms are developed and activated to determine appropriate haemodynamics to the state of maturation of the organism. The fact that circulatory stability is established once augmentation of body weight ceases suggests that one such controlling mechanism is that linking body weight and degree of maturity with the TPR. Although the determinants of the increasing TPR are not known (? nervous influences, ? modification of density and structure, ? humoral and metabolic factors?) the augmentation of body weight probably represents a natural stimulus to the cardiovascular system to increase TPR.

It is possible, furthermore, that the increase of MAP represents the haemodynamic stimulus to reduce the HR, by activating baroreceptors [29]. Since the haemodynamic consequence of the reduction in HR is a progressive fall in CO, it can be deduced that the fall in the latter parameter with growth is neurologically determined and that the arterial baroreceptors may play a critical role, via the fall in HR, in the circulatory remodelling during maturation.

Finally, the fact that the reduction in PV follows that in CO renders it improbable that the PV represents a fundamental determinant of CO during development.

In conclusion, it appears that in terrestrial mammals the augmentation of body weight during growth represents a natural stimulus which initiates the sequence of circulatory changes underlying the haemodynamic modifications of the maturing cardiovascular system.

5. The arterial pressure maturation curve

As already described the BP increase progressively during growth, reaching double its value at birth by maturity, reflecting the gradual increase in TPR. Furthermore longitudinal studies in experimental animals have established the morphology of the BP-time curve in several species [16, 30]. Although longitudinal studies are difficult to perform in growing children several cross-sectional studies have confirmed the concept of a BP maturation curve in humans [31, 32], and have demonstrated striking inter-species similarity in the morphology of the curves despite widely differing body dimensions and final body weight.

Clearly the maturation of BP is but one facet of the complex process of body growth, and it may therefore be unreasonable to presume that as such the factors responsible for total body growth may also determine the modification of BP with time and age.

Body growth is defined as the progressive development of a living being of part of an organism from its earliest stage to maturity, including the attendant increases in size [33]. Comparative physiological studies have led to the broad classification of animals into those whose growth continues throughout their lifecycles (indeterminate) and those whose growth ceases at a genetically predetermined stage of their cycle (determinate) [34]. Most of the higher vertebrates exhibit determinate growth whilst many invertebrates and lower vertebrates growth indeterminately. Indeed terrestrial mammals are presumed to have been forced to abandon indeterminate growth because, lacking the buoyancy of an acquitic environment it became necessary to avoid growing to a weight too heavy to support, and too difficult to nourish. In contrast indeterminate animals generally inhabit more hostile and aggressive environments so that they are liable to succumb to a violent death before having such problems.

The factors determining the ultimate cessation of body growth are legion, but one of the most obvious mechanisms of stopping growth is to limit the elongation of the long bones, achieved in determinate animals by the fusion of the cartilaginous plates and by the diminished secretion of growth hormone by the anterior pituitary soon after the development of sexual maturity.

There is also much experimental evidence which suggests that growth processes are controlled by negative feedback mechanisms both within specific organs (autoregulation) and centrally [35, 36].

Whether or not the maturation of BP is controlled by the same factors as total body growth remains unclear. As indeterminately growing animals (such as the whale) are virtually impossible to study, it is not known whether the BP continues to rise with increasing body dimensions throughout the animals' lifetime. In contrast, longitudinal studies in determinate animals and epidemiological data in humans indicate that coincident upon the arrest of body growth the slope of the BP-time curve is markedly reduced and indeed in some subpopulations reaches a plateau, with subsequent rise, mainly in systolic pressure, in old age largely attributable to diminished compliance of the aortic wall.

The most simple explanation would be that the absolute weight determines the BP and that both increase in parallel during the period of growth.

However, this is not borne out by comparative physiological data, where one finds that species as different in body weight, dimension and aggressiveness as rats and lions have trikingly similar BP values and patterns of BP maturation [37].

This led to the alternative hypothesis that the rate of change of BW, rather than its absolute value provides the natural stimulus to BP maturation. Canine studies provide support for this postulate which implies that BP maturation is indeed ultimately dependent on the determinants of growth of the body as a whole [7].

An alternative interpretation of the phenomena of finite BW and BP maturation is that just as evolutionarily a balance has to be struck between the advantages and disadvantages of increasing body weight and dimensions [34], so a balance is struck between the BP sufficient to provide adequate resting tissue perfusion and the need for a reserve capacity to augment BP and thus tissue perfusion at moments of stress, particularly for fight or flight exertion for survival. Thus, the plateau of the BP curve would represent an evolutionarily superior capacity to vasodilate minimizing cardiac work at rest, by reducing the preload, and maximizing the capacity to augment flow by vasoconstriction on exercise [38]. In this case a continuing rise in BP after growth ceases (hypertension) would be regarded as a more primitive evolutionary stage of BP development.

In essence therefore the argument is whether or not the maturation of blood pressure is a function of time or rather a function of the increase of body weight. Until experiments are designed which allow dissociation of these two variables it is likely that this question will remain unsolved.

In conclusion, the natural history of BP and other haemodynamic factors and their interrelationships have been outlined and their possible dependance on the global growth process discussed. The relevance of such an analysis lies in the opportunity in provided to force errors in the natural maturation curve of blood pressure to force errors in the natural maturation curve of blood pressure to determine their importance in the genesis of hypertension. A similar approach may also prove valuable in defining the factors controlling the regional circulations and their resistances, about which little is known and which clearly cannot be determined by invasive studies in growing children.

References

1. Van Mierof LHS (1970): Blood pressure in chick embryos, Ch. 1, p 27, in: Adams FH, Swan HJC, Hall VE (eds), *Pathophysiology of Congenital Heart Disease. Development of the cardiovascular system,* UCLA Forum Med Sci No 10, Univ California Press, Los Angeles.
2. Patten BM, Krauser TC, Barry A (1948): Valvular action in the embryonic chick heart by localized apposition of endocardial masses. *Anatomical Record* 102: 299.
3. Iberall AS (1975): Growth, forms and function in mammals. *Annals New York Academy of Science* 78.
4. Walsh SZ, Meyer WW, Lind J (1974): Postnatural changes in the pulmonary and systemic circulation, p 129, in: Swinyard (ed), *The Human Fetal and Neonatal Circulation.* Springfield, Illinois: C.C. Thomas.
5. Assali NS (1970): Control of systemic, pulmonary and regional blood flow in the fetal and neonatal periods, Ch 2, p 47, in: Adams FH, Swan HJC, Hall VE (eds), *Pathophysiology of Congenital Heart Disease.* UCLA Forum Med Sci No 10, Univ California Press, Los Angeles.
6. Woods JR, Dandavino A, Brinkman CR, Nurwayhid B, Assali NS (1977): Cardiac output changes during neonatal growth. *Am J Physiol* 234: H520.
7. Magrini F (1978): Haemodynamic determinants of the arterial blood pressure rise during growth in conscious puppies. *Cardiovasc Res* 12: 422.
8. Kloffenstein HS, Rudolph AM (1978): Postnatal changes in the circulation and responses to volume loading in sheep. *Circ Res* 42: 839.
9. Rudolph AM, Heymann MA (1970): Circulatory changes during growth in the fetal lamb. *Circ Res* 26: 289.
10. Guyton AC, Taylor AE, Granger HJ (1975): Synthesis of the total system for the control of body fluid volumes, Ch 21, p 316, in: Guyton AC, Taylor AE, Granger HJ (eds), *Circulatory Physiology,* Volume II: *Dynamics and Control of Body Fluids.* Philadelphia-London-Toronto: W.B. Saunders.
11. Holliday MA (1971): Metabolic rate and organ size during growth from infancy to maturity and during late gestation and early infancy. *Pediatrics* 47: 169.
12. Cayler GG, Rudolph AM, Nadas AS (1963): Systemic blood flow in infants and children with and without heart disease. *Pediatrics* 30: 186.
13. Assali NS, Morris JA (1964): Circulatory and metabolic adjustments of the fetus at birth. *Biology Neonate* 7: 141.
14. Naeye RL, Burlington VT (1961): Arterial changes during the perinatal period. *Archives Pathology* 71: 121.
15. Walsh SZ, Meyer W, Lind J (1974): Neonatal circulation, Section II, Ch 6, p 189, in: Swinyard CA (ed), *The Human Fetal and Neonatal Circulation.* Springfield, Illinois: C.C. Thomas.
16. Boatman DL, Snaffer RA (1965): Function of vascular smooth muscle and its sympathetic innervation in the newborn dog. *J Clin Invest* 44: 241.

17. Friis-Hansen B (1971): Body composition during growth: In vivo measurements and biochemical data correlated to differential anatomical growth. *Pediatrics* 47: 264.
18. Meyer N, Kleibsch N (1963): Die Strukturabwandlung der Pfortader nach der Geburt in ihrer Beziehung zur postnatalen Kreislaufumstelling. *Frankfurter Z Pathol* 73: 188.
19. Little R (1970): Changes in the blood volume of the rabbit with age. *J Physiol* 208: 485.
20. Romero T, Friedman W, Lovell J (1970): The pressure volume relations of the fetal newborn and adult heart. *Circulation* 51–52 (suppl III): 52.
21. Emery JL, Mithal A (1961): Weights of cardiac ventricles at and after birth. *Br Heart J* 23: 313.
22. Riemenschneider MA, Ruttenberg HO, Adams FA (1978): Maturational changes in left and right ventricular electromechanical intervals in the newborn lamb. *Cardiovasc Res* 12: 228.
23. Noods J, Dandavino A, Murayama K, Brinkman LR, Assali NS (1977): Autonomic control of cardiovascular functions during neonatal development and in adult sheep. *Circ Res* 40: 401.
24. Mace SE, Levy MN (1983): Autonomic nervous control of heart rate: Sympathetic-parasympathetic interactions and age related differences. *Cardiovasc Res* 17: 547.
25. Truccone NJ, Levine R (1973): Cardiovascular effects of propranolol in intact puppies and adult dogs. *Pediatric Res* 7: 931.
26. Coppoletta JM, Wolbach SB (1933): Body length and organ weights of infants and children. *Am J Pathol* 9: 55.
27. Philips CE, Deweese JA, Manning JA, Mahoney EB (1960): Maturation of small pulmonary arteries in puppies. *Circ Res* 8: 1268.
28. Levin DL, Rudolph AM, Heymann MA, Phibbs RH (1976): Morphological development of the pulmonary vascular bed in fetal lambs. *Circulation* 53: 144.
29. Dowling SE (1960): Baroreceptor reflexes in newborn rabbits. *J Physiol* 198: 201.
30. Pfeffer MA, Frohlich ED (1973): Hemodynamic and myocardial function in young and old normotensive and spontaneously hypertensive rats. *Circ Res* 32 (suppl I): 28.
31. McLain LG (1976): Hypertension in childhood: A review. *Am Heart J* 92: 634.
32. Report of the Task Force on Blood Pressure Control in Children (1977): *Pediatrics* 159 (suppl).
33. Sinclair D (1978): Nature of growth, Ch 1, p 1, in: *Human Growth after Birth*, 3rd ed. Belfast: Oxford University Press.
34. Goss RJ (1974): *Aging versus Growth. Perspectives in Biology and Medicine*, p 485.
35. Kavanau JL (1964): A model of growth and growth control in mathematical terms, Ch 20, p 353, in: Frost HM (ed), *Bone Biodynamics*, 1st ed. London: Churchill Ltd.
36. Saetren H (1956): A principle of auto-regulation of growth. *Experimental Cell Res* 11: 229.
37. Altman PL, Dittmer DS (1973): *Biological Handbooks: Respiration and Circulation*. Bethesda: Federation of American Societies for Experimental Biology.
38. Harris P (1983): Evolution and the cardiac patient: Review. *Cardiovasc Res* 17: 373.

5. Systemic hemodynamics and aging

CARLO ALICANDRI and GIULIO MUIESAN

The influence of advancing age on cardiovascular function has been the subject of many studies in the last few years. The increase of average life span and proportion of old people in the general population stimulated a number of studies in order to obtain a deeper knowledge of the normal physiology of aged individuals. Cross-sectional and longitudinal studies are used to examine the effects of aging. Both type of studies have some drawbacks. The cross-sectional study is planned to analyze at one time a group of individuals of different ages. In such study, it is difficult to eliminate genetic or environmental differences among groups. Furthermore, the older groups may represent a selected long-lived subset of the younger population. A longitudinal study examines the same individuals as their age advances and, therefore, a very prolonged time is required for studying humans. In such a study among many other obvious obstacles, an important one is the possible changes in methodology, not always easy to differentiate from age changes. In any case, the extent to which these studies may analyze the normal aging process is determined by the level of certainty regarding the absence of disease. This requirement can be difficult to be met, owing to the prevalence of atherosclerosis or occult coronary disease in the old age [1].

The more evident effect of advancing senescence on the cardiovascular system appears to be alterations in the anatomy and dynamic properties of the aorta and systemic vasculature. It has long been known that aging is associated with increased wall thickness and reduced elasticity of the aorta. This is accompanied by an increase in diameter and volume of the aorta, which also becomes elongated and tortuous [2]. The principal physiological consequence of these changes is a disproportional rise in systolic relative to diastolic pressure. Isolated systolic hypertension, characterized by a high systolic but normal diastolic pressure, is, actually, a common finding in the elderly. In some elderly patients the brachial artery may become so rigid that blood pressure

M.E. Safar & F. Fouad-Tarazi (eds.), The heart in hypertension.
© *1989 Kluwer Academic Publishers, Dordrecht –*

readings by cuff sphygmomanometer become unreliable. Such rigid arteries in order to be compressed require much more cuff pressure than the true intra-arterial pressure. This effect may result in 'pseudohypertension', and consequently overtreatment if not recognized [3]. The arterial rigidity may be defined by the ratio of change in arterial pressure ($\triangle P$) over the change in arterial volume ($\triangle V$). In man, the $\triangle P$ can be derived by the pulse pressure (PP) and the $\triangle V$ by the stroke volume (SV). Therefore, the PP/SV ratio can be a clinically useful index of rigidity of the aorta [4]: the higher its value, the higher the aortic rigidity. This method in evaluating aortic rigidity, or its reciprocal, that is aortic compliance, was validated by comparison with the method proposed by Simon et al. [5]. A very good correlation was found between the PP/SV ratio and the Simon's method [6], which estimated the arterial compliance from the analysis of the monoexponential blood pressure time curve during diastole, according to a simple viscoelastic model. Using the PP/SV ratio as an index of aortic rigidity, a positive correlation was noted between aortic rigidity and plasma noradrenaline ($r = 0.62$) in essential hypertensive patients older than 45 years (Figure 1) [6]. In these patients, the acute alpha and beta blockade (induced by labetalol 100 mg i.v., or by propranolol 10 mg i.v., followed by phientolamine 10 mg i.v.) decreased the PP/SV ratio in a significant positive relation to the basal levels of plasma noradrenaline ($r = 0.81$; Figure 2). These data suggested that aortic rigidity can be determined not only by anatomic structural changes, but also by functional factors and that the sympathetic nervous system activity might be one of the factors influencing this functional component of aortic rigidity at least in hypertensive patients older than 45. Simon et al., on the basis of the hemodynamic effect of beta-blockade alone, have suggested that the sympathetic tone may sustain systolic hypertension through beta-receptors stimulation in young hypertensive patients [6]. In elderly patients, otherwise, it has been noted a diminished beta-adrenoceptor mediated response with advancing age [7] ensuing in a relative preponderance of alpha-receptors mediated vasoconstriction [8]. Therefore, even a normal level of sympathetic tone could contribute to intensify the stiffness of arterial wall in the presence of an increased alpha and decreased beta-receptors responsiveness. This effect could be enhanced in the elderly, whose plasma noradrenaline levels at rest have been found to approximately double between the third and eight decades by Zighers et al. [9]. This age-associated increase of plasma noradrenaline levels may also influence the peripheral vasoconstriction. The significant positive correlation found in previous studies between total peripheral resistance and plasma noradrenaline in essential hypertensive patients [10, 11] seems to support this hypothesis. Even in these studies, the acute alpha and beta-blockade induced a decrease of total peripheral resistance, which was significantly related to the basal plasma noradrenaline level (Figure 3). Therefore, the sympathetic tone, through its

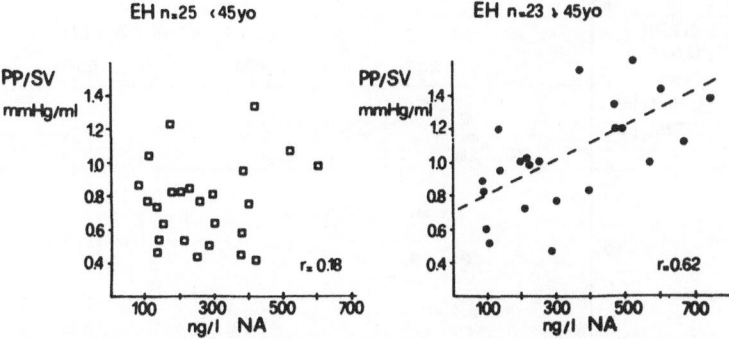

Figure 1. Plasma noradrenaline (NA) versus pulse pressure (PP)/stroke volume (SV) ratio in essential hypertensive patients (EH), 25 younger than 45 years and 23 older than 45.

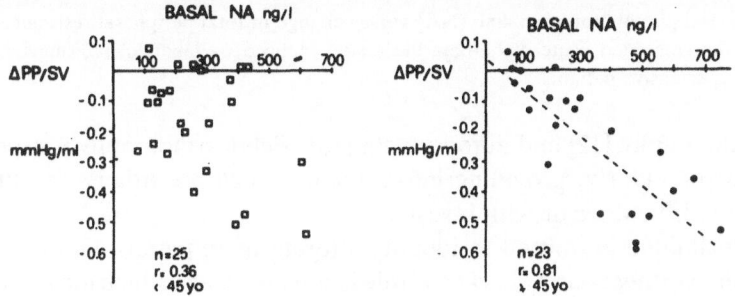

Figure 2. Basal plasma noradrenaline (NA) versus change of pulse pressure (PP)/stroke volume (SV) ratio induced by acute alpha and beta blockade in the same patients as in Figure 1.

influence on aortic rigidity and total peripheral resistance may be one of factors determining both the systolic and diastolic arterial pressure level. This influence may become more evident as age advances, owing to the age-related changes in adrenergic receptors sensitivity [7, 8].

The age associated changes in sympathetic tone and in structure and reactivity of the arterial bed can also greatly increase the impedance to left ventricular ejection and, consequently, may affect cardiac performance. Impedance to left ventricular ejection is a function of the central aortic rigidity, the peripheral resistance, the reflected pressure waves and the inertial properties of the blood. Age changes are associated with the first two factors, which are, at least in part, under the control of sympathetic activity. The aged heart, working against a higher impedance, due to increased aortic stiffness and peripheral resistance, must sustain a higher work load. A higher systolic blood pressure must also be developed, adding more work to the left ventricle. This increased load on the heart may explain the increase in left ventricular wall thickness and cardiac mass with age in both man and woman as shown by

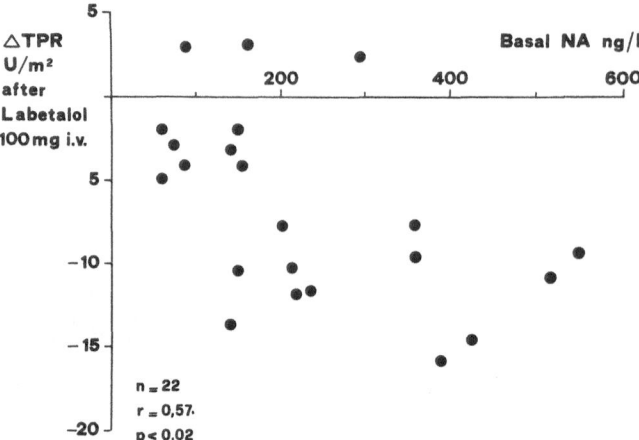

Figure 3. Basal plasma noradrenaline (NA) versus change in total peripheral resistance (TPR) following the combined acute alpha-beta bloàckade induced by labetalol (100 mg i.v.) in 22 essential hypertensive patients.

echocardiography [12] and autopsy data [13]. Echocardiography is especially useful in the elderly, providing informations which are otherwise obtained with many difficulties or with invasive testing.

This technique permitted to identify alterations in passive and active left ventricular stiffness during early diastole in advanced age which may result in a compromised cardiac function in old subjects [14]. The age related increase of sympathetic activity could, theoretically, support this decrease of cardiac performance. However, as with advanced age beta-receptors sensitivity may be reduced and alpha-receptors reactivity increased, the net result of an enhanced sympathetic activity in the aged could be a further increase of impedance to left ejection (through the adrenergic influence on arterial rigidity and peripheral resistance) more than an improvement of cardiac performance. Brandfonbrener et al. [15] first observed a decline of cardiac output with age: an approximately 50 percent decrease in cardiac index from 20 to 80 years of age or an average fall 1% a year from a mean 6.49 L/min in the third decade to 3.87 L/min in the ninth. Stroke volume, also, fell from 85.6 ml to 60.1 ml over the same age span. However, in a less stressful situation (no arterial or venous catheters involved) Rodeheffer et al. [16], measuring cardiac output by gated blood pool scanning over a broad age range of 30 to 80 years, did not observe an age associated change in cardiac output, end diastolic or end systolic volumes, or ejection fraction at rest. During exercise, a decline of cardiac performance has been observed in many studies with advancing age. Although the intrinsic cardiac muscle function evaluated in isolated cardiac muscle showed relatively little age-related change, it has been suggested that alterations in cardiovascular performance with advancing age, observed particularly during exercise, might also be related to a decreased responsiveness to beta-adrenergic stimulation of heart rate, myocardial contractility and arterial vasculature. In the study of Rodeheffer et al., during vigorous exercise, cardiac output was not related to age, while an age-related increase in end-diastolic volume and stroke volume and an age-related decrease in heart rate was noted. The dependence of the age-related increase in stroke volume or diastolic filling was emphasized by the fact that end systolic volume was higher and ejection fraction lower with increasing ge. These results suggested that although aging does not limit cardiac output per se in healthy subjects, the hemodynamic profile accompanying exercise is altered by age and can be, in effect, explained by an age-related diminution in the cardiovascular response to beta-adrenergic stimulation. In a previous study, involving essential hypertensive patients [10, 11], resting cardiac output and stroke volume resulted inversely related to basal plasma noradrenaline level (Figure 4). Similar results were more recently reported by Izzo et al. [17]. These authors noted also a decline of cardiac output with age (cardiac output measured without catheters by a rebreathing method). Partial regression analysis of their data demonstrated independent effect of sympathetic nervous activity and the aging process on cardiac function. These data seem to indicate that increase of catecholamines may be an adaptive response that attempts to sustain cardiac performance. This hypothesis is supported by the effects obtained with acute beta-blockade (propranolol 10 mg i.v.) which reduced cardiac performance (evaluated by the response of left ventricular end-diastolic pressure to the stress of isometric exercise) more in patients with the higher basal level of plasma noradrenaline (personal observation) (Figure 5). The shift in cardiac performance induced by propranolol is an indirect index of sympathetic contribution to cardiac performance [18] and, therefore, could be particularly useful in old patients, in order to evaluate the effective inotropic activity of sympathetic tone, particularly in the presence of a decreased beta-receptors sensitivity and increased plasma noradrenaline levels. It has been proposed that the increased secretion of noradrenaline in elderly normotensive subjects could be a consequence of a reduced baroreceptor sensitivity with aging [19]. Many studies have shown an age-related decline in baroreceptor reflex sensitivity [20, 21]. This reduced baroreflex mechanism would result in a less tonic inhibition of the vasomotor center which is associated to increased neural noradrenaline release and to vagal inhibition. Response of heart rate to various stimuli can give important informations in humans regarding the level of autonomic nervous system activity. Heart rate response following tilting has been recently shown to decrease with advancing age both in normotensives and in essential hypertensive patients [22].

Other age-related differences in heart rate response to various physiological stimuli have been reported. The above mentioned diminished beta-adrenergic

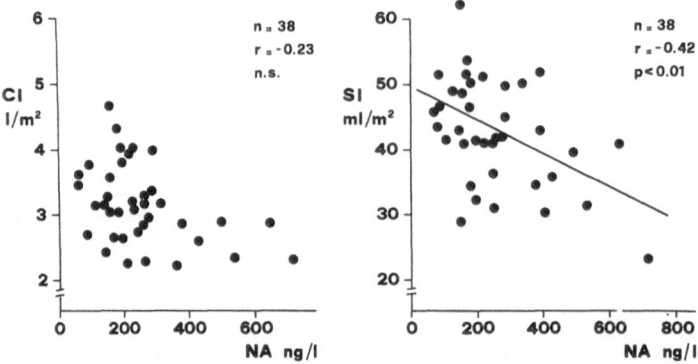

Figure 4. Plasma noradrenaline (NA) versus cardiac index (CI) and stroke index (SI) in essential hypertensive patients.

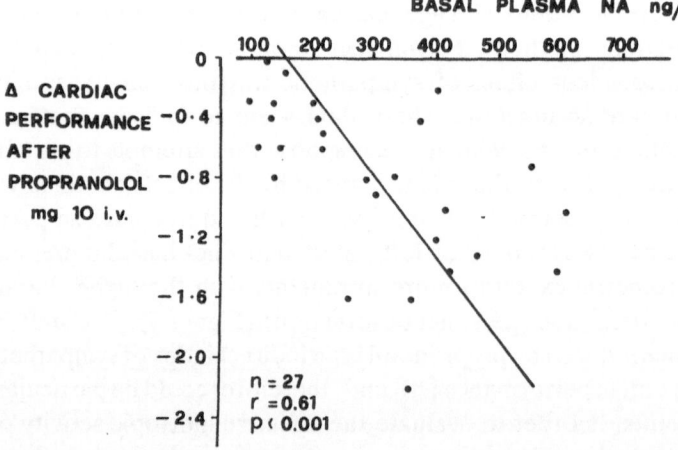

Figure 5. Basal plasma noradrenaline (NA) versus change in cardiac performance induced by propranolol (10 mg i.v.) in essential hypertensive patients. Cardiac performance was evaluated by the change of pulmonary wedge pressure in response to the increase of blood pressure and heart rate induced by static exercise.

responsiveness with age could be responsible of such a decline in heart rate response, but diminution of parasympathetic tone should also be considered. We have shown that parasympathetic control of heart rate, evaluated on the basis of variation of heart period (VHP) [23], declines with age in normotensive subjects, while such a relationship was not observed in essential hypertensive patients. However, the relationship between age and the change in heart rate following propranolol (0.09 mg/kg i.v.) and atropine (0.03 mg/kg i.v.) was significantly negative both in normotensive subjects and hypertensives, but the slope and intercept of the regression line were lower in the hypertensives.

The heart rate reached after the autonomic blockade induced by propranolol and atropine was also inversely related to age in normotensives ($r = -0.73$) and essential hypertensives ($r = -0.79$), but slope and intercept were again lower in essential hypertensives than normotensives. These data indicated that in normal subjects, parasympathetic control of heart rate decreases as age advances independently of the level of sympathetic activity, while such a relationship seems far less evident in essential hypertensive patients. A possible decline with age of intrinsic pacemaker activity both in normotensives and in essential hypertensives was also supposed, although the intrinsic pacemaker activity resulted lower in the hypertensives at all ages, but particularly in the young age. Whether this decline of parasympathetic activity with age could affect systemic hemodynamics is still under study. However, an inverse relationship was noted between parasympathetic tone, evaluated by the VHP, and blood pressure [24]. Furthermore, the increase of parasympathetic tone noted with ACE-inhibition was significantly related to the blood pressure reduction induced by this class of drugs [25].

In conclusion, at least some changes in the heart and the vascular system can be attributed to the aging process. The aortic rigidity and peripheral vasculature resistance are increased, the impedance to left ventricular ejection is greater. These age induced changes do not appear to alter appreciably the overall cardiovascular function in the resting state. Age changes, however, can affect cardiovascular function in stressful conditions. While previous studies have shown a decrease of cardiac performance, more recent studies indicate that cardiac output during exercise does not decrease although the maximal heart rate response to exercise is reduced. This effect can be explained by a higher stroke volume determined by a higher diastolic volume. The sympathetic tone may increase its activity as age advances and this may greatly influence the hemodynamic parameters and mainly aortic rigidity and cardiac performance. The parasympathetic tone, on the contrary, seems to decrease its activity as age advances. The parasympathetic control of heart rate in particular decreases with age, Since heart rate is one of the two principal determinants of cardiac output, it might be expected that a parasympathetic alteration would exert an important effect also on cardiac output and arterial pressure. However, more extended and better controlled studies are certainly needed to fully evaluate the relationship among age, hemodynamics and autonomic nervous system activity.

References

1. Kasser JG, Bruce RA (1969): Comparative effects of aging and coronary heart disease on submaximal and maximal exercise. *Circulation* 39: 759–774.
2. Yin FCP (1980): The aging vasculature and its effects on the heart. In: Weisfeldt ML (ed), *The aging heart.* pp. 137–213. New York: Raven Press.
3. Messerli FH, Ventura HO, Amodeo C (1985): Osler's maneuver and pseudohypertension. *N Eng J Med* 312: 1548–1551.
4. Tarazi RC, Magrini F, Dustan HP (1975): The role of aortic distensibility in hypertension. In: Millez P, Safar M (eds), *International Symposium on Hypertension.* pp. 133–145. Monaco: Boehringer Ingelheim.
5. Simon AC, Safar MA, Loevenson VA, Kheder AM, Levhy BI (1979): Systolic hypertension: hemodynamic mechanism and choice of antihypertensive treatment. *Am J Cardiol* 44: 505–511.
6. Alicandri C, Agabiti-Rosei E, Fariello R, Beschi M, Boni E, Castellano M, Montini E, Romanelli G, Zaninelli A, Muiesan G (1982): Aortic rigidity and plasma catecholamines in essential hypertensive patients. *Clin Exper Hyper-Theory and Practice* A4, pp. 1073–1083.
7. Landen GM, Safar ME, Weiss YA, Miller PL (1976): Isoproterenol sensitivity and total body clearance on propranolol in hypertensive patients. *J Clin Pharmacol* 16: 174–182.
8. Amann FW, Bolli P, Kiowski W, Buehler FR (1981): Enhanced alpha adrenoceptor mediated vasocontriction in essential hypertension. *Hypertension* 3 (suppl. I): I 119–123.
9. Ziegher MG, Lake CR, Kapin IJ (1976): Plasma noradrenaline increases with age. *Nature* 261: 333–335.
10. Agabiti-Rosei E, Alicandri C, Fariello R, Muiesan G (1979): Catecholamines and haemodynamics in fixed essential hypertension. *Clinical Science* 57: 193s–196s.
11. Agabiti-Rosei E, Alicandri C, Beschi M, Boni E, Castellano M, Fariello R, Montini E, Muiesan ML, Romanelli G, Muiesan G (1982): The adreno-sympathetic system in essential hypertension. In: Condorelli M, Zanchetti A (eds), *Hypertension, recent advances and research.* pp. 13–22. Verona: Cortina International.
12. Gerstenblith G, Frederiksen J, Yin FCP, Fortuin NJ, Lakatta EG, Weisfeldt ML (1977): Echocardiography assessment of a normal adult aging population. *Circulation* 56: 273–278.
13. Linzbach AJ, Akuamoa-Boating EA (1973): Die Alternsveranderungen des Menschlichen Herzen. *Klin Wochenschr* 51: 156–160.
14. Weitfeld MC, Gerstenblith G, Lakatta EG (1985): Alteration in circulatory function. In: Andres R, Bierman EL, Hazzard WR (eds), *Principles of Geriatric Medicine*, pp. 248–279. New York: McGraw-Hill.
15. Brandfonbrener M, Landowne M, Shock NW (1955): Changes in cardiac output with age. *Circulation* 12: 557–566.
16. Rodeheffer RJ, Gerstenblith G, Becker LC, Fleg JL, Weisfeldt ML, Lakatta EG (1984): Exercise cardiac output is maintained with advancing age in healthy human subjects: cardiac dilation and increased stroke volume compensate for a diminished heart rate. *Circulation* 69: 203–213.
17. Izzo JC, Smith RJ, Larrabee PS, Kallay MC (1987): Plasma norepinephrine and age as determinants of systemic hemodynamics in men with established essential hypertension. *Hypertension* 9: 415–419.
18. Alicandri C, Fouad FM, Tarazi RC, Bravo EL, Greenstreet RL (1983): Sympathetic contribution to cardiac response to stress in hypertension. *Hypertension* 5: 147–154.
19. Shimada K, Kitazumi T, Sadakane N, Ogura H, Ozawa T (1985): Age related changes of baroreflex function, plasma norepinephrine, and blood pressure. *Hypertension* 7: 113–117.

20. Lakatta EG (1980): Age-related alterations in the cardiovascular response to adrenergic mediated stress. *Fed Proc* 39: 3173–3177.
21. Bertel O, Buehler FR, Kiowski W, Lutold BE (1980): Decreased beta adrenoceptor responsiveness as related to age, blood pressure and plasma catecholamines in patients with essential hypertension. *Hypertension* 2: 130–138.
22. London GM, Weiss YA, Pannier BP, Laurent SL, Safar M (1987): Tilt test in essential hypertension. Differential response in heart rate and vascular resistance. *Hypertension* 10: 29–34.
23. Alicandri C, Boni E, Fariello R, Zaninelli A, Minotti F, Cantalamessa A, Muiesan G (1987): Parasympathetic control of heart rate and age in essential hypertensive patients. *J Hyperten* 5 (suppl. 5): S345–S347.
24. Fariello R, Boni E, Zaninelli A, Cantalamessa A, Alicandri C, Muiesan G (1986): Is there a parasympathetic influence on arterial pressure? *Cardiologia* 31: 603–607.
25. Boni E, Alicandri C, Fariello R, Zaninelli A, Cantalamessa A, Muiesan G (1986): *Effect of enalapril on parasympathetic activity*. Proceedings of 11th Scientific Meeting of the International Society of Hypertension, Heidelberg, F.R.G., August 31 – September 6, 1986, p. 242. In: *Cardiovascular Drugs and Therapy* (in press).

6. The hemodynamics of borderline hypertension

BRENT M. EGAN and STEVO JULIUS

Introduction

The hemodynamic history of borderline hypertension is rich with the contributions of numerous investigators over the past five decades. This is a particularly propitious time to review the literature, since it comes near the end of a long transition period from basic descriptive hemodynamic investigations of cardiac output, mean arterial pressure, and calculated peripheral resistance to studies of more subtle abnormalities in cardiovascular compliance, regional hemodynamic regulation, receptor specific hemodynamic events, and the cellular basis of hemodynamic derangements. In the following pages these considerable accomplishments are summarized and an attempt is made to synthesize the information into a unifying concept on the hemodynamic pathogenesis and progression of borderline hypertension.

The review is made difficult more by the plasticity of the definition of borderline hypertension than by the purported lability of the blood pressure. As the definition of mild hypertension has changed, much of what constituted borderline hypertension has fallen under the umbrella of mild hypertension. This review encompasses literature which predominantly reflects the traditional definition of borderline hypertension, e.g., average blood pressures < 160/100 with either intermittent or sustained blood pressures > 140/90. One additional complicating factor is the multiplicity of terms for this condition including transient hypertension, prehypertension, and labile hypertension. Among these, only labile hypertension continues to receive mention. Labile hypertension is an appropriate term if limited in scope to describing subjects with fluctuation of blood pressure above and below some arbitrary dividing line. Labile hypertension is, however, an unfortunate term which implies increased blood pressure variability. As will be discussed, the blood pressure outside the laboratory setting in borderline hypertension is not excessive.

M.E. Safar & F. Fouad-Tarazi (eds.), The heart in hypertension.
© 1989 Kluwer Academic Publishers, Dordrecht –

Blood pressure regulation in borderline hypertension

Before engaging in a discussion of hemodynamic mechanisms in borderline hypertension, a preliminary review of blood pressure regulation in borderline hypertension may provide important background for subsequent comments. Blood pressure variability in borderline hypertension continues to receive intense interest, largely because of a longstanding and widely accepted hypothesis that repeated pressor episodes induce structural cardiovascular changes which result in established hypertension. Blood pressure variability is difficult to assess, since peaks in blood pressure may be missed by infrequent measurement or minimized by viewing variability only as the standard deviation about the mean. Nevertheless, spontaneous fluctuation of blood pressure does not appear excessive in those with borderline hypertension [1, 2, 3].

The response of blood pressure to provocative stimulation in a laboratory setting suggests that reactivity is greater in borderline hypertensive patients compared to normal controls. Data also indicate that greater reactivity in the laboratory to stressors including cold [4, 5], exercise [6], mental arithmetic [7] and orthostasis [8] is independently predictive of future hypertension. The evidence suggesting that borderline hypertensive subjects are more reactive to stimuli including mental stress [9, 10], orthostatic stress [11, 12] perhaps reflecting increased sympathetic drive [13, 14], exercise [15, 16], and cold [17] is substantial but not uniform [18–35].

In our studies, blood pressure in borderline hypertension is regulated normally during exercise [26, 27], volume loading [35], upright tilt [33], and cardiac autonomic blockade [36] around a higher set point. In other words, although baseline blood pressure is higher, the change in pressure from that higher 'set point' in response to several stimuli is not excessive. The objective is not to refute the excellent studies showing increased variability under carefully defined conditions but rather to suggest that hypertension does not invariably develop through the summation of repeated pressor episodes. Some evidence suggests that the nervous system may induce sustained elevation of blood pressure without excessive lability [37, 38]. Furthermore, even when excessive variability in response to a specific laboratory stress is predictive of subsequent hypertension, the factors raising the set point for blood pressure may also be associated with abnormal regulation of pressure. For example, the intraleukocyte sodium level is predictive of not only increased pressor reactivity to mental and physical stressors [39] but also the subsequent development of hypertension [40]. Consequently, increased pressor reactivity may be coincidentally rather than causally related to subsequent hypertension. The absence of sustained hypertension in animals following baroreflex ablation, which increases blood pressure variability [41, 42], supports the viewpoint that blood pressure lability is not an independently sufficient requisite for permanent hypertension.

Baroreflex sensitivity. Hypothetically, increased blood pressure variability in borderline hypertension could reflect diminished carotid baroreflex sensitivity (BRS), since BRS is a known determinant of blood pressure variability [43, 44]. Conceivably, a primary abnormality in BRS is one potential cause of borderline hypertension. Furthermore, reduced BRS has been reported in borderline hypertension [45]. However, other data suggest that variables which may participate in the genesis of borderline hypertension including electrolyte balance [46, 47], neurogenic factors [48], and the renin-angiotensin system [43, 49] influence BRS. Additional evidence suggests that BRS is normal but 'reset' to regulate arterial pressure at a higher level [50]. In an attempt to resolve some of the confusion, one study noted that BRS was normal in borderline hypertensive subjects with systolic blood pressure < 140 mmHg but reduced in those whose systolic pressure exceeded that level [51]. Based on the available literature, any diminution of BRS in borderline hypertension likely reflects abnormalities in variables such as arterial compliance [52], neurohumoral balance, or electrolyte metabolism.

Blood flow and vascular resistance in borderline hypertension

Historical perspective

Although the majority of patients with essential hypertension has normal cardiac output and elevated peripheral resistance, exceptions were noted beginning nearly a half-century ago. In 1939, Wezler and Boger, who estimated cardiac output from complex formulas of pulse pressure and arterial elasticity, suggested that some patients had 'cardiac output hypertension' while most had 'resistance' hypertension [53]. Five years later in 1944, Goldring and Chasis, using more contemporary methods, confirmed that increased total peripheral resistance was indeed the hallmark of hypertension [54]. In 1949, Werko and Lagerlof investigated a small number of relatively young patients with predominantly systolic hypertension in whom peripheral resistance was normal [55]. Widimsky et al., in 1958, evaluated a larger group of young patients in whom blood pressure was maintained by an elevated cardiac output [31]. In 1962, Eich and coworkers identified increased cardiac output levels in borderline hypertensive patients over a wide age range [56]. These original observations indicated that the hemodynamic pathophysiology of borderline hypertension was distinct from that in established hypertension. These works stimulated subsequent descriptive, mechanistic, and natural history studies to better define the borderline hypertensive disorder.

High cardiac output in borderline hypertension

Elevated cardiac output in a substantial fraction of subjects with borderline hypertension has widespread international documentation from studies in Argentina [57], Czechoslavakia [31, 56], France [58–62], Germany [63–65], Japan [66, 67], Norway [68,69], Soviet Union [16], Sweden [24, 28], United States [27, 35,70–76], and Uruguay [15]. The prevalence of high cardiac output varied from approximately 15–50% of the borderline hypertensive subjects. In general, cardiac outputs were highest in younger subjects and those with elevated pressure at the time of hemodynamic investigation.

Reproducibility of the elevated cardiac output. On repeated measurements during the same study, cardiac output declined more yet remained higher in the hyperkinetic group compared to control subjects [33, 56]. Long-term follow-up studies of hyperkinetic (high cardiac output) borderline hypertensive subjects ranging from months to two decades indicated a common trend: cardiac output declined and total peripheral resistance increased in all studies [77], while blood pressure either remained constant [78, 79, 80] or increased [81, 82].

Physiologic basis for the increased cardiac output. On initial analysis, the high cardiac output could be explained by elevated heart rate and/or stroke volume. A higher heart rate was the mechanism in a majority of studies [16, 29, 34, 63, 64, 65, 68, 69, 72], followed by increases of both heart rate and stroke volume [27, 31, 54, 57, 65, 74], while only rarely was an isolated increase of stroke volume [67, 85] responsible for the elevated cardiac output. In order to better understand the physiological basis for the increased cardiac output a more detailed discussion is required.

Blood volume distribution and venous compliance. One prominent theory of hypertension proposes that elevated arterial pressure is initiated by volume expansion which subsequently raises cardiac output [86]. The elevated cardiac output elicits an autoregulatory increase of vascular resistance which reduces flow toward normal at the expense of a higher blood pressure level [87, 88]. Volume-induced increases of cardiac output in borderline hypertension were discussed [89] and a positive relationship between cardiac output and blood volume was repeatedly verified [57, 63, 72, 74, 90, 91, 92], especially in the established hypertensive patient. However, in the subject with borderline hypertension, the cardiopulmonary blood volume serves as the better corre-late of cardiac output [62, 74]. While central blood volume is often increased in borderline hypertension [62, 74, 84], documentation for an absolute expansion of either blood or plasma volume in borderline hypertension is absent. On the contrary, several reports noted either normal [57, 70, 72] or decreased [58, 92, 93] blood or plasma volume in borderline hypertensive patients.

Venous distensibility, which is reduced in borderline hypertensive patients [94], may contribute in two ways to a relative volume expansion. First, reduced peripheral venous capacitance may contribute to redistribution of the blood volume [95]. However, not all patients with reduced venous compliance have increased central blood volume. More importantly, a normal or even slightly reduced absolute value for blood volume may represent a virtual, or relative, expansion in the setting of a restricted capacitance system. While venous alpha-adrenergic tone may contribute to reduced venous compliance, other factors such as venous structure and/or myogenic tone are likely responsible for the differences in venous distensibility observed in borderline hypertension [94]. Other evidence indicates a link between sodium-potassium cotransport abnormalities and the decreased venous distensibility in this group [96].

The dynamic relationship of the peripheral venous abnormality to central hemodynamics was demonstrated in two ways. First, during the Valsalva maneuver, patients with borderline hypertension exhibit a smaller decrease in left atrial size on echocardiography in relationship to the rise in peripheral venous pressure [97]. Second, borderline hypertensive subjects, especially those with low plasma renin activity, pool less blood in their lower extremities and have smaller reductions in right atrial pressure in response to thigh cuff inflation compared to normotensive subjects [98]. The abnormal venous dis-tensibility affects central hemodynamic variables which in turn have neuro-humoral consequences. The greater preservation of central blood volume, especially in the low-renin borderline hypertensives [98, 99], during simulated orthostatic stress (thigh cuff inflation) minimizes the unloading of cardiopul-monary receptors which are important in the neurogenic regulation of renin release in man [100, 101]. Consequently, reduced venous distensibility may constitute an important component of diminished renin responsiveness in some borderline-mild hypertensive subjects.

Neurogenic factors in high cardiac output borderline hypertension

Heart rate. An increased heart rate is responsible for at least a portion of the elevated cardiac output in the majority of studies. Studies of the 'hyperkinetic' subgroup which utilized pharmacologic probes to assess autonomic tone pro-vide convincing evidence that the relative baseline tachycardia is neurogen-

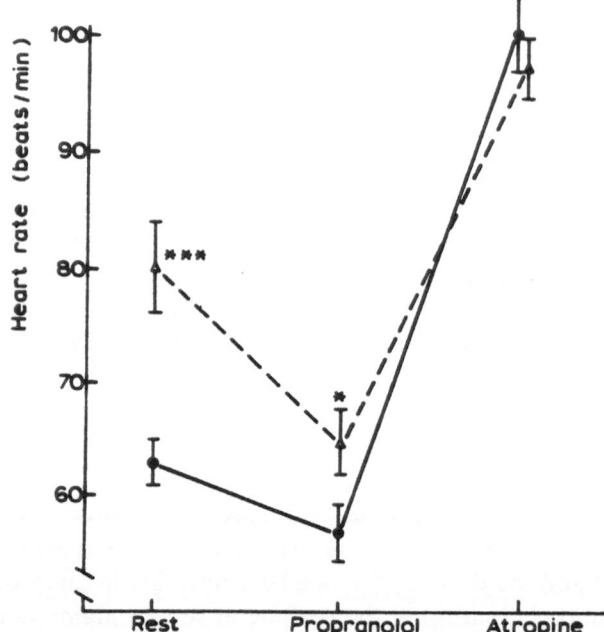

Figure 1. Heart rate is shown for the hyperkinetic borderline hypertensive subjects ($\triangle$---$\triangle$) and normotensive controls (●——●). Compared to controls, heart rate is higher in hyperkinetic subjects at baseline and declines more yet remains higher after intravenous propranolol at 0.2 mg/kg. Following addition of atropine at 0.04 mg/kg intravenously, heart rate increases less in hyperkinetic patients and is no longer different from the normotensive controls. Data = mean ± SE; *** $p < 0.001$; * $p < 0.05$.

ically mediated. In these subjects, heart rate declines more following beta-adrenergic blockade with propranolol but remains higher than in normotensives. Addition of atropine to abolish cardiac parasympathetic tone produces a smaller rise of heart rate in the borderline hypertensive as compared to normotensive subjects. Following the combined cardiac autonomic blockade heart rate is similar in the two groups (Figure 1). Consequently, in the patients with increased cardiac output levels, the higher heart rate represents both increased cardiac beta-adrenergic and decreased cardiac parasympathetic tone [95, 102].

Stroke volume. An increased stroke volume, frequently associated with the elevated heart rate, contributes to the increased cardiac output in many of the patients with the hyperkinetic state. As noted, a redistribution of the blood volume toward the central circulation is an important factor elevating stroke volume. However, the ratio of stroke volume to central blood volume is also increased in the hyperkinetic subjects [103]. In these subjects, the autonomic

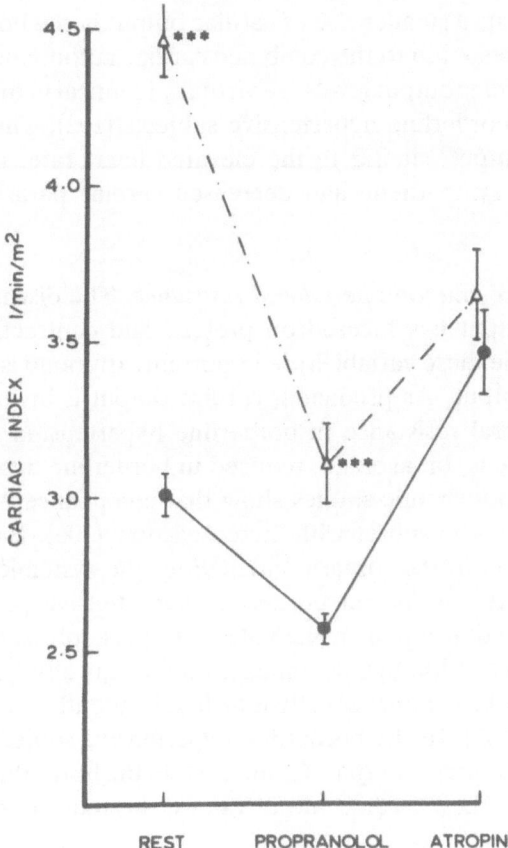

Figure 2. Cardiac index at supine baseline is higher in hyperkinetic borderline hypertensive subjects (△–•–△) compared to nomotensive controls (●———●). Cardiac index declines more but remains higher after propranolol. After addition of atropine, cardiac index increases less in the hyperkinetic group and is no longer distinguishable from the normal controls. Data = mean ± SE; *** p < 0.001 (patients vs. controls).

nervous system is responsible for the increased cardiac contractility [95], since combined blockade with propranolol and atropine normalizes the stroke volume to central blood volume relationship.

Cardiac output. Since the elevated heart rate and increased contractility are both related to an autonomic imbalance, one might predict that the elevated cardiac output in borderline hypertension similarly reflects autonomic factors. Compared to normotensive controls, the hyperkinetic borderline hypertensive patients manifest a greater decline in cardiac output in response to propranolol. Despite the greater decline, cardiac output remains higher in the borderline hypertensive subjects following propranolol. Addition of atropine to propranolol elicits a smaller rise of cardiac output in the borderline hypertensive group. In response to the combined cardiac autonomic blockade with the two agents, cardiac output levels are virtually identical in the normotensive and hyperkinetic borderline hypertensive subjects [102]. Therefore, the increased cardiac output, similar to the elevated heart rate, represents both increased cardiac sympathetic and decreased cardiac parasympthetic tone (Figure 2).

Arterial compliance and total peripheral resistance. The discussion of factors raising cardiac output has focused on preload and contractile state of the myocardium. While these variables are important, afterload is also a determinant of cardiac output. As predicted, cardiac output is inversely related to calculated peripheral resistance in borderline hypertension [27]. Although arterial compliance is, on average, reduced in borderline hypertension [104, 105], regional hemodynamic studies show that compliance is normal in the borderline hypertensive subset with increased flow [106]. Based on this intriguing observation in the forearm circulation, the systemic hemodynamic data in the Ann Arbor file on borderline hypertensive patients were re-evaluated. The relationship of stroke volume to pulse-pressure served as the index of compliance. Although the index is mathematically related to cardiac output through stroke volume, SV : PP is an independently confirmed index of compliance [105, 107]. In the borderline hypertensive subjects, SV : PP was inversely related to cardiac output. Of interest, in the borderline hypertensive subjects with the highest cardiac output values, this index of compliance was

Table 1. Systemic arterial compliance in borderline hypertension.

	Normotensive	Borderline hypertensive cardiac output[a]		
	(285)	Low (16)	Normal (100)	High (69)
Age, yrs	26 ± 6	28 ± 2	28 ± 1*	26 ± 1
SAP, mmHg	119 ± 3	129 ± 4*	132 ± 1*	135 ± 2*
DAP, mmHg	64 ± 1	72 ± 2*	75 ± 1*	74 ± 1*
CO, L/min	5.6 ± 0.1	4.4 ± 0.1*	5.9 ± 1.1	8.6 ± 0.2*
SV/PP, ml/mmHg	1.67 ± 0.02	1.30 ± 0.08*	1.58 ± 0.03*	1.84 ± 0.05*

[a] Subjects with borderline hypertension were divided into three groups based on cardiac output as a percentile of the normotensives distribution: (1) Low = < 20th percentile, (2) Normal = 20–80th percentile, (3) = > 80th percentile.
Data = mean ± SE; p = value determined by ANOVA; * p = <0.01 vs. normotensive.
CO = cardiac output.
DAP = diastolic intra-arterial pressure.
SAP = systolic intra-arterial pressure.
SV/PP = stroke volume/pulse pressure, an index of compliance.

'supernormal' (Table 1). Consequently, the high cardiac output was apparently facilitated by an absolute increase of arterial compliance.

In summary, the high cardiac output in borderline hypertension represents, on balance, a number of factors including reduced venous compliance, redistribution of the blood volume toward the central circulation, increased cardiac contractility, increased heart rate, normal or even possibly supernormal arterial compliance, and reduced total peripheral vascular resistance. Determining which of these factors are primarily and which are only secondarily related to the cardiac output level may provide important clues on the etiology of the hyperkinetic borderline hypertensive condition.

Normal cardiac output borderline hypertension

Although the subset of borderline hypertensive patients with high cardiac output has received the majority of attention, in most studies a preponderance of individuals with borderline hypertension had normal cardiac output. Long-term studies unequivocally document that some of these patients represent a later stage in the transition from the high output phase [69, 79, 81]. However, it is not established that all of the normal cardiac output group evolved from the high output phase. Furthermore, cardiac autonomic blockade normalizes cardiac output in the hyperkinetic group without normalizing blood pressure. Consequently, even in the hyperkinetic group, the hemodynamic dysregulation extends beyond the cor.

Despite the normal cardiac output and minimal blood pressure elevation, the 'normokinetic' group has evidence for multiple hemodynamic abnormalities. For example the ratio of stroke volume to central blood volume is reduced possibly reflecting reduced cardiac compliance. Following cardiac autonomic blockade with propranolol and atropine, cardiac output is lower in 'normokinetic' borderline hypertensive as compared to normotensive subjects. Consequently, the mildly increased heart rate in the normokinetic borderline hypertensive patients at baseline, which reflects principally diminished parasympathetic tone, is apparently required to maintain the normal cardiac output at rest [108]. The normokinetic group also has decreased regional [100] and systemic arterial compliance as well as increased peripheral vascular resistance [108] which may further limit stroke volume. Perhaps more significantly, data suggest that the borderline hypertensive subjects with lower cardiac output values progress to established hypertension more rapidly than do their 'hyperkinetic' cohort [69, 81].

Sodium sensitivity, neurogenic mechanisms, and hemodynamics
in borderline hypertension

The blood pressure levels of subjects with borderline hypertension are more responsive to dietary salt manipulation than are the blood pressure values in normotensive controls [109]. Despite the greater blood pressure response, data indicate that changes in body weight are not excessive in the salt-sensitive as compared to salt-resistant normotensive, borderline hypertensive [110], and hypertensive subjects [111]. Furthermore, the cardiac output, on average, does not rise excessively in salt-sensitive subjects [110]. The principal hemodynamic problem in the borderline hypertensive subject whose blood pressure increases during the salt challenge is inadequate vasodilation to counterbalance the rise in blood flow during the sodium challenge [109, 110]. In fact, some of the borderline hypertensive subjects raise blood pressure during a high salt diet entirely through vasoconstriction [109]. Conversely, the salt-resistant subjects respond to a dietary salt challenge with significant vasodilation in the forearm [112], renal [113], and systemic circulation [109]. Consequently, the rise in flow is counterbalanced by a fall in resistance; blood pressure may even decline in the salt-resistant subjects on a high salt diet. Although these studies examined the short-term effects of salt loading, an excessive increase of cardiac output in salt-sensitive subjects during the initial hours of the study, prior to the first measurements, could conceivably induce a rapid autoregulatory response of the vascular resistance which was inapparent a few days later.

Proposed mechanisms whereby salt influences hemodynamics
through the sympathetic nervous system

Salt-sensitive humans do not reduce sympathetic drive normally during a salt challenge [111, 114]. In Dahl salt-sensitive rats, increased adrenergic vasoconstriction accounts for approximately 50% of the rise in peripheral resistance during a salt challenge [115]. These findings are consistent with observations by the same investigators in humans with borderline hypertension. In the borderline hypertensive subjects, increased dietary salt raises baseline forearm vascular resistance and augments reflex (neurogenic) forearm vasoconstriction to lower body negative pressure [116] and cold stress [117]. Other data link the rate of proximal renal tubular sodium reabsorption to alpha-adrenergic reactivity [118]. Of interest, the proximal tubular sodium reabsorption correlates with red cell sodium-lithium countertransport [119] which is elevated in subjects with borderline hypertension [120]. These data suggest that salt in conjunction with membrane transport disorders raises vascular alpha-tone.

The increased vascular alpha-tone, in turn, participates in the inappropriate adjustment of peripheral resistance to flow in salt-sensitive animals and humans. While the precise mechanism of the sodium-induced rise in vascular alpha-tone is unknown, in selected rats, sodium induces a rise in alpha-receptor number [121], alpha-receptor affinity [122], and neural norepinephrine release per nerve impulse [123].

Transition from predominantly neurogenic high cardiac output
to principally non-neurogenic normal cardiac output borderline hypertension

The strongest evidence for sympathetic nervous system overactivity in hypertension occurs in young patients with mild disease [124, 125, 126]. Conversely, it is difficult to obtain consistent evidence for an important contribution of the sympathetic nervous system to hypertension in older subjects with more significant blood pressure elevation. This could indicate either that the hyperkinetic phase does not evolve into established hypertension or that a transition to a predominantly 'non-neurogenically' mediated hypertension occurs. Several lines of evidence suggest that the hyperkinetic phase does not always resolve spontaneously. First, elevated heart rate combined with a borderline blood pressure elevation increases the future likelihood of established essential hypertension. Furthermore, normotensive individuals with an elevated resting heart rate are also at higher risk for future hypertension when compared to their normotensive cohort with normal heart rates [127]. More convincingly, the transition from high to normal cardiac output associated with an increase of blood pressure is well documented [69, 79].

In the initial stages, the manifestations of sympathetic overactivity are predominantly cardiac with increased heart rate [98, 110] and increased cardiac contractility [102, 128, 129]. The normal peripheral resistance, which is not appropriately reduced (adjusted) to the level of blood flow, is the only apparent effect of increased sympathetic drive to the vasculature. The increased vascular alpha-tone at this early stage, which predominantly reflects increased sympathetic drive (plasma norepinephrine), is confirmed by an enhanced vasodilator response to phentolamine as shown in Figure 3 [85, 130]. However, only in the subgroup with high-renin, where evidence for neurogenic overactivity is greatest, is systemic blood pressure normalized following combined autonomic blockade with propranolol, atropine, and phentolamine [37, 85]. Since cardiac output is positively correlated to oxygen consumption, an autoregulatory stimulus for increased vascular resistance is not obvious [27, 131].

The decline in cardiac output over time may be explained without invoking classical autoregulation. Cardiac beta-receptor sensitivity declines [102, 108,

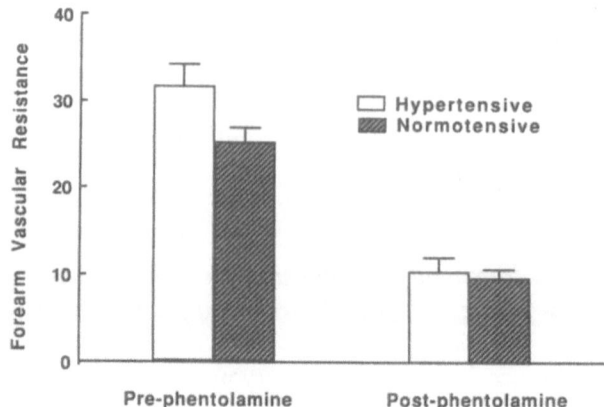

Figure 3. Forearm vascular resistance at baseline (pre-phentolamine) is higher in subjects with mild hypertension compared to weight-matched normotensive controls, $p < 0.04$. After regional (intra-arterial) phentolamine at 0.012 mg/100 ml forearm volume/min × 10 minutes (post-phentolamine) regional resistance levels are no longer significantly different [130].

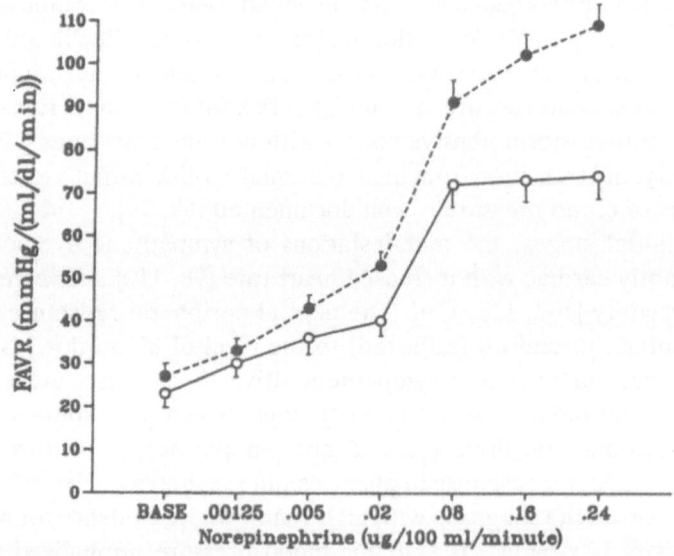

Figure 4. Forearm vascular resistance (FAVR, mean ± SE) is shown for mild hypertensive patients (●---●) and normotensive controls (○——○) at baseline and in response to regional (intra-arterial) norepinephrine. Resistance response at the lowest dose (sensitivity) is not greater in the hypertensives. However, the slope of the response and maximum response are greater in the hypertensives. This response pattern is most consistent with a structural vascular amplication [143, 145].

132], in response to the increased sympathetic drive [133] which would tend to reduce both heart rate [108] and the increased stroke volume : central blood volume [95, 103]. Cardiac hypertrophy reflecting both increased myocardial workload [134] and increased sympathetic drive [135, 136] may impair ventricular diastolic function [137], thereby reducing stroke volume. Abnormalities of diastolic function unexplained by cardiac hypertrophy [138] as well as increased afterload reflecting decreased arterial compliance and increased arteriolar resistance would also serve to limit stroke volume. The increased blood pressure [139, 140] and elevated sympathetic drive [141, 142] may, in addition, contribute to vascular hypertrophy. However, the vascular changes substantially amplify alpha-adrenergic vasoconstriction [143–145] as depicted in Figure 4. Furthermore, an elevated arterial pressure, perhaps through an effect on the vascular endothelium [146, 147] may contribute to increased alpha-receptor sensitivity as a function of higher arterial blood pressure [148]. The elevated vascular resistance at this later phase could be perpetuated with normal levels of sympathetic drive. Consequently, borderline hypertension, initially characterized by a neurogenic hyperdynamic state, could be sustained subsequently without increased autonomic drive at comparatively normal levels of blood flow accompanied by increased peripheral resistance [36,149].

References

1. Kanell WB, Sorlie P and Gordon T (1979): Labile hypertension: A faulty concept? The Framingham Study. *Circulation* 61: 1183–1187.
2. Horan MJ, Kennedy HL, Padgett NE (1981): Do borderline hypertensive patients have labile blood pressure? *Ann Int Med* 94(Part 1): 466–468.
3. Pickering TG, Harshfield GA, Blank S, James GD, Laragh JH, Clark L, Denby L, Pregibon D (1986): Behavioral determinants of 24-hour blood pressure patterns in borderline hypertension. *J Cardiovasc Pharmacol* 8(suppl 5): S89–92.
4. Hines EA (1951): The significance of hyperreactivity in the natural history of essential hypertension, in: *A Symposium on Essential Hypertension:* An Epidemiologic Approach to the Elucidation of Its Natural History in Man, pp 256–263. Boston: Wright & Potter Printing Co.
5. Wood DL, Sheps SG, Elveback LR, Schirger A (1984): Cold pressor test as a predictor of hypertension. *Hypertension* 6: 301–306.
6. Dlin RA, Hanne N, Silverberg DS, Bar-Or O (1983): Follow-up of normotensive men with exaggerated blood pressure response to exercise. *Am Heart J* 106: 316–320.
7. Falkner B, Kushner H, Onesti G, Angelakos ET (1981): Cardiovascular characteristics in adolescents who develop essential hypertension. *Hypertension* 3: 521–527.
8. Payen DM, Safar ME, Levenson JA, Totomokouo JA, Weiss YA (1982): Prospective study of predictive factors determining borderline hypertensive individuals who develop sustained hypertension: Prognostic value of increased diastolic orthostatic blood pressure tilt-test response and subsequent weight gain. *Am Heart J* 103: 379–383.

9. Nestel PJ (1969): Blood pressure and catecholamine excretion after mental stress in labile hypertension. *Lancet* 1: 692–694.

10. Falkner B, Onesti G, Angelakos ET, Fernandes M, Langman C (1979): Cardiovascular response to mental stress in normal adolescents with hypertensive parents. Hemodynamics and mental stress in adolescents. *Hypertension* 1: 23–30.

11. Esler MD, Nestel PJ (1973): Sympathetic responsiveness to head-up tilt in essential hypertension. *Clin Sci* 44: 213–226.

12. Hull DH, Wolthuis RA, Cortese T, Longo MR Jr, Triebwasser JH (1977): Borderline hypertension versus normotension: Differential response to orthostatic stress. *Am Heart J* 94: 414–420.

13. Frohlich ED, Tarazi RC, Ulrych M, Dustan HP, Page IH (1967): Tilt test for investigating a neural component in hypertension. *Circulation* 36: 387–393.

14. Eide I, Campese V, Stein D, Eide K, DeQuattro V (1978): Clinical assessment of sympathetic tone: Orthostatic blood pressure responses in borderline primary hypertension. *Clin Exper Hypertension* 1(1): 51–65.

15. Folle LE, Dighiero J, Sadi I, Pommerenck C, Elena R (1970): Hemodynamic response to exercise after beta-adrenergic blockade in normal and labile hypertensive patients. *Cardiology* 55: 105–113.

16. Kramer AA, Shkhvatsabaya LV, Eventov AZ, Pershakova LP (1972): Peculiarities of the central and renal hemodynamics in patients with hypertensive disease at its early stage. *Kardiologiya* 12: 31–40.

17. Thacker EA (1940): A comparative study of normal and abnormal blood pressures among university students, including the cold pressor test. *Am Heart J* 20: 89–97.

18. Shapiro AP (1961): An experimental study of comparative responses of blood pressure to different noxious stimuli. *J Chronic Dis* 13: 293–311.

19. Thomas CB, Stanley JA, Kendrick MA (1961): Observations on some possible precursors of essential hypertension and coronary artery disease, VII: The subjective reaction to the cold pressor test as expressed in the verbal response. *J Chronic Dis* 14: 355–365.

20. Cuddy RP, Smulyan H, Keighley JF, Markason CR, Eich RH (1966): Hemodynamic and catecholamine changes during a standard cold pressor test. *Am Heart J* 71: 446–465.

21. Eich RH, Jacobsen EC (1967): Vascular reactivity in medical students followed for 10 years. *J Chronic Dis* 20: 583–592.

22. Konig K, Reindell H, Steim H, et al. (1959): Beitrag zur hamodynamik hypertoner regulationsstorungen [Contribution to the hemodynamics of the hypertone regulation]. *Z Kreislaufforsch* 48: 923–939.

23. Maidorn K, Mellevovicz H (1963): Arterial blood pressure during an ergometric lead. *Z Kreislaufforsch* 52: 53–63.

24. Sannerstedt R (1966): Hemodynamic response to exercise in patients with arterial hypertension. *Acta Med Suppl* 458: 1–83.

25. Levy AM, Tabakin BS, Hanson JS (1967): Hemodynamic responses to graded treadmill exercise in young untreated labile hypertensive patients. *Circulation* 35: 1063–1072.

26. Conway J, Julius S, Amery A (1968): Effect of blood pressure level on the hemodynamic response to exercise. *Hypertension* 16: 79–85.

27. Julius S, Conway J (1968): Hemodynamic studies in patients with borderline blood pressure elevation. *Circulation* 38: 282–288.

28. Sannerstedt R (1969): Hemodynamic findings at rest and during exercise in mild arterial hypertension. *Am J Med Sci* 258: 70–79.

29. Sannerstedt R, Julius S (1972): Systemic haemodynamics in borderline arterial hypertension: Responses to static exercise before and under the influence of propranolol. *Cardiovasc Res* 6: 318–403.

30. DeCarvalho JGR, Messerli FH, Frohlich ED (1979): Mitral valve prolapse and borderline hypertension. *Hypertension* 1(5): 518–522.
31. Widimsky VJ, Fejfarova HM, Fejfar Z, Dejdar R, Exnerova M, Pirk F (1958): Der jugendliche Hochdruk [Juvenile hypertension]. *Arch Kreislaufforsch* 28: 100–124.
32. Brod J (1963): Haemodynamic basis of acute pressor reactions and hypertension. *Br Heart J* 25: 227–245.
33. Sannerstedt R, Julius S, Conway J (1970): Hemodynamic responses to tilt and beta-adrenergic blockade in young patients with borderline hypertension. *Circulation* 42: 1057–1064.
34. Molzahn M, Dissmann TH, Halim S, Lohmann FW, Oelkers W (1972): Orthostatic changes of haemodynamics, renal function, plasma catecholamines and plasma renin concentration in normal hypertensive man. *Clin Sci* 422: 209–222.
35. Julius S, Pascual AV, Sannerstedt R, Mitchell C (1971): Relationship between cardiac output and peripheral resistance in borderline hypertension. *Circulation* 43: 382–390.
36. Julius S (1987): Hemodynamic, pharmacologic and epidemiologic evidence for behavioral factors in human hypertension, in: Julius S and Bassett DR (eds), *Handbook of Hypertension*, Vol 9: *Behavioral Factors in Hypertension*, Ch 4, pp 59–74. Amsterdam: Elsevier Science Publishers.
37. Esler M, Julius S, Zweifler A, Randall O, Harburg E, Gardiner H, DeQuattro V (1977): Mild high-renin essential hypertension. Neurogenic human hypertension? *New Engl J Med* 296: 405–411.
38. Schneider RH, Egan BM, Johnson EH, Drobny H, Julius S (1986): Anger and anxiety in borderline hypertension. *Psychosomat Med* 48(3/4): 242–248.
39. Ambrosioni E, Costa FV, Borghi C, Montebugnoli L, Giordani MF, Magnani B (1982): Effects of moderate salt restriction on intralymphocytic sodium and pressor response to stress in borderline hypertension. *Hypertension* 4: 789–794.
40. Borghi C, Costa FV, Boschi S, Mussi A, Ambrosioni E (1986): Predictors of stable hypertension in young borderline subjects: A five-year follow-up study. *J Cardiovasc Pharm* 8(suppl 5): S138–141.
41. Cowley AW, Liard JF, Guyton AC (1973): Role of the baroreceptor reflex in daily control of arterial blood pressure and other variables in dogs. *Circ Res* 32: 564.
42. Talman WT, Alonso DR, Reis DJ (1980): Impairment of baroreceptor function and chronic lability of arterial pressure produced by lesions of A2 catecholamine neurons of rat brain: Failure to evolve into hypertension, in: Sleight P (ed), Baroreceptors and hypertension, pp 448 *ff.* Oxford: Oxford University Press.
43. Watson RDS, Stallard TJ, Flinn RM, Littler WA (1980): Factors determining direct arterial pressure and its variability in hypertensive man. *Hypertension* 2: 333–341.
44. Conway J, Boon N, Davies C, Vann Jones J, Sleight P (1984): Neural and humoral mechanisms involved in blood pressure variability. *J Hypertension* 2: 203–208.
45. Takeshita A, Tanaka N, Kuroiwa NM, et al. (1975): Reduced baroreceptor sensitivity in borderline hypertension. *Circulation* 51: 738–742.
46. Skrabal F, Auböck J, Hörtnagl H, Braunsteiner H (1980): Effect of moderate salt restriction and high potassium intake on pressor hormones, response to noradrenaline and baroreceptor function in man. *Clin Sci* 59: 157s–160s.
47. Ferrario CM, Tramposch A, Kawano Y, Brosnihan KB (1987): Sodium balance and the reflex regulation of baroreceptor function. *Circulation* 75(suppl I): I–141–148.
48. Takeshita A, Tanaka S, Nakamura M (1978): Effects of propranolol on baroreflex sensitivity in borderline hypertension. *Cardiovasc Res* 12: 148–151.
49. Ibsen H, Egan B, Julius S (1983): Baroreflex sensitivity during converting enzyme inhibition with Enalapril (MK—421) in normal man. *J Hypertension* 1(suppl 2): 222–224.

50. Julius S (1976): Neurogenic component in borderline hypertension, in: Julius S and Esler M (eds), *The Nervous System in Arterial Hypertension*, pp 301–330. Springfield, Ill.: Charles C. Thomas.

51. Eckberg DL (1979): Carotid baroreflex function in young men with borderline blood pressure elevation. *Circulation* 59: 632–636.

52. Randall OS, Esler MD, Bulloch GF, Maisel AS, Ellis CN, Zweifler AJ, Julius S (1976): Relationship of age and blood pressure to baroreflex sensitivity and arterial compliance in man. *Clin Sci Mol Med* 51: 357s–360s.

53. Wezler K, Boger A (1939): Die dynamik des arteriellen systems: Der arterielle blutdruck und seine komponenten [The dynamics of the arterial system: Arterial pressure and its components]. *Ergeb Physiol* 41: 292–606.

54. Goldring W, Chasis H (1944): *Hypertension and Hypertensive Disease*. New York, N.Y.: The Commonwealth Fund.

55. Werko L, Lagerlof B (1949): Studies on the circulation in man (IV). Cardiac output and blood pressure in the right auricle, right ventricle and pulmonary artery in patients with hypertensive cardiovascular disease. *Acta Med Scand* 133: 427–436.

56. Eich RH, Peters RJ, Cuddy RP, Smulyan H, Lyons RH (1962): The hemodynamics in labile hypertension. *Am Heart J* 63: 188–195.

57. Finkielman S, Worcel M, Agrest A (1965): Hemodynamic patterns in essential hypertension. *Circulation* 31: 356–368.

58. Safar ME, Weiss YA, Levenson JA, et al. (1973): Hemodynamic study of 85 patients with borderline hypertension. *Am J Cardiol* 31: 315–319.

59. Safar M, Milliez P (1972): Hemodynamic findings in human arterial hypertension. *Rev Eur Etud Clin Biol* 27: 147–154.

60. Tourniaire A, Blum J, Tartulier M, Lestaevel M (1972): Hypertension arterielle labile – varietes hemodynamiques. *Nouv Presse Med* 1: 255–256.

61. Safar ME, Hornych AF, Levenson JA, Simon ACh, London GM, Bariety JL, Milliez PL (1981): Central hemodynamics and plasma prostaglandin E_2 in borderline and sustained essential hypertensive patients before and after indomethacin. *Clin Sci* 61: 323s–325s.

62. Safar ME, Weiss YA, London GM, Frachowiak RF, Milliez PL (1974): Cardiopulmonary blood volume in borderline hypertension. *Clin Sci Mol Med* 47: 153–164.

63. Dissmann T, Gotzen R, Molzahn M, Lohmann FW, Schwab M (1970): Blood circulation mechanics in essential and renovascular hypertension. *Arch Kreislaufforsch* 63: 226–256.

64. Molzahn M, Dissmann TH, Gotzen R, Lohmann FW (1971): The effects of acute and chronic diminution of cardiac output on blood pressure in early hypertension. Hemodynamic alterations after beta-receptor blockade. *Klin Wochenschr* 49: 476–484.

65. Juchama Von R, Wertz U (1969): Central hemodynamics of the hyperkinetic syndrome under blockade with beta receptors. *Muench Med Wochenschr* 111: 2567–2571.

66. Kuramoto K, Murata K, Yazaki Y, Ikeda M, Nakao K (1968): Hemodynamics in the juvenile hypertension with special reference to the response to propranolol. *Jap Circ J* 32: 981–987.

67. Miura Y,, Kobayashi K, Sakuma H, Tomioka H, Acachi M, Yoshinaga K (1978): Plasma noradrenaline concentrations and haemodynamics in the early stage of essential hypertension. *Clin Sci Mol Med* 55: 69s–71s.

68. Lund-Johansen P (1967): Hemodynamics in early essential hypertension. *Acta Med Scand* suppl 482: 1–100.

69. Lund-Johansen P (1986): Hemodynamic patterns in the natural history of borderline hypertension. *J Cardiovasc Pharm* 8(suppl 5): S8–14.

70. Bello CT, Sevy RW, Harakal C (1965): Varying hemodynamic patterns in essential hypertension. *Am J Med Sci* 250: 24–35.

71. Frohlich ED, Tarazi RC, Dustan HP (1969): Re-examination of the hemodynamics of hypertension. *Am J Med Sci* 257: 9–23.
72. Frohlich ED, Kozul VJ, Tarazi RC, Dustan HP (1970): Physiological comparison of labile and essential hypertension. *Circ Res* 46(suppl 1): 55–69.
73. Julius S, Pascual AV, London R (1971): Role of parasympathetic inhibition in the hyperkinetic type of borderline hypertension. *Circulation* 44: 413–418.
74. Messerli FH, DeCarvalho JGR, Christie B, Frohlich ED (1978): Systemic and regional hemodynamics in low, normal and high cardiac output borderline hypertension. *Circulation* 58: 441–448.
75. Messerli FH, Frohlich ED, Suarez DH, Reisin E, Dreslinski GR, Dunn FG, Cole FE (1981): Borderline hypertension: Relationship between age, hemodynamics and circulating catecholamines. *Circulation* 64(4): 760–764.
76. Sullivan JM, Prewitt RL, Josephs JA (1983): Attenuation of the microcirculation in young patients with high-output borderline hypertension. *Hypertension* 5: 844–851.
77. Eich RH, Cuddy RP, Smulyan H (1966): Hemodynamics in labile hypertension: A follow-up study. *Circulation* 34: 299–307.
78. Eliasch H, Varnauskas E, Werko L (1971): Minutvolym och perifert motstand vid hypertoni-enlongitudinell studie, in: Hansson L (ed): *Hypertoni och arteriosklerosfragor*, pp 17–19. Goteborg, Sweden: Lindgren.
79. Weiss YA, Safar ME, London GM (1978): Repeat hemodynamics determinations in borderline hypertension. *Am J Med* 64: 382–387.
80. Julius S, Quadir H, Gajendragadkar S (1979): Hyperkinetic stage: A precursor of hypertension? A longitudinal study of borderline hypertension, in: Gross F, Strasser T (eds): *Mild hypertension: Natural history and management*, pp 116–126. Bath, UK: Pittman Medical.
81. Lund-Johansen P (1979): Hemodynamic observations in mild hypertension, in: Gross F, Strasser T (eds): *Mild hypertension: Natural history and management*, pp 19–34. Bath, UK: Pittman Medical.
82. Andersson OK, Sannderstedt T, Beckman M (1983): Essential hypertension: Implications for pathogenesis from repeated hemodynamic investigations in young men with elevated blood pressure. *J Hypertension* 1(suppl 2): 91–93.
83. Ibrahim MM, Tarazi RC, Dustan HP, Bravo EL (1973): Cardioadrenergic factor in essential hypertension: Clinical recognition. *Circulation* 48(suppl 4): 180.
84. Ellis CN, Julius S (1973): Role of central blood volume in hyperkinetic borderline hypertension. *Br Heart J* 35: 450–455.
85. Esler M, Julius S, Randall OS, Ellis CN, Kashima T (1975): Relation of renin status to neurogenic vascular resistance in borderline hypertension. *Am J Cardiol* 36: 708–715.
86. Borst JGG, Borst-de Geus A (1963): Hypertension explained by Starling's theory of circulatory homeostasis. *Lancet* 1963/1: 677–682.
87. Coleman TG, Granger HJ, Guyton AC (1971): Whole-body circulatory autoregulation and hypertension. *Circ Res* 28–29(suppl 2): 76–86.
88. Guyton AC, Coleman TG (1967): Long-term regulation of the circulation: Interrelationships with body fluid volumes, in: Reeve EG, Guyton AC (eds): *Physical Bases of Circulatory Transport: Regulation and Exchange*, p 179. W.B. Saunders Co.
89. Ledingham, JM (1971): The etiology of hypertension. *Practitioner* 202: 5–19.
90. Kuramoto K, Murata K, Yazaki Y, Ikeda M, Nakao K (1968): Hemodynamics in the juvenile hypertension with special reference to the response to propranolol. *Jap Circ J* 32: 981–987.
91. Birkenhager WH, Van Es LS, Houwing A, Lamers HJ, Mulder AH (1968): Studies on the lability of hypertension in man. *Clin Sci* 35: 445–456.

92. Julius S, Pascual AV, Reilly K, London R (1971): Abnormalities of plasma volume in borderline hypertension. *Arch Intern Med* 127: 116–119.

93. Dissman TH, Gotren R, Muller B, Neuber K (1967): Plasma and red blood cell volume in incipient essential hypertension. *Verh Dtsch Ges Inn Med* 73: 604–607.

94. Takeshita A, Mark AL (1979): Decreased venous distensibility in borderline hypertension. *Hypertension* 1(3): 202–206.

95. Julius S, Esler M (1975): Autonomic nervous cardiovascular regulation in borderline hypertension. *Am J Cardiol* 36: 685–696.

96. Weder AB, Fitzpatrick MA, Torretti BA, Hinderliter AL, Egan BM, Julius S (1987): Red blood Li$^+$-Na$^+$ countertransport, Na$^+$-K$^+$ cotransport, and the hemodynamics of hypertension. *Hypertension* 9: 459–466.

97. Robertson D, Shand DG, Hollifield JW, Nies AS, Frolich JC, Oates JA (1979): Alterations in the responses of the sympathetic nervous system and renin in borderline hypertension. *Hypertension* 1(2): 118–124.

98. Fitzpatrick MA, Hinderliter AL, Egan BM, Julius S (1986): Decreased venous distensibility and reduced renin responsiveness in hypertension. *Hypertension* 8(suppl II): II–36–43.

99. Egan B, Fitzpatrick MA, Julius S (1987): The heart and the regulation of renin. *Circulation* 75(suppl I): I–130–133.

100. Kiowski W, Julius S (1978): Renin response to stimulation of cardiopulmonary mechanoreceptors in man. *J Clin Invest* 62: 656–663.

101. Egan B, Julius S, Cottier C, Osterziel KJ, Ibsen H (1983): The role of cardiovascular receptors on the neural regulation of renin release in normal man. *Hypertension* 5: 779–786.

102. Julius S (1976): Abnormalities of autonomic nervous control in borderline hypertension. *Schweiz med Wschr* 106: 1698–1705.

103. Tarazi RC, Ibrahim MM, Dustan HP, Ferrario C (1974): Cardiac factors in hypertension. *Circ Res* 34–35(suppl I): I–213–221.

104. Ferguson JJ, Julius S, Randall OS (1984): Stroke volume-pulse pressure relationships in borderline hypertension: A possible indicator of decreased arterial compliance. *J Hypertension* 2(suppl 3): 397–399.

105. Ventura H, Messerli FH, Oigman W, Suarez DH, Dreslinski GR, Dunn FG, Reisin E, Frohlich ED (1984): Impaired systemic arterial compliance in borderline hypertension. *Am Heart J* 108: 132–136.

106. Simon A, Levinson J, Bouthier J, Maarek B (1987): Hemodynamic basis of early modifications of the large arteries in borderline hypertension. *J Hypertension* 5: 179–184.

107. Tarazi RC, Magrini F, Dustan HP (1975): The role of aortic distensibility of hypertension, in: Miller P, Safar MD (eds), *International Symposium on Hypertension, Monaco*, p. 133. Boehringer Ingelheim.

108. Julius S, Randall OS, Esler MD, Kashima T, Ellis C, Bennett J (1975): Altered cardiac responsiveness and regulation in the normal cardiac output type of borderline hypertension. *Circ Res* 36–37(suppl I): I–199–207.

109. Sullivan JM, Ratts TE, Taylor JC, Kraus HD, Barton BR, Patrick DR, Reed SW (1980): Hemodynamic effects of dietary sodium in man: A preliminary report. *Hypertension* 2: 506–514.

110. Sullivan JM, Prewitt RL, Ratts TE, Josephs JA, Connor MJ (1987): Hemodynamic characteristics of sodium-sensitive human subjects. *Hypertension* 9: 398–406.

111. Campese VM, Romoff MS, Levitan D, Saglikes Y, Freidler R, Massry S (1982): Abnormal relationship between sodium intake and sympathetic nervous system activity in salt-sensitive patients with essential hypertension. *Kidney Int* 21: 371–378.

112. Kirkendall WM, Connor WE, Abboud FM, Rastogi SP, Anderson TA, Fry M (1972): Effect of dietary sodium on the blood pressure of normotensive man, in: Genest J (ed), *In-*

ternational Symposium on Renin-Angiotensin-Aldosterone-Sodium in Hypertension, pp 360–373. Springer-Verlag.

113. Redgrave J, Rabinowe S, Hollenberg W, et al. (1985): Correction of abnormal renal blood flow response to angiotensin II by converting enzyme inhibition in essential hypertensives. *J Clin Invest* 75: 1285.

114. Fujita T, Henry WL, Bartter FC, Lake CR, Delea CS (1980): Factors influencing blood pressure in salt-sensitive patients with hypertension. *Am J Med* 69: 334–344.

115. Takeshita A, Mark AL (1978): Neurogenic contribution to hindquarter vasoconstriction during high sodium intake in Dahl strain of genetically hypertensive rats. *Circ Res* 43(suppl I): I–86–91.

116. Mark AL, Lawton WJ, Abboud TM, Fitz AE, Connor WE, Heistad DD (1975): Effects of high and low sodium intake on arterial pressure and forearm vascular resistance in borderline hypertension. *Circ Res* 36–37(suppl I): I–194–198.

117. Takeshita A, Imaizumi T, Ashihara T, Nakamura M (1982): Characteristics of responses to salt loading and deprivation in hypertensive subjects. *Circ Res* 51: 457–464.

118. Skrabal F, Herholz H, Neumayr M, Hamberger L, Ledochocowski M, Sporer H, Hortnagl H, Schwartz S, Schonitzer D (1984): Salt sensitivity in humans is linked to enhanced sympathetic responsiveness and to enhanced proximal tubular reabsorption. *Hypertension* 6: 152–158.

119. Weder AB (1986): Red cell lithium-sodium countertransport and renal lithium clearance. *N Engl J Med* 314: 198–201.

120. Weder AB, Fitzpatrick MA (1986): Lithium-sodium countertransport: Physiological moorings for red cell transport disorders in hypertension. *J Cardiovasc Pharm* 8(suppl 5): S76–81.

121. Pettinger W, Sanchez A, Saavedra J, Haywood JR, Gandler T, Rodes T (1982): Altered renal alpha$_2$-adrenergic receptor regulation in genetically hypertensive rats. *Hypertension* 4(suppl II): II–188–192.

122. Lin C, Lu H, Lin K (1982): Adrenergic receptors and increased reactivity of aortic smooth muscle in renal hypertensive rats. *J Autonomic Nerv Sys* 5: 253–264.

123. Folkow B, Ely DL (1987): Dietary sodium effects on cardiovascular and sympathetic neuroeffector functions as studied in various rat models. *J Hypertension* 5: 383–395.

124. Julius S, Esler M, Randall OS (1975): Role of the autonomic nervous system in mild human hypertension. *Clin Sci Mol Med* 48: 243s–252s.

125. Goldstein DS (1983): Plasma catecholamines and essential hypertension: An analytical review. *Hypertension* 5: 86–99.

126. Esler M, Jennings G, Biviano B, Lambert G, Hasking G (1986): Mechanism of elevated plasma noradrenaline in the course of essential hypertension. *J Cardiovasc Pharmacol* 8(suppl 5): S39–43.

127. Levy RL, White PD, Stroud WD, Hillman CC (1945): Transient tachycardia: Prognostic significance alone and in association with transient hypertension. *J Am Med Assoc* 129: 585–588.

128. Cousineau D, DeChamplian J, LaPointe L (1978): Circulating catecholamines and systolic time intervals in labile and sustained hypertension. *Clin Sci Mol Med* 55: 65s–68s.

129. Lehner JP, Safar ME, Dimitriu VM, Simon A, Carrez JB, Plainfosse MT (1979): Systolic time intervals and echocardiographic findings in borderline hypertension. *Europ J Cardiol* 9(4): 319–331.

130. Egan B, Panis R, Hinderliter A, Schork N, Julius S (1987): Mechanism of increased alpha-adrenergic vasoconstriction in human essential hypertension. *J Clin Invest* 80: 812–817.

131. Lund-Johansen P (1980): State-of-the-art: Hemodynamics in essential hypertension. *Clin Sci* 59: 343s–354s.

132. Bertel O, Bühler FR, Kiowski W, Lutold BD (1980): Decreased beta-adrenocepter responsiveness as related to age, blood pressure, and plasma catecholamines in patients with essential hypertension. *Hypertension* 2: 130–138.

133. Trimarco B, Volpe M, Ricciardelli B, Picotti GB, Galva MD, Petracca R, Condorelli M (1983): Studies of the mechanisms underlying impairment of beta-adrenoceptor-mediated effects in human hypertension. *Hypertension* 5: 584–590.

134. Messerli FH (1983): Clinical determinants and consequences of left ventricular hypertrophy. *Am J Med* 75(3A): 51–55.

135. Corea L, Bentivoglio M, Verdecchia P, Motolese M (1984): Plasma norepinephrine and left ventricular hypertrophy in systemic hypertension. *Am J Cardiol* 53: 1299–1303.

136. Egan B, Colfer H, Buda A, Julius S (1984): Evidence that the sympathetic nervous system contributes to cardiovascular hypertrophy in patients with borderline hypertension. *Clin Res* 32: 331A.

137. Shapiro LM, McKenna WJ (1984): Left ventricular hypertrophy: Relation of structure to diastolic function in hypertension. *Br Heart J* 51: 637–642.

138. Dianzumba SB, DiPette DJ, Cornman C, Weber E, Joyner CR (1986): Left ventricular filling characteristics in mild untreated hypertension. *Hypertension* 8(suppl I): I–156–160.

139. Conway J (1963): A vascular abnormality in hypertension: a study of blood flow in the forearm. *Circulation* 27: 520–529.

140. Takeshita A, Mark AL (1980): Decreased vasodilator capacity of forearm resistance vessels in borderline hypertension. *Hypertension* 2: 610–616.

141. Bevan RD (1975): Effect of sympathetic denervation on smooth muscle cell proliferation in the growing rabbit ear artery. *Circ Res* 37: 14–19.

142. Egan B, Julius S (1985): Vascular hypertrophy in borderline hypertension: Relationship to blood pressure and sympathetic drive. *Clin Exp Hypertens* A7: 243–255.

143. Folkow B (1978): Cardiovascular structural adaption: Its role in the initiation and maintenance of primary hypertension. *Clin Sci Mol Med* 55: 3s–22s.

144. Sivertsson R, Olander R (1968): Aspects of the nature of the increased vascular resistance and increased 'reactivity' to noradrenaline in hypertensive subjects. *Life Sci* 7(Part I): 1291–1297.

145. Egan BM, Panis R, Hinderliter A, Schork N (1988): Vascular structure enhances regional resistance responses in mild hypertension. *J Hypertension* 6(1): 41–48.

146. Lockette W, Otsuka Y, Carretero O (1986): The loss of endothelium-dependent vascular relaxation in hypertension. *Hypertension* 8(suppl II): II–61–66.

147. Matsuda H, Kuon E, Holtz J, Busse R (1985): Endothelium-mediated dilations contribute to the polarity of the arterial wall in vasomotion induced by α_2-adrenergic agonists. *J Cardiovasc Pharm* 7: 680–688.

148. Phillip Th, Distler A, Cordes U (1978): Sympathetic nervous system and blood-pressure control in essential hypertension. *Lancet* 1978/2: 959–963.

149. Egan BM (1987): Changed sympathetic tone and responsiveness in the course of human essential hypertension, in: Julius S and Bassett DR (eds), *Handbook of Hypertension, Vol 9: Behavioral Factors in Hypertension*, Ch 15, pp 216–225. Amsterdam: Elsevier Science Publishers.

7. Systemic hemodynamics in sustained essential and reno-vascular hypertension

MICHEL E. SAFAR, GÉRARD M. LONDON and YVES A. WEISS

Before investigating the control of cardiac output in human hypertension, it is important to analyze the mean value of this parameter in different forms of hypertensive vascular disease. This is a difficult problem, due to the paucity of data in the literature [1–8]. This chapter will limit itself to patients with chronic, sustained, uncomplicated essential or reno-vascular hypertension [7]. 'Chronic' implies that the duration of the disease is over three years, in patients aged between 20 and 60 years. 'Sustained' implies that the ambulatory diastolic pressure is consistantly greater than 100 mmHg or that the diastolic pressure is above 90 mmHg on the third day of hospitalization. 'Essential' implies that plasma and urinary electrolytes, urinary catecholamines and timed intravenous pyelography are constantly within normal limits. 'Uncomplicated' means that there is no history of stroke, congestive heart failure or any vascular complication, and that plasma creatinine is less than 1.4 mg%. 'Reno vascular' means that uni- or bilateral stenosis of the renal artery has been diagnosed on the basis of arteriographic findings and that the diagnosis has been confirmed by significant blood pressure reduction after surgery [3].

Accepting all of these criteria, it will be shown in this chapter, that (1) cardiac output remains within the normal range in men with sustained essential or reno-vascular hypertension, and (2) the control mechanisms affecting cardiac output are different in hypertensives compared with age- and sex-matched normotensive subjects. Several aspects have been previously published [7].

Mean value of systemic hemodynamics in sustained essential and reno-vascular hypertension

Essential hypertension. Most studies have been performed with patients at rest

M.E. Safar & F. Fouad-Tarazi (eds.), The heart in hypertension.
© *1989 Kluwer Academic Publishers, Dordrecht –*

in the supine position. Compared with controls of the same age and sex, cardiac output, expressed in ml/min per m² body surface area (i.e. cardiac index), is normal in patients with uncomplicated sustained essential hypertension [1–7], implying an increase in systemic vascular resistance (Table 1). Oxygen consumption is normal or slightly increased. The arterio-venous oxygen difference is elevated, due to a reduction in venous red cell oxygen content [2, 5]. Heart rate is slightly increased [3, 7]. Stroke volume is normal. Blood flow in the liver and lower limbs remains within normal limits, whereas renal blood flow is reduced [8–10].

In the upright position, studied with head-up tilt, cardiac output decreases, whereas heart rate increases and stroke volume decreases to the same extent as in normal subjects (Fig. 1). Systemic vascular resistance increases more than in normotensive controls following tilting. In the absence of congestive heart failure, mean and diastolic blood pressure are slightly increased in the upright position, suggesting that the vasoconstrictive mechanisms that act to maintain blood pressure are amplified in hypertensives compared with controls [4]. In contrast, the hemodynamic response of heart rate to tilting is the same as in controls.

During exercise, cardiac output remains adapted to the metabolic needs of the tissues [2, 5]. However, the slope of the curve relating cardiac output (or stroke volume) to oxygen consumption is reduced [2, 5]. This finding has been attributed to early heart failure [5], but the alterations in ventricular geometry due to cardiac hypertrophy seem to play a more important role [11].

Table 1. Systemic hemodynamics in male subjects with sustained essential and reno-vascular hypertension compared with age- and sex-matched normal subjects. Personal data extended from [26]. Variance analysis of the three subgroups.

	Normotensives (n = 21) (1)	Essential hypertensives (n = 35) (2)	Renal Artery stenosis (n = 30) (3)	p value (1)↔(2)	(1)↔(3)	(2)↔(3)
Age (years)	41 ± 2	40 ± 2	40 ± 2	NS	NS	NS
Systolic arterial pressure (mmHg)	135 ± 3	191 ± 4	214 ± 6	<0.001	<0.001	<0.01
Diastolic arterial pressure (mmHg)	76 ± 2	107 ± 2	116 ± 3	<0.001	<0.001	<0.05
Mean arterial pressure (mmHg)	96 ± 2	135 ± 3	149 ± 3	<0.001	<0.001	<0.02
Heart rate (b/min)	74 ± 2	78 ± 2	75 ± 2	NS	NS	NS
Cardiac index (ml/min/m²)	3668 ± 108	3536 ± 100	3466 ± 146	NS	NS	NS
Total vascular resistance (dynes/sec · cm⁻⁵ m²)	2151 ± 72	3227 ± 109	3680 ± 184	<0.001	<0.001	<0.05

± 1 standard error of the mean.

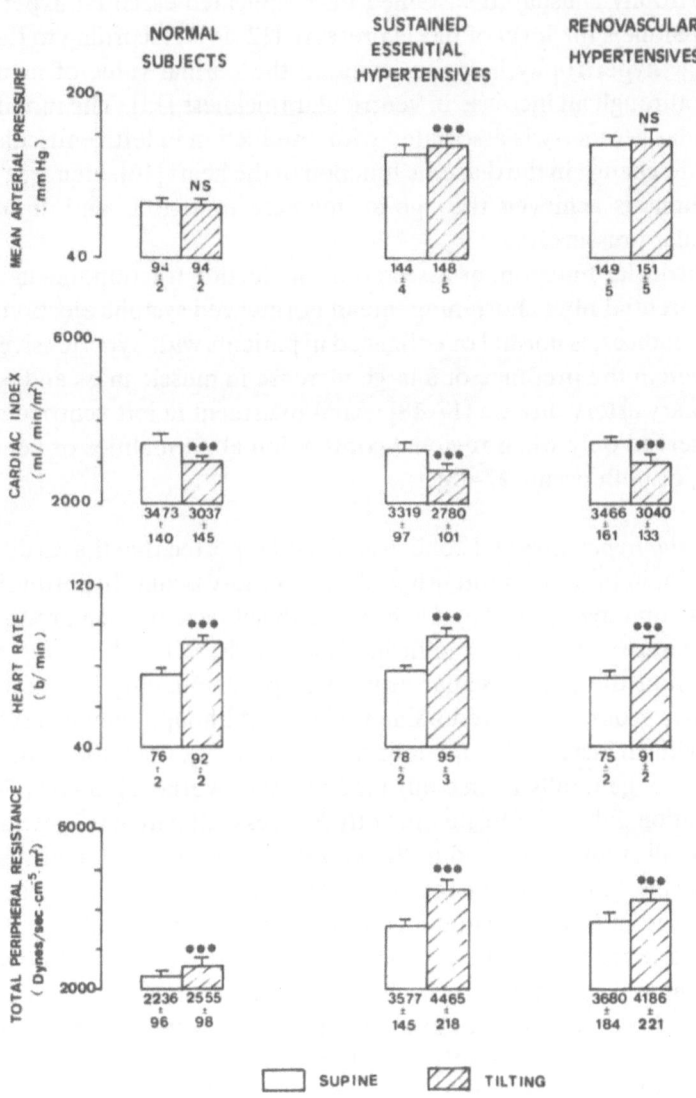

Figure 1. Hemodynamic response to tilting in patients with sustained essential and reno-vascular hypertension compared with age-matched normal subjects. All subjects are male. Personal data extended from [26].

Investigations based on echocardiography have shown that symmetric cardiac hypertrophy is usual in sustained uncomplicated essential hypertension and even parallels the level of blood pressure [12–14]. According to Laplace's law, cardiac hypertrophy helps to maintain the normal value of myocardial wall stress through an increase in ventricular thickness [15]. The modification in ventricular geometry is associated with a reduction in left ventricular compliance and a change in the diastolic function of the heart [16]. Hence, a normal stroke volume is achieved through an increase in systolic and diastolic intraventricular pressures.

Left ventricular function, as assessed from ejection fraction, mean velocity of circumferential fiber shortening, mean normalized systolic ejection rate or isovolumic indices, is normal or enhanced in patients with hypertensive hypertrophy, even in the presence of a large increase in muscle mass and concomitant coronary artery disease [17–18]. An impairment in left ventricular function is observed only when regional contraction abnormalities or ventricular dilatation, or both occur [17–18].

Reno-vascular hypertension. Frohlich et al. [19] reported that the cardiac index was $3.00 \, ml/min/m^2$ in normotension, 3.31 in reno-vascular hypertension and 2.66 in essential hypertension. There were 15 subjects in each group and all differences were statistically significant. It should be noted, however, that the composition of the reno-vascular group was predominantly female whereas the other two groups were predominantly male. Although similar results were obtained with an increased number of subjects [20–22], the findings on cardiac index have not generally been confirmed by other workers [23–27] (Table 1). Tilting position did not differ significantly from essential hypertensive subjects (Fig. 1). In all studies reported in the literature, systemic vascular resistance was significantly increased in reno-vascular hypertensives and these results were observed in both the supine and upright positions. Under such conditions, the basic problem in these patients is to evaluate the contribution of the renin angiotensin system to the mechanisms of the increase in vascular resistance. Hemodynamic studies before and after surgery indicate that the blood pressure reduction is consistently associated with a decrease in vascular resistance (Fig. 2) [22]. However, this finding does not clearly demonstrate that the renin-angiotensin system is the only factor contributing to the blood pressure level for several reasons. First, the decrease in pressure after surgery does not exhibit an 'all or nothing' response, and furthermore is strongly correlated with the pre-operative blood pressure (Fig. 3). This may be observed with any drug treatment in hypertension [28]. Second, in hypertensive patients cured or improved by surgery, blood pressure increases with ageing much more rapidly than in normotensive controls (Fig. 4) [28], suggesting that factors others than the renin-angiotensin system govern the mechanism of reno-vascular hyper-

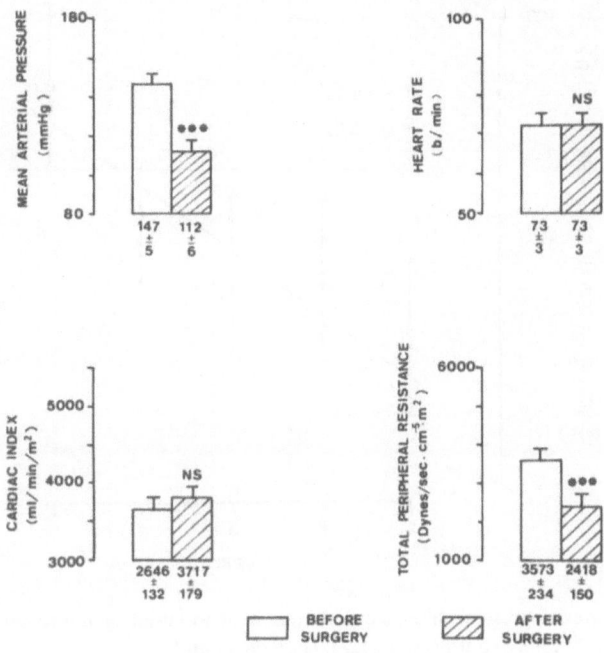

Figure 2. Hemodynamic response to surgical treatment in 19 patients with reno-vascular hypertension. (Personal data)

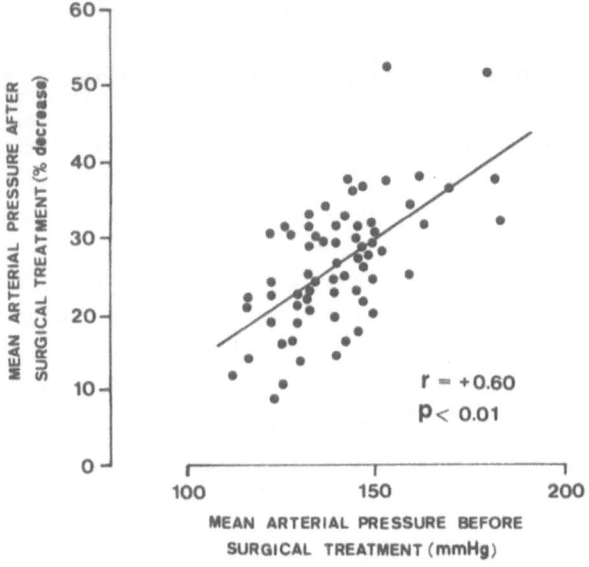

Figure 3. Correlation between mean arterial pressure before and after surgical treatment in cured and improved reno-vascular hypertensives [28]. (Personal data)

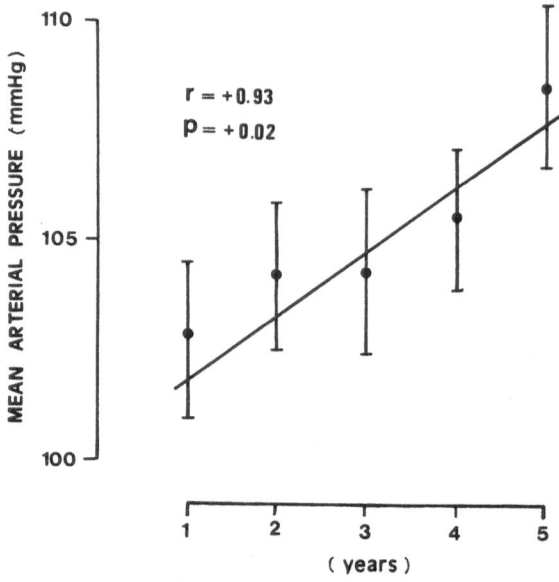

Figure 4. Mean arterial pressure after surgical treatment in cured or improved reno vascular hypertensive patients followed for 5 years [28]. (Personal data)

tension in man. Indeed, genetic factors have been postulated as playing a role in this form of hypertension [28].

Cardiac output control in sustained essential hypertension

Humoral and hemodynamic parameters in hypertension may be characterized in two different ways [7]. Experimental animals have been studied using longitudinal protocols. This approach will identify time-dependent phenomena at the onset of hypertension, but it employs animal models which may not be totally relevant to man. A second approach utilizes cross-sectional clinical studies. These protocols allow comparisons to be made between groups of patients with established hypertension, but tend to obscure details related to the duration and severity of the disease. With regard to both types of protocol, studies of cardiac output control reported in the literature are unique in that both cross-sectional and longitudinal studies have been performed in man, as previously related [7].

The relationship between blood volume and cardiac output: A cross-sectional study. Only a small number of correlations of cardiac output with different hemodynamic and humoral variables have been evaluated in cross-sectional studies of normal subjects and hypertensive patients [29]. Cardiac output is, in general, negatively correlated with blood pressure but age could possibly influence the correlation [29]. Regardless of the factors governing cardiac output, heart rate has been found to be strongly correlated to cardiac index in borderline hypertensives [30–31]. On the other hand, blood volume is significantly and positively correlated with cardiac output in hypertensives [31–32], mainly in obese patients. However, this result has not been universally observed [29, 33], often because of the small number of subjects studied.

In order to better evaluate the correlations of cardiac output with heart rate and blood volume, a population of 196 men (98 normotensives and 98 hypertensives of the same age) was investigated [31, 34]. The mean value of cardiac output was comparable in the normotensive and hypertensive ranges and, as expected, higher in patients with borderline blood pressure elevation. In this study, the correlations between heart rate and cardiac output, and between blood volume and cardiac output, were studied at different blood pressure levels, and gave the most consistent findings. The results were not dependent on correction of blood volume and cardiac output for body size, and showed that: (1) the positive and significant correlation observed between heart rate and cardiac output in the normotensive range became insignificant in the hypertensive range, and (2) the positive correlation observed between blood volume and cardiac output was more significant in the hypertensive than in the normotensive range.

These results were amplified by studying the slopes of the heart rate-cardiac output and blood volume cardiac output relationships, rather than the correlation coefficients [31, 34]. The slope of the curve relating heart rate to cardiac output was steeper in normotensives than in hypertensives, suggesting that, within the normotensive range, the contribution of heart rate to the control of cardiac output is more important. Disregarding the considerable role of the autonomic nervous system in the regulation of cardiac output in normal subjects and borderline hypertensives, it has been suggested that the steeper slope observed in the normotensive range reflects a predominance of neurogenic influences. On the other hand, the slope of the curve relating blood volume to cardiac output was found to be significantly steeper in hypertensives than in normotensives, suggesting that, within the hypertensive range, the contribution of blood volume to the control of cardiac output is more important. However, regarding this latter finding, the term 'contribution of blood volume' remains to be interpreted [7].

Whatever the mechanisms involved, the changes in the significance of the correlations of cardiac output with heart rate and blood volume suggest that the relationship between cardiac output and the metabolic needs of the tissues may be altered in hypertensives. Indeed, cross-sectional studies of the correlation between cardiac output and oxygen consumption in normotensive and hypertensive subjects have confirmed this possibility [35–36]. The positive correlation observed at rest between cardiac output and oxygen consumption in normotensive subjects [35–36] disappears in hypertensives. In these patients, a higher oxygen consumption is required to achieve the same cardiac output as in normal subjects.

The blood volume-cardiac output relationship in borderline hypertension: A longitudinal study. A longitudinal survey of 37 young men with borderline hypertension, followed-up for 47 months without treatment, provided the opportunity to investigate changes in cardiac output control in this category of patients [37]. In agreement with the findings of other workers [38], a primary increase in cardiac output was followed by a secondary increase in total peripheral resistance associated with a reduction in cardiac output; systolic blood pressure then increased further. The reduction in cardiac output was associated with changes in cardiac output control. At the beginning of the survey, the heart rate-cardiac output correlation was significant, whereas the blood volume-cardiac output correlation was not, suggesting a dominant neurogenic control. However, at the end of the survey, the blood volume-cardiac output correlation was significant whereas the heart rate-cardiac output correlation was not, suggesting that, at this time, the contribution of 'volume' factors is predominant. Again, the term 'contribution of volume factors' remains to be interpreted. One possibility is that predominant beta-adrenoceptor-mediated adrenergic functions in the development phase are replaced later by alpha-adrenoceptor-mediated vasoconstriction or structural alterations of the arterial wall or both [39].

In the case of the curve relating cardiac output to oxygen consumption, Lund-Johansen [35,38] has shown that, during long term follow-up, cardiac output remained adapted to oxygen consumption and, therefore, to the metabolic needs of the tissues. However, this author also observed that the hemodynamic pattern was different at rest and on exercise. At rest, the steady state curve relating cardiac output to oxygen consumption was shallower at the end than at the beginning of follow-up [35, 38]. During exercise, a higher oxygen consumption was required at the end of long-term follow-up to achieve the same cardiac output level as that observed at initial examination. This finding indicates that the relationship between cardiac output and oxygen consumption alters with time.

In conclusion, the modifications in hemodynamic pattern observed in the same population of subjects followed over a period of time resembled those found in the cross-sectional study of cardiac output control described above.

The blood volume-cardiac output relationship after rapid dextran infusion: An acute experiment. Cross-sectional and long-term longitudinal studies have thus shown that the curve relating cardiac output to blood volume is steeper in hypertensives than in normotensives [34, 37]. This relationship has been further explored in normotensive and hypertensive patients under conditions of volume expansion caused by rapid iso-onkotic dextran infusion [40–41]. Indeed both cardiac performance and venous compliance may modulate the slope of the volume flow curve.

In studying vascular compliance in human hypertension, most investigations have been based on the estimation of pressure-volume relationships in segments of cutaneous veins and/or forearm vascular beds [42]. The results suggest an increased venous tone in hypertensives. However, for a quantitative evaluation of the role of capacitance vessels, determination of the pressure-volume relationship of the total systemic venous bed is of greater interest. In animals, this is carried out during cardiac arrest, the curve relating blood volume to mean circulatory pressure being determined [43]. In man, although the heart is beating, a similar relationship, between total blood volume and central venous pressure, can be observed during volume expansion [44]. With the use of rapid dextran infusion, the role of reflex phenomena and delayed compliance can be greatly minimized. However, the pressure changes in the central veins are not due entirely to the elastic properties of the vascular bed. The left ventricle in diastole is also involved. In addition, secondary effects of blood volume changes on arterial hemodynamics and venous tone also contribute to produce variations in central venous pressure. For this reason, the term 'effective compliance' is used [44].

Following rapid dextran infusion, it has been found that for the same volume expansion, hypertensives respond by a higher increase in cardiac output, stroke volume and central venous pressure than normotensives [40–41]. Since the curves relating cardiac output to central venous pressure, i.e., cardiac function curves, were similar in both controls and hypertensives [40–41], an alteration in cardiac performance is an unlikely explanation for the greater increase in central venous pressure observed in hypertensives. It seems more probable that the response to volume expansion is due to a reduction in the 'effective compliance' of the vascular bed, as defined above [40–41]. This has been confirmed by studies in spontaneously hypertensive rats [45–46]. Since arterial compliance is an insignificant fraction of total compliance [47] and intrathoracic vascular compliance has been found to be normal in hypertensives [48], it follows that there must be a reduction in compliance of the left ventricle in diastole, and of peripheral veins, in patients with sustained essential hypertension.

In conclusion, the normal value of cardiac output in patients with sustained essential and reno-vascular hypertension clearly indicates that homeostatic mechanisms act to maintain the metabolic needs of the tissues. However, a combination of cross-sectional and longitudinal studies in hypertensive humans has clearly demonstrated that the homeostatic mechanisms are different from those of normal subjects, requiring a higher energy cost in the presence of cardiac hypertrophy and decreased vascular compliance.

References

1. Conway J, Julius S, Amery A (1978): Effect of blood pressure level on the haemodynamic response to exercise. *Cir Res* 16: 79–85.
2. Sannerstedt R (1969): Hemodynamic findings at rest and during exercise in mild arterial hypertension. *Am J Med Sci* 258: 70–76.
3. Frohlich ED, Tarazi RC, Dustan HP (1969): Re-examination of the hemodynamics of hypertension. *Am J Med Sci* 257: 9–15.
4. London GM, Weiss YA, Pannier BP, Laurent St, Safar ME (1987): Tilt test in essential hypertension: Differencial responses in heart rate and vascular resistance. *Hypertension* 10: 29–34.
5. Lund-Johansen P (1973): Hemodynamic alterations in essential hypertension, in: Onesti G, Kim KE, Moyer JH (eds). *Hypertension Mechanisms and Management*, pp 43–49. New York: Grune and Stratton.
6. Birkenhager WH, Schalekamp MADH, Krauss HX, et al. (1972): Systemic and renal haemodynamics, body fluids and renin in benign essential hypertension with special reference to natural history. *Europ J Clin Invest* 2: 115–121.
7. Safar ME (1989): *Clinical Research in Essential Hypertension,* pp 33–38. Stuttgart – New York: Schaltauer Publishers.
8. Brod J, Fencl V, Hejl Z, et al. (1962): General and regional hemodynamic patterns underlying essential hypertension. *Clin Sci* 23: 339–347.
9. Amery A, Bossaert H, Verstraete M (1969): Muscle blood flow in normal and hypertensive subjects. *Am Heart J* 78: 221–229.
10. Temmar MM, Safar ME, Levenson JA, Toto Moukouo JM, Simon ACh (1981): Regional blood flow in borderline and sustained, essential hypertension. *Clin Sci* 60: 653–658.
11. Tarazi RC, Ferrario CM, Dustan HP (1976): The heart in hypertension, in: Genest J, Koiw E, Kuchel O (eds), *Hypertension Physiopathology and Treatment,* pp 738–749. New York: McGraw Hill.
12. Dunn FC, Chandraratna PN, Basta LL, et al. (1976): Pathophysiological assessment of hypertensive heart disease by echocardiography. *Am J Cardiol* 37: 133–139.
13. Karliner JS, Williams D, Gorwitt J, et al. (1977): Left ventricular performance in patients with left ventricular hypertrophy by systemic arterial hypertension. *Br Heart J* 39: 1239–45.
14. Savage DD, Drayer JIM, Henri WL, et al. (1979): Echocardiographic assessment of cardiac anatomy and function in hypertensive subjects. *Circulation* 59: 623–632.
15. Yin FCP (1981): Ventricular wall stress. *Circ Res* 49: 829–842.
16. Merillon JP, Motte G, Masquet C, et al. (1982): Inter relation entre les propriétés physiques du système artériel et la performance ventriculaire gauche lors du vieillissement et dans l'hypertension artérielle, in: Brutsaert DL (ed), *L'hypertrophie ventriculaire gauche,* pp 95–104. Paris: Masson.
17. Strauer BE (1979): Ventricular function and coronary hemodynamics in hypertensive heart disease. *Am J Cardiol* 44: 999–1006.
18. Olivari MT, Fiorentini C, Polese A, et al. (1978): Pulmonary hemodynamic and right ventricular function in hypertension. *Circulation* 57: 1185–1196.

19. Frohlich ED, Ulrych M, Tarazi RC, Dustan HP, Page IH (1968): A hemodynamic comparison of essential and renovascular hypertension. *Circulation* 35: 289–294.
20. Frohlich ED, Ulrych M, Tarazi RC, Dustan HP, Page IH (1968): Hemodynamics of renal arterial diseases and hypertension. *Am J Med Sci* 29: 255–261.
21. Frohlich ED, Tarazi RC, Dustan HP (1969): Re-examination of the hemodynamic of hypertension. *Am J Med Sci* 9: 257–268.
22. Tarazi RC, Frohlich ED, Dustan HP (1973): Contribution of cardiac output of renovascular hypertension in man. *Am J Cardiol* 31: 600–606.
23. Brod J (1960): Essential hypertension: Hemodynamic observations with a bearing on its pathogenesis. *Lancet* 1960/2: 773–775.
24. Brod J, Hejl Z, Hornych A, Jirka J, Slechta V (1966): Hemodynamic changes underlying renovascular hypertension. *Proc. of Third International Congress of Nephrology*. Washington, D.C.
25. Brod J, Hejl Z, Ulrych M, Fencl V, Jirka J (1961): Hemodynamic basis of renal hypertension. *Cesk Fysiol* 10: 228–239.
26. London GM, Safar ME (1989): Renal hemodynamics in patients with sustained essential hypertension and in patients with unilateral stenosis of the renal artery. *Am J Hypertension* 2: 244–252.
27. Kioschos JM, Kirkendall WM, Valenca MR, Fitz AE (1967): Unilateral renal hemodynamics and characteristics of dyedilution cuves in patients with essential hypertension and renal disease. *Circulation* 35: 229–235.
28. Ben Maiz H, Safar M, Weiss Y, Ben Ayed HB, Milliez P (1977): Renovascular hypertension: The role of nonspecific factors in the antihypertensive effect of surgery. *Clin Nephrol* 7(1): 26–30.
29. Birkenhager WH, De Leeuw PW, Schalekamp MADH (1982): *Control Mechanisms in essential hypertension*, 2nd ed, pp 33–37. Amsterdam: Elsevier Biomedical Press.
30. Conway J, Julius S, Amery A (1968): Effect of blood pressure level on the hemodynamic response to exercise. *Circ Res* 16: 79–84.
31. Safar ME, Chau NPh, London GM, Weiss YA, Milliez PL (1976): Control of cardiac output in essential hypertension. *Am J Cardiol* 38: 332–336.
32. Safar ME, Weiss YA, London GM, Frackowiak RF, Milliez PL (1974): Cardiopulmonary blood volume in borderline hypertension. *Clin Sci Mol Med* 47: 153–164.
33. Dustan HP, Tarazi RC, Mujais S (1981): A comparison of hemodynamic and volume characteristics of obese and non obese hypertensive patients *Inter J Obesity* 5 (suppl 1): 19–25.
34. Chau NPh, Safar ME, Weiss YA, London GM, Simon ACh, Milliez PL (1978): Relationship between cardiac output, heart rate and blood volume in essential hypertension. *Clin Sci Mol Med* 54: 175–180.
35. Lund-Johansen P (1966): Central hemodynamics in essential hypertension *Acta Med Scand* 180 (suppl 606): 10–12.
36. London GM, Safar ME, Bouthier JL, Gitelman RM (1984): Cardiac output, oxygen consumption and renal blood flow in essential hypertension. *Clin Science* 67: 313–319.
37. Weiss YA, Safar ME, London GM, Simon ACh, Levenson JA, Milliez PL (1978): Repeat hemodynamic determinations in borderline hypertension. *Am J Med* 64: 382–387.
38. Lund-Johansen P (1980): State-of-the-Art: Hemodynamics in essential hypertension. *Clin Sci* 59: 343s–354s.
39. Amann FW, Bolli P, Kiowski W, et al. (1981): Enhanced alpha-adreno-receptor metiated vasoconstriction in essential hypertension. *Hypertension* 3 (suppl 1): 119–123.
40. London GM, Safar ME, Simon ACh, Alexandre JM, Levenson JA, Weiss YA (1978): Total effective compliance, cardiac output and fluid volumes in essential hypertension. *Circulation* 57: 995–1000.

41. Safar ME, London GM, Levenson JA, Simon ACh, Chau NPh (1979): Rapid Dextran infusion in essential hypertension. *Hypertension* 1: 615–623.
42. Walsh JA, Hyman C, Maronde RF (1969): Venous distensibility in essential hypertension. *Cardio Vasc Res* 3: 338–345.
43. Guyton AC, Coleman TG, Granger HJ (1972): Circulation: Overall regulation *Am Rev Physiol* 34: 13–29.
44. Echt M, Duveling J, Gauer OH, et al. (1974): Effective compliance of the total vascular bed and the intrathoracic compartment derived from changes in central venous pressure induced by volume changes in man. *Circ Res* 33: 61–72.
45. Trippodo NC, Yamamoto J, Frohlich ED (1981): Whole-body venous capacity and effective total tissue compliance in SHR. *Hypertension* 3: 104–112.
46. Rickstein SE, Yao T, Ljung B, et al. (1980): Distensibility of left atrium in normotensive and spontaneously hypertensives rats. *Acta Physiol Scand* 110: 1–6.
47. Safar ME, London GM (1987): Arterial and venous compliance in sustained essential hypertension. *Hypertension* 10: 133–139.
48. London GM, Safar ME, Payen DM, Gitelman RC, Guerin AM (1982): Total, peripheral and intrathoracic effective compliance of the vascular bed in normotensive and hypertensive patients. *Contro Nephrol* 30: 144–153.

8. Systemic hemodynamics in primary aldosteronism

EMMANUEL L. BRAVO

Administration of mineralocorticoids and salt lead to significant increases in arterial pressure. The rise in arterial pressure is not uniformly associated with cardiac output or blood volume changes. The final common pathway responsible for the elevated arterial pressure is generally accepted to be an increase in peripheral vascular resistance. The sequence of events leading from excess mineralocorticoids and salt to the elevated peripheral vascular resistance continues to be the subject of intensive investigation.

Studies in primary aldosteronism

Cardiac output characteristics. Patients with primary aldosteronism have a higher cardiac index compared to age- and sex-matched essential hypertensive patients. However, individual values may vary from a low of 2.58 to a high of 4.04 liters/min/M^2 [1]. Subdivision of cardiac index values around an average of ± 10% revealed that the distribution curve is skewed towards higher values in primary aldosteronism and towards lower values in two other groups of essential hypertension (Figure 1).

The increased cardiac output correlates positively with intravascular volume (Figure 2). However, differences in cardiac output among patients with primary aldosteronism and patients with essential hypertension cannot be attributed to differences in intravascular volume since patients with either the hypovolemic or hypervolemic form of essential hypertension have a lower cardiac output than normovolemic patients with primary aldosteronism.

In these patients, cardiac output is inversely correlated with arterial pressure (Figure 3). This indicates that changes in peripheral resistance is probably more important than the elevated cardiac output in the maintenance of hypertension. In two other types of 'high-output' hypertension (i.e. renovascular

M.E. Safar & F. Fouad-Tarazi (eds.), The heart in hypertension.
© *1989 Kluwer Academic Publishers, Dordrecht –*

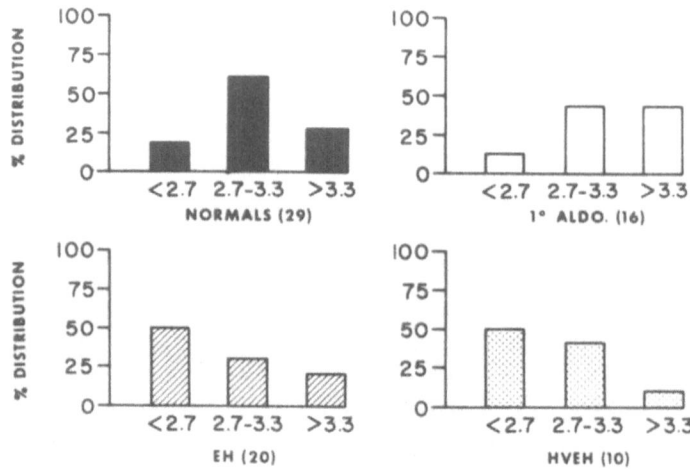

Figure 1. Distribution of cardiac index within three hypertensive groups: primary aldosteronism (1° Aldo), hypovolemic essential hypertension (EH), and hypervolemic essential hypertension (HVEH).

Reproduced from Tarazi et al. [1] by courtesy of the *New England Journal of Medicine.*

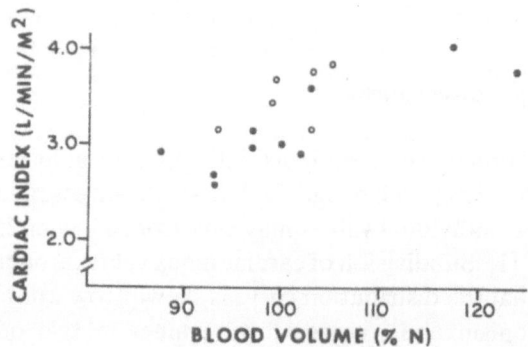

Figure 2. Correlation between total blood volume and cardiac index in 16 patients with primary aldosteronism. $r = 0.721$; $p < 0.01$; ● men; ○ women.

Reproduced from Tarazi et al. [1] by courtesy of *New England Journal of Medicine.*

hypertension and those associated with end-stage kidney disease) chronic hypertension is primarily a function of increased peripheral resistance rather than increased cardiac output [2, 3].

Other cardiac characteristics. Aside from having a higher cardiac index (3.30 vs. 2.85; $p < 0.01$) patients with primary aldosteronism have higher heart rates (83 vs. 73: $p < 0.02$) and a more rapid rate of left ventricular ejection (158 vs. 140; $p < 0.02$) than patients with essential hypertension. While increases in intravascular volume could explain the elevated cardiac output,

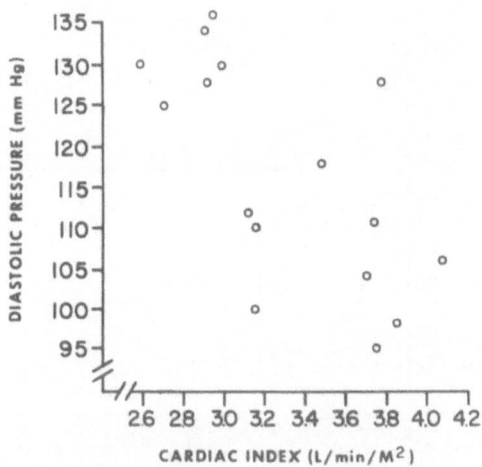

Figure 3. Inverse correlation between cardiac index and diastolic blood pressure in 16 patients with primary aldosteronism. r = 0.661; p < 0.01.
Reproduced from Tarazi et al. [1] by courtesy of the *New England Journal of Medicine.*

enhanced cardiac performance cannot be excluded. Some reports suggest a strong cardiotonic or digitalis-like effect of aldosterone [4, 5]. However, other workers have failed to find any inotropic action of aldosterone on isolated cardiac tissue [6]. Increased activity of the sympathetic nervous system could explain the enhanced cardiac performance. Against this possibility are studies suggesting that mineralocorticoid hypertension in human beings is not associated with enhanced sympathetic nervous activity, but rather with some decrease in that activity [7–11]. Mineralocorticoids stimulate an early increase in membrane permeability that results in a rapid increase in sodium influx [12, 13]. This, in turn, leads to increased intracellular calcium and may account for the increased myocardial contractility.

Blood volume characteristics. Mineralocorticoids lead to fluid retention and might be expected to increase intravascular volume. Early studies have reported hypervolemia in primary aldosteronism but this abnormality is not a universal finding (Figure 4) [1, 14]. Many have either low or normal intravascular volume and there is no correlation between arterial pressure and plasma or total blood volume in either men or women with untreated primary aldosteronism. In contrast, there is a significant inverse correlation between volume and total peripheral resistance (r = −0.61; p < 0.02) similar to that reported in essential hypertension, renal arterial disease, and normal subjects (Figure 5). These results might suggest that intravascular volume as such plays no role in the hypertension of primary aldosteronism. This conclusion, however, must be qualified by two observations. First, the correlation between volume and

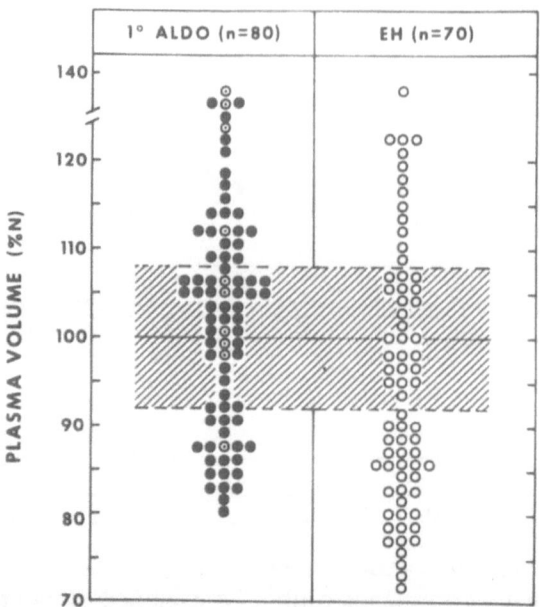

BASAL PLASMA VOLUME VALUES

Figure 4. Plasma volume distribution during normal dietary sodium intake. Values are expressed as percent of normal. For patients with primary aldosteronism (1° Aldo), solid circles represent adenomas (n = 70) and open circles with dotted centers represent hyperplasia (n = 10). The cross-hatched area represents the variability of the method (± 8%), EH: essential hypertension. In primary aldosteronism, there are as many patients who are hypovolemic (25%) as there are hypervolemic (30%).

Reproduced from Bravo et al. [14] by courtesy of the *American Journal of Medicine*.

resistance in primary aldosteronism and in essential hypertension is similar only in its sign (negative) and slope; the two groups differ significantly in the levels of intravascular volume. For any level of peripheral resistance, plasma volume is always greater in primary aldosteronism. Second, with diuretic therapy, the arterial pressure response is directly and significantly related to the magnitude of intravascular volume alterations [15].

Pathogenetic mechanisms in mineralocorticoid hypertension

The volume expansion that results from sodium retention has been proposed as the pivotal factor in the pathogenesis of this type of hypertension via the resulting increase in cardiac output [16]. It is reasoned that the initial increase in circulatory blood volume enhances venous return, thereby augmenting cardiac-filling pressure and cardiac performance. The increase in total peripheral resistance to maintain the elevated arterial pressure occurs later, follow-

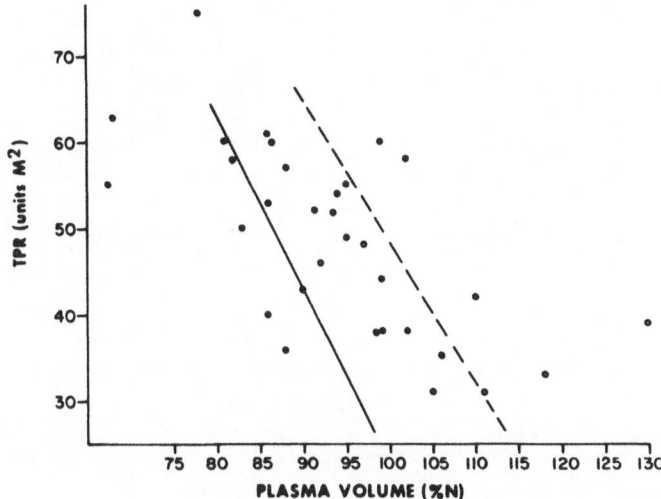

Figure 5. Correlation between plasma volume and total peripheral resistance (TPR) in patients with primary aldosteronism and those with hypovolemic essential hypertension. The slopes of the regression equations defining the two lines are not significantly different from each other, but the intercepts are. O--O: primary aldosteronism (n = 16; r = −0.531; p < 0.05) ●———●: essential hypertension (n = 16; r = −0.610; p < 0.02).
Reproduced from Tarazi et al. [1] by courtesy of the *New England Journal of Medicine.*

ing vascular autoregulation. This hypothesis is not supported by a number of observations. Mineralocorticoid hypertension in the dog produces no consistent increases in cardiac output, even though consistent increases in extracellular fluid volume occur during the initial increase in blood pressure [17]. In these studies, prevention of rises in cardiac output by β-adrenoreceptor blockade does not prevent the development of hypertension. Similar findings were reported by Terris and co-workers [18] in the DOCA-hypertensive pig and by Conway and Hatton [19] in the DOCA-salt hypertensive dog.

Gradual and progressive increases in salt intake elevate arterial pressure in metyrapone-treated dogs but not in a time-control group [20]. Changes in cardiac output and extracellular fluid volume are virtually identical in both groups at all levels of sodium repletion (Figure 6). Arterial pressure elevations in metyrapone-treated dogs occur because of either a rise in peripheral vascular resistance or an inability to vasodilate in the face of increasing flow.

These observations strongly suggest that changes in cardiac output and fluid volumes are not the main factors responsible for the rise in pressure. The rise in arterial pressure is clearly resistance-mediated from the early stages. Also, of considerable importance is the demonstration that the rise in arterial pressure is not time-dependent but is related entirely to the amount of sodium given.

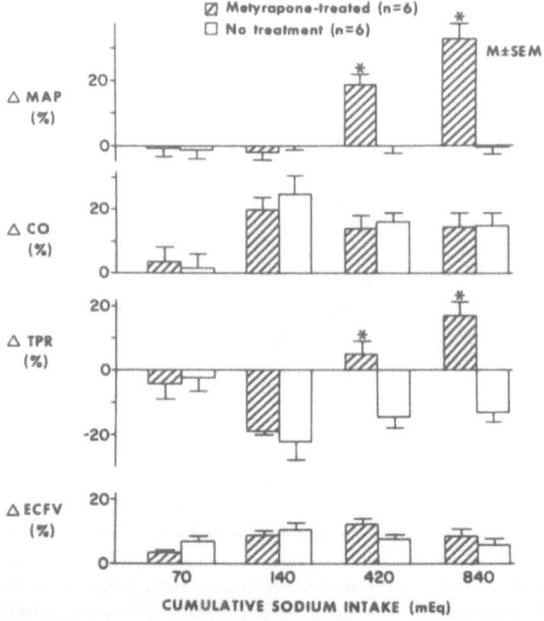

Figure 6. The relationships between increases in mean arterial pressure (MAP) changes in cardiac output (CO), changes in total peripheral resistance (TPR), changes in extracellular fluid volume (ECV) and the amount of cumulative sodium intake over 7 days. Asterisk represents values that are significantly different ($p < 0.05$) from the control animals.

Summary and conclusions

Evidence from hemodynamic studies in patients with primary aldosteronism and from sequential hemodynamic studies in conscious animals (dogs, pigs) treated with mineralocorticoids suggest that the early increases in extracellular fluid volume and cardiac output may contribute but do not predetermine the rise in arterial pressure. There is ample evidence, for instance, that mineralocorticoid-induced elevations in arterial pressure can occur without an increase in cardiac output, and is not inhibited with cardiac β-adrenoreceptor blockade. Changes in vascular smooth muscle, leading to enhanced contractility and increased resistance appears to be the primary contributor to both the initial vasoconstrictive response and the sustained and progressive hypertensive state.

References

1. Tarazi RC, Ibrahim MM, Bravo EL, Dustan HP (1973): Hemodynamic characteristics of primary aldosteronism. *NEJM* 289: 1330.
2. Tarazi RC, Frohlich ED, Dustan HP (1973): Contribution of cardiac output to renovascular hypertension in man: relation to surgical treatment. *Am J Cardiol* 31: 600.
3. Kim KE, Onesti G, Schwartz AB, Chinitz JL, Swartz C (1972): Hemodynamics of hypertension in chronic end-stage renal disease. *Circulation* 46: 456.
4. Ballard K, Lefer A, Sayers G (1960): Effect of aldosterone and of plasma extracts on a rat heart-lung preparation. *Am J Physiol* 199: 221.
5. Tanz RD (1962): Studies on the inotropic action of aldosterone on isolated cardiac tissue preparations: including the effects of pH, ouabain and SC-8109. *J Pharmacol Exp Ther* 135: 71.
6. Lefer AM, Sayers G (1965): Antagonism of the inotropic action of ouabain by aldosterone. *Am J Physiol* 208: 649.
7. Bravo EL, Tarazi RC, Dustan HP, Fouad FM (1985): The sympathetic nervous system and hypertension in primary aldosteronism. *Hypertension* 7: 90.
8. Distler A, Barth C, Liebau H, Vecsei P, Wolf HP (1970): The effect of tyramine, noradrenaline, and angiotensin on the blood pressure in hypertensive patients with aldosteronism and low plasma renin. *Eur J Clin Invest* 1: 196.
9. Biglieri EG, McIlroy MB (1966): Abnormalities of renal function and circulatory reflexes in primary aldosteronism. *Circulation* 33: 78.
10. Philipp T, Luth B, Wucherer G, Distler A (1983): Mechanism of mineralocorticoid-induced hypertension in man, in: Kaufman W, Wambach HA, Meurer KA (eds), *Mineralocorticoid Hypertension*, p. 129. New York: Springer-Verlag.
11. Chobanian AV, Volicer L, Tiffit CP, Gavras H, Liang CS, Faxon D (1979): Mineralocorticoid-induced hypertension in patients with orthostatic hypotension. *NEJM* 301: 68.
12. Bohr DF, Harris AL, Guthe CC, Webb RC (1984): Hypertension: multiple membrane malfunctions, in: Villarreal H, Sambhi MP (eds), *Topics in Pathophysiology of Hypertension*, pp. 100 ff. The Hague: Martinus Nijhof Publishers (Series DICM, Volume 30).
13. Webb RC (1984): Vascular changes in hypertension, in: Antonaccio MJ (ed), *Cardiovascular Pharmacology*, p. 2115. New York: Raven Press.
14. Bravo EL, Tarazi RC, Dustan HP, Fouad FM, Textor SC, Gifrd RW Jr., Vidt DG (1983): The changing clinical spectrum of primary aldosteronism. *Am J Med* 74: 641.
15. Bravo EL, Dustan HP, Tarazi RC (1973): Spironolactone as a non-specific treatment for primary aldosteronism. *Circulation* 48: 491.
16. Guyton AC, Coleman TG, Bower JD, Granger JH (1970): Circulatory control in hypertension. *Circ Res* 27 (suppl 2): 135.
17. Bravo EL, Tarazi RC, Dustan HP (1977): Multifactorial analysis of chronic hypertension by electrolyte-active steroids in trained, unanesthetized dogs. *Circ Res* 40 (suppl I) I-140.
18. Terris J, Berecek KH, Cohen EL, Stanley JC, Whitehouse WM Jr, Bohr DF (1976): Desoxycorticosterone hypertension in the pig. *Clin Sci Mol Med* 51 (suppl III): 303s.
19. Conway FJ, Hatton R (1978): Development of deoxycorticosterone acetate hypertension in the dog. *Circ Res* 43 (suppl 1): 82.
20. Onoyama K, Bravo EL, Tarazi RC (1979): Sodium, extracellular fluid volume, and cardiac output changes in the genesis of mineralocorticoid hypertension in the intact dog. *Hypertension* 1: 331.

9. Systemic hemodynamics in patients with pheochromocytoma

M.E. SAFAR, Y.A. WEISS, J.L. CUCHE and G.M. LONDON

Paroxysmal hypertension, tachycardia, orthostatic hypotension and reduced blood volume are classical hemodynamic features of patients with pheochromocytoma [see review in 1]. In contrast with these well-known findings, systemic hemodynamics have been poorly investigated. Normal, increased or slightly decreased values of cardiac output have been reported in series including a small number of patients [2–4]. In a previous study, we have reported the mean values of blood pressure, cardiac output and blood volume in a group of 14 males with pheochromocytoma [3]. In the present review, we have extended the results to the comparison of males and females. Particular attention has been paid to the hemodynamic response following orthostasis and the effects of surgical treatment.

Basic methodological concepts

The hemodynamic characteristics of hypertension associated with pheochromocytoma are classically inferred from the effects that catecholamines have on the circulation when infused intravenously into normal subjects [5–6]. Thus, epinephrine-secreting tumors are expected to increase arterial pressure, heart rate, cardiac output, stroke volume and left ventricular ejection time, whereas norepinephrine-secreting tumors might be expected to raise arterial pressure and increase total peripheral resistance while reducing heart rate and cardiac output slightly by reflex mechanisms. These hemodynamic findings may possibly be observed in the presence of paroxysmal hypertension. However, it is well accepted that tumors rarely secrete only one of the two hormones, and that the expected hemodynamic alterations would tend to result from the combined effects of these, depending on the relative proportions of the concentration of the circulating catecholamines. For this reason, it is important to

M.E. Safar & F. Fouad-Tarazi (eds.), The heart in hypertension.
© *1989 Kluwer Academic Publishers, Dordrecht –*

investigate patients with pheochromocytoma in the absence of paroxysmal hypertension.

In the present review, a hemodynamic study was performed in 14 males and 13 females with pheochromocytoma, aged between 20 and 67 years. Their clinical characteristics are listed in Table 1. Patients were hospitalized during a 10-day period, during which they received a 110 mEq/day sodium diet. All treatment was discontinued at least 1 month before the study. At the time of the investigation, 19 patients had a diastolic blood pressure greater than or equal to 90 mmHg, whereas 8 patients had a diastolic pressure below this value. Orthostatic hypotension was present in 10 patients and disorders of glucose regulation in 14 patients. Fundoscopic examination revealed haemorrhages, exudates and/or papillary oedema in 6 cases. Mild to severe left ventricular hypertrophy was observed in 12 patients. Creatinine clearance was in all cases greater than or equal to 80 ml/min. None of the patients had cardiac, neurologic or renal involvement. In the 27 subjects, the pre-operative diagnosis was made on the basis of urinary vanyl mandelic acid determination and confirmed by the operative finding of a benign adrenal medullary tumor on histological examination.

Hemodynamic investigations were performed with patients in the supine and erect positions, as described elsewhere [7]. In 4 patients, a second investigation was carried out 3 months after surgery, in the absence of antihypertensive therapy. The 14 males with pheochromocytoma were compared with two groups of age-matched male subjects: 33 normal controls and 65 patients with sustained essential hypertension. The two control groups were investigated under the same conditions as patients with pheochromocytoma [8]. Their clinical characteristics are summarized in Table 1. The 13 females

Table 1. Clinical characteristics of males and females with pheochromocytoma, compared with two control populations: 33 normal male subjects and 65 male patients with essential hypertension. (Personal data)

	Pheochromocytoma		Normal subjects	Essential hypertensives
	Men	Women		
Number of patients	14	13	33	65
Age (years)	40 ± 4	41 ± 4	36 ± 3	38 ± 2
Weight (kg)	69 ± 3	49 ± 2	65 ± 2	75 ± 2
Height (cm)	171 ± 2	158 ± 2	170 ± 1	171 ± 1
Body surface area (m²)	1.81 ± 0.05	1.48 ± 0.04	1.76 ± 0.03	1.87 ± 0.02
Normotensive*: Hypertensive	7:7	1:12	33:0	0:33

± 1 standard error of the mean.
* Diastolic pressure < 90 mmHg.

with pheochromocytoma were compared with the group of males with pheochromocytoma.

Systemic hemodynamics in the supine position

Table 2 shows the results of investigations of systemic hemodynamics in men
with pheochromocytoma compared with age- and sex-matched controls.
When compared with normal subjects, patients with pheochromocytoma had
a significant increase in blood pressure ($p < 0.001$), heart rate ($p < 0.001$) and
total peripheral resistance ($p < 0.001$), with no change in cardiac index, stroke
index or blood volume. When compared with essential hypertensives, they
had a significant increase in heart rate ($p < 0.02$).

Table 3 indicates that hemodynamic parameters were nearly identical in
men and women with pheochromocytoma. In women, the stroke index and
hematocrit were slightly reduced ($p < 0.05$).

Figure 1 summarizes the hemodynamic differences between normotensive
and hypertensive men with pheochromocytoma. Hypertensives had higher
values of total peripheral resistance ($p < 0.001$) and lower values of cardiac
index ($p < 0.05$). Heart rate was similar in the two groups of patients.

Figure 2 shows the relationship between blood volume and, respectively,
diastolic pressure and cardiac output, in males with pheochromocytoma. The
correlation between cardiac output and blood volume was strongly significant

Table 2. Supine hemodynamics in 14 males with pheochromocytoma, 33 normal male subjects and
65 male patients with essential hypertension. Variance analysis was performed. (Personal data)

	Normal subjects (1)	Essential hypertensives (2)	Men with pheochromocytoma (3)	p value (1)–(3)	(2)–(3)
SAP (mmHg)	124 ± 2	188 ± 4	171 ± 12	< 0.001	NS
DAP (mmHg)	72 ± 2	109 ± 2	93 ± 7	< 0.001	NS
MAP (mmHg)	90 ± 2	134 ± 2	122 ± 8	< 0.001	NS
CI (ml/min/m²)	3321 ± 102	3258 ± 68	3528 ± 237	NS	NS
HR (b/min)	72 ± 2	78 ± 2	88 ± 6	< 0.001	< 0.02
SI (ml/min²)	45 ± 2	44 ± 3	42 ± 3	NS	NS
TPR (Dynes/ sec · cm⁻⁵ · m²)	2118 ± 256	3143 ± 223	2962 ± 276	< 0.001	NS
PV (ml/kg)	44 ± 1	39 ± 2	41 ± 2	NS	NS
TBV (ml/kg)	78 ± 2	69 ± 2	75 ± 2	NS	NS
Ht (%)	43 ± 1	43 ± 1	45 ± 2	NS	NS

± 1 standard error of the mean.
Abbreviations: see Figure 1.

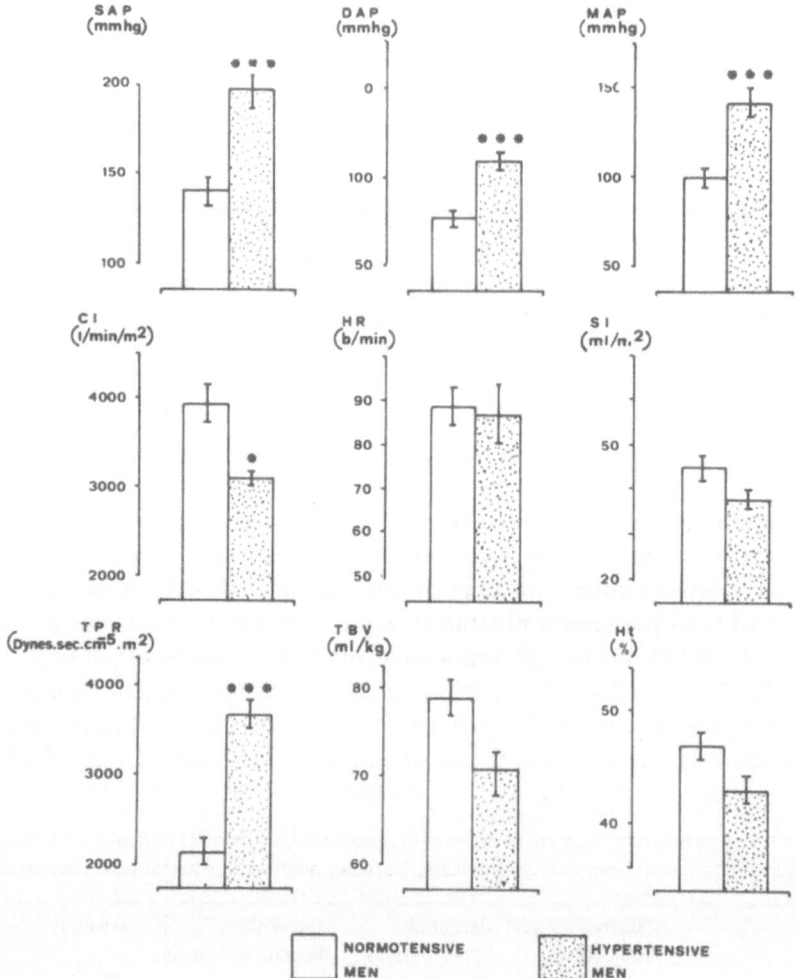

Figure 1. Hemodynamic parameters in 7 normotensive and 7 hypertensive men with pheochromo-
cytoma (Personal data).
* p < 0.05; *** p < 0.001. SAP = Systolic arterial pressure; DAP = Diastolic arterial pressure;
MAP = Mean arterial pressure. CI = Cardiac index; HR = Heart rate; SI = Stroke index.
TPR = Total peripheral resistance; PV = Plasma volume; TBV = Total blood volume; Ht =
Hematocrit.

(r = +0.70). On the other hand, a significant negative correlation was observed between blood volume and diastolic pressure (r = −0.64). In patients with
pheochromocytoma, the relationship between blood volume and blood pressure, and between blood volume and cardiac output was consistently within
the confidence limits of the curves of control subjects [8]. Finally, the study
clearly shows that systemic hemodynamics are similar in patients with pheo-

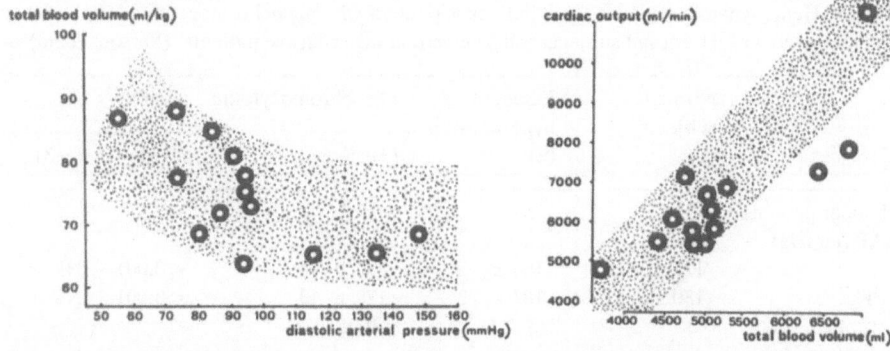

Figure 2. Relationship between blood volume and diastolic pressure, and between blood volume and cardiac output, in men with pheochromocytoma. The black area corresponds to the confidence limits of the curves observed in controls [8]. With the permission of *Clinical Science.*

Table 3. Supine hemodynamics in 14 men and 13 women with pheochromocytoma. (Personal data)

	Men	Women
SAP (mmHg)	171 ± 12	194 ± 13
DAP (mmHg)	93 ± 7	106 ± 7
MAP (mmHg)	122 ± 8	128 ± 3
CI (ml/min/m²)	3528 ± 237	3060 ± 193
HR (b/min)	88 ± 6	100 ± 6
SI (ml/m²)	42 ± 3	32 ± 2*
TPR (Dynes/sec · cm⁻⁵ · m²)	2962 ± 276	3846 ± 457
PV (ml/kg)	41 ± 2	43 ± 2
TBV (ml/kg)	75 ± 2	70 ± 2
Ht (%)	45 ± 2	40 ± 1*

*p < 0.05.
± 1 standard error of the mean.
Abbreviations: see Figure 1.

chromocytoma, and in patients with essential hypertension with the exception of heart rate.

Hemodynamic response to tilt

Table 4 summarizes the hemodynamic response to tilt in patients with pheochromocytoma, in normal subjects and in patients with sustained essential hypertension. In patients with pheochromocytoma, the responses of diastolic pressure, cardiac index and total peripheral resistance were the same as in controls. However, following tilt, there was a significant reduction in systolic

Table 4. Hemodynamic response to tilt in 10 male patients with pheochromocytoma. The patients are compared with 11 normal subjects and 57 essential hypertensive patients. (Personal data)

	Normal subjects (1)	Essential hypertensives (2)	Pheochromocytoma (3)	p value (1–3)	(2–3)
Number patients	11	57	10		
SAP (mmHg)					
S	127 ± 2	186 ± 3	184 ± 14	<0.001	NS
T	130 ± 5	182 ± 3	170 ± 13	<0.001	NS
p value	NS	NS	<0.05		
DAP (mmHg)					
S	68 ± 2	109 ± 2	102 ± 7	<0.001	NS
T	73 ± 4	114 ± 2	102 ± 7	<0.001	NS
p value	NS	NS	NS		
MAP (mmHg)					
S	89 ± 2	132 ± 2	132 ± 7	<0.001	NS
T	94 ± 4	133 ± 2	124 ± 6	<0.001	NS
p value	NS	NS	<0.05		
CI (ml/min/m^2)					
S	3371 ± 105	3534 ± 71	3164 ± 114	NS	NS
T	2958 ± 161	2825 ± 76	2604 ± 118	NS	NS
p value	<0.001	<0.001	<0.01		
HR (b/min)					
S	72 ± 1	76 ± 1	87 ± 7	<0.05	<0.05
T	85 ± 2	86 ± 2	100 ± 5	<0.05	<0.02
p value	<0.01	<0.01	<0.01		
SI (ml/m^2)					
S	47 ± 2	46 ± 1	38 ± 3	NS	NS
T	35 ± 2	33 ± 1	27 ± 2	<0.01	<0.01
p value	<0.001	<0.001	<0.01		
TPR (Dynes/ sec · cm^{-5} · m^2)					
S	2173 ± 72	3128 ± 88	3376 ± 242	<0.001	NS
T	2625 ± 140	3849 ± 117	3832 ± 253	<0.001	
p value	<0.001	<0.001	<0.05		

± 1 standard error of the mean.
Abbreviations: see Figure 1.
S = supine position; T = tilting position; p = p value between supine and tiling position or between patients and controls.

and mean arterial pressure in patients with pheochromocytoma (p < 0.05). In the erect position, stroke index was lower than in controls (p < 0.001).

Patients with pheochromocytoma were divided into two groups: those with and those without orthostatic hypotension, as compared with the response of normal subjects [9]. The supine hemodynamics of the two subgroups were similar (Table 5). However, Figure 3 indicates that, in patients with orthostatic

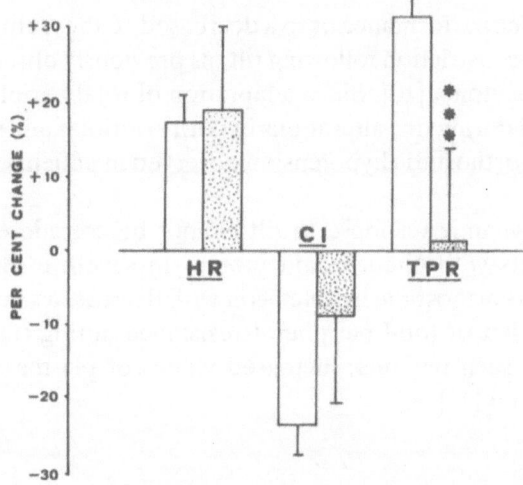

Figure 3. Hemodynamic response to tilt in 5 patients with ▨ and 5 patients without □ orthostatic hypotension. (Personal data)
HR = Heart rate; CI = Cardiac index; TPR = Total peripheral resistance.

hypotension, the increment of total peripheral resistance during tilt was significantly reduced ($p < 0.001$), in comparison with patients without orthostatic hypotension.

Finally, a predominant orthostatic systolic hypotension was observed in patients with pheochromocytoma. This was associated with 3 abnormalities: reduced blood volume, decreased stroke volume and impaired adaptation of total peripheral resistance during tilt. The reduced blood volume alone could not explain the fall in blood pressure during tilt, since blood volume was similar in patients with pheochromocytoma and in patients with sustained essential hypertension but without orthostatic hypotension (Table 4). The reduced stroke volume is a better explanation for the predominant systolic orthostatic hypotension. The decreased stroke volume could be due either to a

Table 5. Pheochromocytoma: Supine hemodynamics in 5 patients with and 5 patients without orthostatic hypotension. (Personal data)

	Without orthostatic hypotension	With orthostatic hypotension
Number patients	5	5
MAP (mmHg)	129 ± 15	135 ± 9
CI (ml/min/m²)	3323 ± 224	2994 ± 67
HR (b/min)	80 ± 7	95 ± 16
PV (ml/kg)	43 ± 1	41 ± 2

± 1 standard error of the mean.
Abbreviations: see Figure 1.

reduction in cardiac performance or to a decreased venous return caused by an alteration in venoconstriction following tilt, as previously observed in patients with pheochromocytoma [10]. Since adaptation of total peripheral resistance was also impaired during tilt, alterations in both arteriolar and venous reflexes could explain the orthostatic hypotension observed in patients with pheochromocytoma.

Such a hemodynamic response to tilt cannot be considered as a specific pattern in patients with pheochromocytoma. In severe essential hypertensives, spontaneous orthostatic hypotension with decreased stroke volume and impaired adaptation of total peripheral resistance during tilt has also been described [9]. In such patients, increased values of plasma catecholamines have been observed [11].

Hemodynamic changes following surgery

Our experiance with regard to systemic hemodynamics before and after surgery is limited to 4 patients. Before surgery, 3 patients were hypertensives and 1 patient was normotensive (Fig. 4). Blood pressure fell after surgery, but

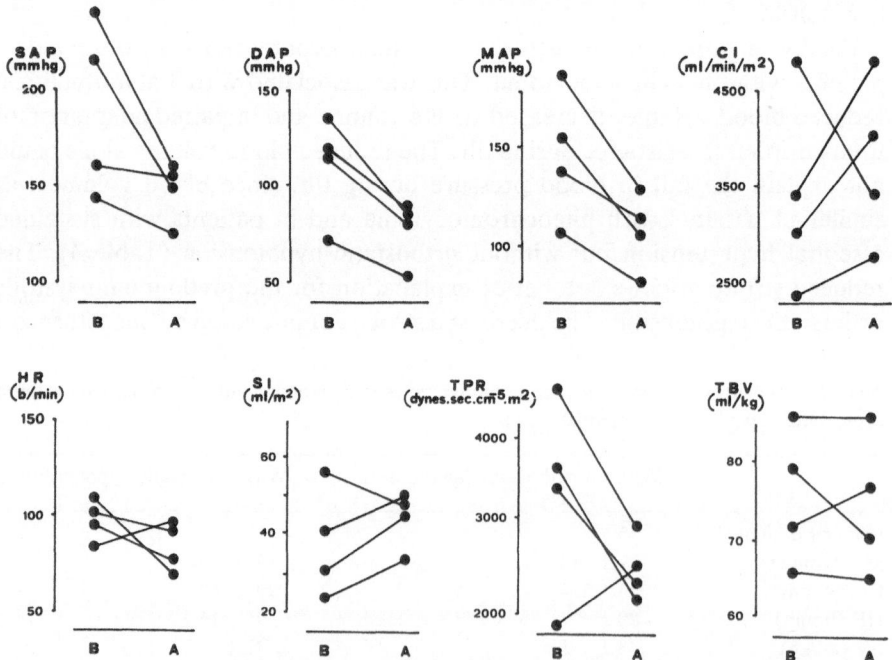

Figure 4. Hemodynamic parameters before (B) and after (A) surgery in 4 patients with pheochromocytoma. Abbreviations: see Fig. 1. (Levenson et al. [3], with the permission of Clinical Science)

mean arterial pressure remained above 100 mmHg in the 3 patients who were previously hypertensives. Total peripheral resistance decreased in 3 cases and increased in 1 case. In the 4 subjects, heart rate decreased markedly, suggesting a dissociation between heart rate and the pressure changes. After surgery, heart rate fell consistently, whereas mean arterial pressure remained slightly elevated in the previously hypertensive patients. Thus, the tachycardia better reflected the increased production of catecholamines than the elevated blood pressure itself.

Conclusion

The present review has shown that systemic hemodynamics are similar in patients with pheochromocytoma and in those with essential hypertension. In this regard, it is relevant to note that the incidence of pheochromocytoma is low in the general population, whereas essential hypertension is common. Thus, it is possible that the observed association between the tumor and (essential) hypertension was due to chance alone. The results observed following surgery do not exclude this possibility: in the studied patients, whereas heart rate returned toward normal values, the high blood pressure of the previously hypertensive patients was improved but not completely normalized by surgery, as observed by others [12–13]. Thus, the complex relationships between pheochromocytoma and high blood pressure are still difficult to explain and require further investigations.

References

1. Sjoerdsma A, Engelman K, Waldmann T, Cooperman LH, Hammond W (1966): Pheochromocytoma: Current concepts of diagnosis and treatment. *Ann Inter Med* 65: 1302–1326.
2. Guedon J, Bonvalet JP, Legrain M (1967): Le débit cardiaque dans l'hypertension artérielle, in: *Actualités Néphrologiques de l'Hôpital Necker*, pp 333. Paris: Flammarion.
3. Levenson JA, Safar ME, London GM, Simon ACh (1980): Haemodynamics in patients with pheochromocytoma. *Clin Sci* 58: 349–356.
4. Dustan HP, Tarazi RC, Bravo EI (1974): Physiologic characteristics of hypertension, in: Laragh JH (ed), *Hypertension Manual*, p. 233. New York: DunDonnelley.
5. Eckstein JW, Abboud FM (1962): Circulatory effects of sympathetic amines. *Am Heart J* 119: 63–76.
6. Innes IR, Nickerson M (1965): Drugs acting in post ganglionic adrenergic nerves endings and structures innervated by them, in Goodman LS, Gilman (ed), *The Pharmacological Basis of Therapeutics*, 3rd ed, pp 477–520. New York: Macmillan.
7. Safar M, Weiss Y, Levenson JA, London G, Milliez PL (1973): Hemodynamic study of 85 patients with borderline hypertension. *Am J Cardiol* 31: 315–319.
8. Safar ME, Chau NPh, Weiss YA, London GM, Simon ACh, Milliez PL (1976): The pressure-

volume relationship in normotensive and permanent essential hypertensive patients. *Clin Sci Mol Med* 50: 207–212.

9. Frohlich ED, Tarazi RC, Ulrych M (1967): Tilt test for investigating a neural component in hypertension: Its correlation with clinical characteristics. *Circulation* 36: 387–393.
10. Engelman K, Zelis R, Waldmann T, Mason DT, Sjoerdsma A (1968): Mechanisms of orthostatic hypotension in pheochromocytoma. *Circulation* 37 (suppl VI): 72.
11. Kopin IJ (1979): Plasma catecholamines in human and experimental hypertension, in: Meyer Ph, Schmitt H (eds), *Nervous System and Hypertension*, p. 267. Willey-Flammarion.
12. Tcherdakoff Ph, Simoni G, Milliez P (1974): Caractères évolutifs du phéochromocytome. *Nouvelle Presse Médicale*, 3: 861–864.
13. Manger WM, Gifford RW (1977): Pheochromocytoma, pp 304–344. New York – Heidelberg – Berlin: Springer Verlag Publisher.

10. Systemic hemodynamics
in renal parenchymal disease

MICHEL CHAIGNON and JACQUES GUÉDON

Hypertension is the most frequent complication of chronic renal disease. Nearly 80 percent of patients developing end stage renal failure will exhibit hypertension, regardless of their primary renal disease. Atherosclerosis and its cardiovascular complications continue to be identified as the leading cause of mortality in patients undergoing chronic dialysis. Advances in the past decade have greatly improved our understanding of the hemodynamic basis of hypertension in chronic renal failure; its study is no longer restricted to the determination of systemic hemodynamics; more accurate assessment of cardiac performance, loading condition of the heart, distribution of blood volume, vascular compliance, renal hemodynamics has helped draw a comprehensive view of the multiple factors involved during the progression of renal disease.

1. Systemic hemodynamics and renal disease

The hypertension of acute glomerulonephritis has been characterized by an elevated cardiac output; in a later phase, the renal disease was associated with normal cardiac output and elevated peripheral resistances [1]. With the improvement of the disease, blood pressure and peripheral resistances decreased together while cumulative sodium balance returned to normal.

Hypertension can develop at the early stage of chronic renal disease. The hemodynamic studies have revealed that the rise in blood pressure was related to an elevated cardiac output followed by a progressive increase in peripheral vascular resistance while cardiac output returned to normal [2].

It is conceivable that renal hypertension is initiated by an increase in cardiac output and maintained by a later rise in peripheral resistance; this pattern has been observed in dogs after partial nephrectomy leaving one third of the renal mass when fed a high sodium diet.

M.E. Safar & F. Fouad-Tarazi (eds.), The heart in hypertension.
© *1989 Kluwer Academic Publishers, Dordrecht –*

The hypertension araising from renal disease does not present an uniform pathophysiologic picture; this is due to the various factors involved in the hypertensive process [3]. Among the possible patterns, two extreme types can be observed in renal hypertension: at one extreme is a volume dependent type and at the other is a pattern characterized by increased peripheral resistance, reduced plasma volume and activation of the renin-angiotensin system; in between are a number of hemodynamic patterns with elements of both in various proportion (Figure 1).

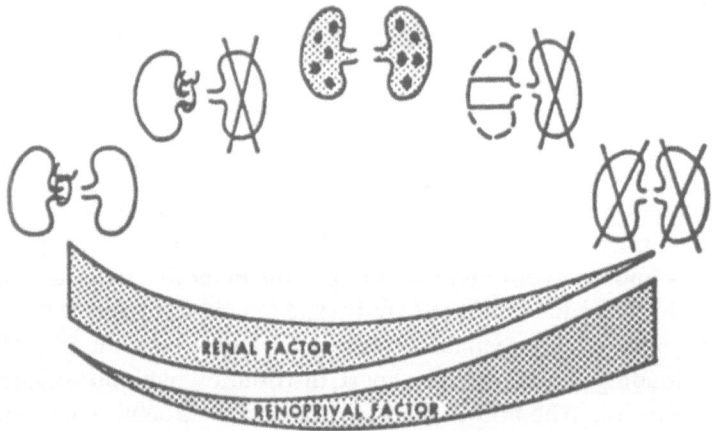

Figure 1. Renal and renoprival mechanisms in various types of 'renal' hypertension. At one extreme is the renal mechanism activated by critical narrowing of one renal artery, the other remaining intact, at the other, removal of both kidneys leads to a renoprival volume-dependent state. In between these two extremes, both renal and renoprival factors participate in different combinations in the development of hypertension, depending on the amount of renal tissue lost and on impairment of circulation through the remainder. With the permission of Tarazi and Gifford [3].

In end stage renal disease, the hemodynamic studies have shown an increase in cardiac output in hypertensive as well as in normotensive patients. Correction of the anemia led to reduce cardiac output to normal level with a concomitant increase in peripheral resistance and blood pressure [4]. When hemodialysis is started, the cardiac hemodynamics is mainly related to the level of hydration explaining the large variety of hemodynamic results [5]; the extracellular volume plays an important role in determining the cardiac output level; the strong correlation observed between stroke volume and total blood volume before and after dialysis indicates that intravascular volume is a major determinant of cardiac hemodynamics in dialysis patients [6] (Figure 2). However, various cardiac abnormalities can interfere with the schema, in relation to a possible coronary artery disease, pericarditis, left ventricular

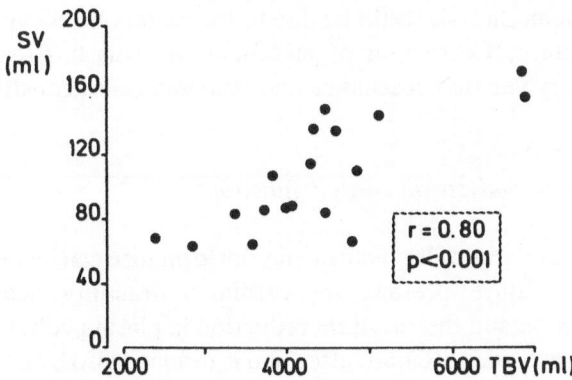

Figure 2. Relationship between total blood volume (TBV) and stroke volume (SV) before hemodialysis.

hypertrophy secondary to hypertension which are responsible for the variety of the hemodynamic patterns [7].

Secondary hyperparathyroidism is a frequent complication of the uremic state; in a recent study, inadequate left ventricular hypertrophy has been observed in dialysis patients and related to the severity and progression of secondary hyperparathyroidism [8]; parathyroidectomy has been shown improve the left ventricular function suggesting that parathormone may be a potent uremic toxin and could affect the heart.

2. Systemic hemodynamics and hemodialysis

2.1 *Effects of hemodialysis on cardiac hemodynamics and blood volume*

In patients without signs of cardiac decompensation and/or evidence of coronary artery disease, studies have demonstrated a significant decrease in diastolic and systolic left ventricular dimensions following the dialysis session [9]; stroke volume and cardiac output were reduced after dialysis. The decrease in cardiac output was not explained by a decrease in cardiac performance; in several studies, the ejection fraction was unchanged after dialysis; thus reduction in stroke volume was basically the result of fluid loss; however, it was found in a prospective study that the reduction in the left ventricular end diastolic volume was greater than expected from the contraction of blood volume; thus, it has been suggested that the hemodynamic changes following hemodialysis are not a simple consequence of volume loss but may also be related to the redistribution of blood volume [6]. The lack of veino-constriction following hemodialysis could be due to the metabolic changes associated with the procedure. Correction of metabolic acidosis has been shown to reduce pulmonary vascular resistance and systemic veino-constriction.

2.2 *Effects of hemodialysis on cardiac function*

The major determinants of left ventricular performance can be affected by the hemodialysis procedure: preload, myocardial contractility, heart rate, after load. Ultrafiltration and the resultant reduction in plasma volume is expected to reduce left ventricular preload; afterload is reduced also by hemodialysis; a decrease in blood pressure is commonly observed during the procedure; acetate has been found to induce vasodilatation; however various patterns of change in total peripheral resistance are observed; the dialysis procedure could therefore be compared to a volume depletion study with uniform decrease in preload and variable alteration in resistance to ejection.

In patients without cardiac complications, the ejection fraction was found in the normal range before dialysis; this index did not change after dialysis confirming previous observations. It has been suggested that the ejection fraction may not change when both preload and afterload are decreased simultaneously. However mean velocity of circumferential fiber shortening (mean V_{CF}) was significantly increased suggesting that dialysis did improve left ventricular contractility [10].

In a study performed with three different types of dialysis, it has been possible to separate the effects of the change in cardiac filling volume, the removal of uremic toxins, the metabolic changes induced by dialysis on left ventricular function; it was concluded that the increase in contractility of the left ventricle was independant of the alteration in left ventricular filling volume [11].

The increased left ventricular contractility has been related to the humoral changes induced by hemodialysis. Among the possibilities, the changes in plasma calcium and potassium levels have been proposed as possible factors [10]; indeed, the central role of plasma ionized calcium concentration has been confirmed [12].

2.3 *Hemodialysis and blood pressure control*

Severe hypotension during hemodialysis can occur in some patients despite careful attention to fluid balance. As the fall in blood pressure is usually controlled by infusion of saline or colloid solutions, the initial hypothesis naturally related hypotension to hypovolemia; it was found that hypotensive patients started the dialysis procedure with a lower blood volume than the others [13] although this result was not confirmed in others studies.

In some patients, because of a poor adaptation to moderate fluid depletion, severe hypotensive episodes could occur despite a moderate volume and low rate of ultrafiltration and a small decrease in cardiac output; these findings have suggested a lack of an adequate increase in peripheral vascular resistance during hemodialysis. In a study of two groups of dialysed patients, both blood volume and cardiac output fell equally in those with post-dialysis hypotension and in those with stable arterial pressure indicating an altered response of peripheral vaso-constriction in the hypotensive group [14]. Indeed, it was confirmed that the normal hemodynamic response to volume depletion could be impaired during hemodialysis [15]; abnormalities of the autonomic nervous system have been reported [13]; in addition, several factors can interfere with the peripheral vascular tone; among them, the vasodilatory effect of acetate has been emphasized and the beneficial effect of bicarbonate instead of acetate has been reported [16].

3. Systemic hemodynamics and renal transplantation

Renal transplantation may have a beneficial effect on cardiac hemodynamics in normotensive patients; in a study after an average of nine months after renal transplantation, the mean left ventricular diameter, both systolic and diastolic, was reduced to normal, although the mean cardiac index remained high because of the open arteriovenous fistula [17]. Several factors contributed to the improvement in left ventricular size including reduction in preload and afterload, correction of anemia, equilibration of water and sodium balance. Reduction of afterload brought about a significant decrease in left ventricular wall thickness and mass after renal transplantation; other results suggested an improvement in left ventricular function [18]. These data confirm that cardiac alterations induced indirectly by chronic renal failure can be reversed by adequate corrections of the renal disorders.

However, a high incidence of hypertension is observed in most surveys of stable transplantation. Many factors are able to induce hypertension in renal transplant patients; it is of the greatest importance to differenciate the role of the native kidneys, an allograft renal artery stenosis or a drug induced hypertension (ciclosporine); for the latter, there is evidence that ciclosporine induces renal vasoconstriction as well as systemic peripheral vasoconstriction which is reversible when the drug is discontinued at least in the first year after renal transplantation [19].

4. Hemodynamics and the development of renal failure

Experimental studies have shown that the reduction in renal mass induced an increase in perfusion and filtration in the remaining nephrons [20]; it has been suggested recently that these long term hemodynamic alterations might be deleterous: the permanent hypertension and hyperperfusion in the glomerulus induce a progressive sclerosis of the glomerular capillaries. This hypothesis may help a better understanding of the mechanisms of progressive nephronic reduction such as it is observed during diabetes, arterial hypertension and chronic nephropathies. For instance, in the diabetic glomerulosclerosis, it has been clearly shown that hypertension accelerated the deterioration of renal function while the antihypertensive treatment delayed glomerular lesions [21]. The increase in glomerular capillary pressure is the results of the redistribution of afferent and efferent arteriolar resistances: in spontaneous hypertensive rats, where pre-capillary resistance is elevated, the glomerular capillary pressure is maintained within normal range and the development of glomerular sclerosis is delayed. By contrast, in Dahl sodium sensitive rats, the glomerular capillary pressure is elevated (in relation to low precapillary resistance) and severe glomerular sclerosis is observed for a comparable level of systemic blood pressure [20]. Therefore, it is reasonable to speculate that any treatment which reduce glomerular hypertension and hyperfiltration might protect the nephrons from sclerosis. However, long term controlled studies are needed to confirm these experimental results.

5. Conclusions

Cardiac complications are the most frequent causes of death in long term dialysis patients. A specific uremic cardiac involvement has been suggested; however hypertension and/or coronary artery disease which are frequently associated with end stage renal failure must be considered as a primary cause of altered cardiac function. Prevention of accelerated artherosclerosis and calcium disorders, treatment of hypertension and overhydration are required for preservation of cardiac hemodynamics in these patients.

References

1. Birkenhager WH, Schalekamp MAD, Schalekamp-Kuyken MPA, Kolsters G, Krauss XH (1970): Interrelations between arterial pressure, fluid-volumes, and plasma-renin concentration in the course of acute glomerulonephritis. *Lancet* 1970/1: 1086.

2. Brod J (1974): Hemodynamic basis of hypertension in chronic renal disease, in: Villarreal H (ed), *Proceedings of the Fifth Int. Congress of Nephrology*, Vol 3, p. 60. New York: S. Karger.
3. Tarazi RC, Gifford RW (1979): Systemic arterial pressure, in: Sodeman WA Jr and Sodeman TM (eds), *Pathologic Physiology*, 6th ed, pp 198–229. Philadelphia: Saunders.
4. Kim KE, Onesti G, Schwartz AB, Chinitz JL, Swartz C (1972): Hemodynamics of hypertension in chronic end-stage renal disease. *Circulation* 46: 456–464.
5. Golf S, Lunde P, Abrahamsen AM, Oyri A (1983): Effect of hydration state on cardiac function in patients on chronic haemodialysis. *Br Heart J* 49: 183–186.
6. Chaignon M, Chen WT, Tarazi RC, Bravo EL, Nakamoto S (1981): Effect of hemodialysis on blood volume distribution and cardiac output. *Hypertension* 3 (3): 327–332.
7. Friedman HS, Shah BN, Kim HG, Bove LA, Del Monte MM, Smith AJ (1981): Clinical study of the cardiac findings in patients on chronic maintenance hemodialysis: The relationship to coronary risk factors. *Clin Nephrol* 16 (2): 75–85.
8. London GM, Fabiani F, Marchais SJ, De Vernejoul MC, Guerin AP, Safar ME, Metivier F, Llach F (1987): Uremic cardiomyopathy: An inadequate left ventricular hypertrophy. *Kidney Int* 31: 973–980.
9. MacDonald IL, Uldall R, Buda AJ (1981): The effect of hemodialysis on cardiac rhythm and performance. *Clin Nephrol* 15 (6): 321–327.
10. Chaignon M, Chen WT, Tarazi RC, Nakamoto S, Salcedo E (1982): Acute effects of hemodialysis on echographic-determined cardiac performance: Improved contractility resulting from serum increased calcium with reduced potassium despite hypovolemic-reduced cardiac output. *Am Heart J* 103 (3): 374–378.
11. Nixon JV, Mitchell JH, MacPhaul JJ, Henrich WL (1983): Effect of hemodialysis on left ventricular function: Dissociation of changes in filling volume and in contractile state. *J Clin Invest* 71: 377–384.
12. Henrich WL, Hunt JM, Nixon JV (1984): Increased ionized calcium and left ventricular contractility during hemodialysis. *New Engl J Med* 310: 19–23.
13. Lilley JJ, Golden J, Stone RA (1976): Adrenergic regulation of blood pressure in chronic renal failure. *J Clin Invest* 57: 1190–1200.
14. Chaignon M, Chen WT, Tarazi RC Nakamoto S, Bravo EL (1981): Blood pressure response to hemodialysis. *Hypertension* 3 (3): 333–339.
15. Rouby JJ, Rottembourg J, Durande JP, Basset JY, Degoulet P, Glaser P, Legrain M (1980): Hemodynamic changes induced by regular hemodialysis and sequential ultrafiltration hemodialysis: A comparative study. *Kidney Int* 17: 801–810.
16. Graefe U, Milutinovitch J, Follette WC, Vizzo JE, Babb AL, Scribner BH (1978): Less dialysis induced morbidity and vascular instability with bicarbonate in dialysate. *Ann Intern Med* 88: 332–336.
17. Ikaheimo M, Linnaluoto M, Huttunen K, Takkunen J (1982): Effects of renal transplantation on left ventricular size and function. *Br Heart J* 47: 155–160.
18. Lai KN, Barnden L, Mathew TH (1982): Effect of renal transplantation on left ventricular function in hemodialysis patients. *Clin Nephrol* 18 (2): 74–78.
19. Luke RG (1987): Hypertension in renal transplant recipients. *Kidney Int* 31: 1024–1037.
20. Meyer TW, Anderson S, Rennke HG, Brenner BM (1987): Reversing glomerular hypertension stabilizes established glomerular injury. *Kidney Int* 31: 752–759.
21. Zatz R, Anderson S, Meyer TW, Rentz-Dunn B, Rennke HG, Brenner BM (1987): Lowering of arterial blood pressure limits glomerular sclerosis in rats with renal ablation and in experimental diabetes. *Kidney Int* 31 (suppl 20): S123–S129.

11. Hemodynamics in patients with overweight and hypertension

EFRAIN REISIN and EDWARD D. FROHLICH

Several epidemiological studies, cross-sectional [1–3] and longitudinal [1, 4–6], have shown that obesity and hypertension are two directly related pathological disorders at any age [1, 7], and the overweight condition is a predicting and predisposing factor for future development of elevated systolic and diastolic pressures [4–6]. More recent studies, however, have concluded that in determining the risk profile of obese subjects, assessment of body fat distribution is important [8–11]. Thus, considerably evidence suggests that fat distribution is a relatively constant characteristic of human beings, even after major weight changes [8, 9]. By a variety of techniques, such as skinfold thickness measurements [10], circumference measurements [10–12], and computed tomography [13], estimates of fat distribution in different body regions support the concept that an increased waist-hip circumference ratio (upper-body obesity or hypertrophic obesity) shows a preponderance of fat in the abdominal region. This specific type of obesity, in contrast to subjects having low waist-hip circumference ratios (lower-body obesity or hyperplastic obesity), is associated with increased risk of hypertension, impaired glucose tolerance, and hyperinsulinemia [14–17]. This finding is true across race and gender groups and is independent of age [16, 17].

The underlying mechanisms accounting for the elevated arterial pressure in the obese population are not fully understood. However, studies have been concerned with changes in metabolic, endocrine, and hemodynamic functions that have been associated with obesity and hypertension [18–23] (Figure 1). Modifications of these mechanism, promoted by weight reduction, are important attempts to elucidate a better understanding of the pathophysiology of this association. Not surprisingly, most of these mechanisms have been studied in the obese-hypertensive population, and not specifically in those obese patients with increasing fat accumulation in the upper part of their bodies and who have an increased risk of hypertension.

M.E. Safar & F. Fouad-Tarazi (eds.), The heart in hypertension.
© *1989 Kluwer Academic Publishers, Dordrecht –*

This discussion is concerned primarily with those pathophysiologic mechanisms that seem to be involved in obesity hypertension, emphasizing the difference between upper- and lower-body obesity (when reported) and the changes produced by weight reduction. The rational for this reasoning is supported by the thesis that even a moderate decrease in weight has been shown to be associated with improvement in hypertension [18–21].

Part One: Mechanisms in obesity-hypertension

1 *Metabolic and endocrine alterations in obesity-hypertension*

1.1 *The renin-angiotensin-aldosterone system.* The precise role of the renin-angiotensin-aldosterone system in obesity-hypertension remains unclear. Plasma renin activity (PRA) may be unchanged [22] or reduced [20, 23] in inverse proportion to weight. Reduction of plasma renin activity could be a consequence of increased sodium intake, increased total body sodium, water retention, and the expanded intravascular volume that follows the increase in body weight [23]. This inverse correlation between blood volume and plasma renin activity was shown previously in essential hypertensive patients and normal subjects [24].

In some studies, plasma levels of aldosterone, related to the low plasma renin activity, were considered to be inappropriately elevated in the obese hypertensive patients [23]; and, when both plasma renin activity and aldosterone levels were measured in a group of patients with essential hypertension and various weights, the levels of plasma renin activity correlated inversely with the increase of relative body weight but not with urinary sodium excretion. Nevertheless, serum aldosterone levels were not influenced by relative body weight; and the aldosterone/PRA ratio was found to increase progressively with the increase in weight [23]. Recent data have shown significantly high plasma aldosterone concentrations in obese adolescents [25], and high aldosterone secretion in obese adults (whether expressed in absolute values or indexed by body surface area) [26]. These studies suggest that hyperaldosteronism associated with obesity may participate in the hypertension of obesity through sodium and water retention and an expansion of intravascular volume of the obese hypertensive patients [23]. However, the renin-angiotensin-aldosterone differences between the upper- and lower-body obesity patients remains unknown.

1.2 *Steroid changes.* According to one study [27], upward shifts in body-fat deposition and insulin resistance occurs in the presence of cortisol excess. Other investigators have shown that the excretion of metabolites of cortisol is greater in the obese population, even when the data were corrected for body surface area [28]. Nonetheless, other investigators have found that glucocorticoid secretion is normal if expressed in terms of milligrams of 17-hydrosteroids per gram of urinary creatinine [29]. These studies, however, have generally excluded patients who have hypertension, and whether this mechanism affects the finding of insulin resistance in obesity-hypertension as described is merely speculative [30].

Abnormal levels of adrenal androgens have also been associated with obesity [31]. More recently, one report suggested that an imbalance in androgenic/estrogenic activity could play an important role in abdominal fat distribution and associated metabolic abnormalities [32].

Centripetal fat distribution characteristic in upper-body-obese patients has been reported to be a direct function of the level of serum dehydroepiandrosterone sulphate (DHEA-S) in overweight women [33]. And serum DHEA-S levels have also been reported to be increased in persons with hypertension and upper-body obesity [33].

1.3 *Adrenergic and thyroid changes.* Previous studies have shown that overfeeding is associated with increased sympathetic activity, as indicated by norepinephrine turnover [34, 35], an extremely sensitive index of adrenergic participation [36]. This increased sympathetic activity has been attributed to high insulin levels having an adrenergic stimulatory effect [32], a link that can explain the higher association of upper-body obesity with hypertension. Other studies have shown that overfeeding increases the concentration of triiodothronine, increasing the reactivity of the tissues to catecholamines as a consequence [37, 38].

Some investigators, comparing a small group of borderline hypertensive obese patients with lean hypertensive controls, found in the former group higher levels in plasma norepinephrine, epinephrine, and norepinephrine in response to changes in posture and isometric handgrip exercise [39]. Others, however, found no differences in plasma levels of norepinephrine or excretion rates of norepinephrine or epinephrine in obese hypertensives when compared with obese normotensives [40].

These findings suggested to Landsberg and Young that changes in sympathetic activity could account for the increased incidence of arrhythmias, angina pectoris, and hypertension in patients with obesity [35].

1.4 *Sodium and Na$^+$-K$^+$-ATPase.* Many epidemiological studies have shown an increased prevalence of hypertension in populations whose sodium intake is excessive [41–44]. Some have proposed that in obese patients, increased sodium intake and higher caloric intake are the underlying factors promoting hypertension [45].

Various theories may explain the mechanisms involved in sodium-dependent blood pressure elevation: (a) passive waterlogging of the vessel wall [46], (b) increased sensitivity to catecholamines [47], (c) increased angiotensin II receptor sensitivity [48], and (d) reduced active-ion-exchange transport mechanisms involving sodium and potassium [49]. Some studies [50, 51] have concentrated on active ion transport mechanisms inasmuch as the Na^+-K^+-activated adenosine triphosphatase (Na^+-K^+-ATPase) may be responsible for as much as 20% to 50% of total cellular thermogenesis, which may be impaired in obesity. Decreased Na^+-K^+-ATPase activity has been found in red blood cells of obese adolescents and adults [52, 53], but not by all investigators [54]. This diminished enzyme activity should result in increased intracellular sodium concentration, decreased cellular thermogenesis, lower energy expenditure, and a consequent increase in body weight [50, 51].

The relationship between the Na^+-K^+ pump and increased blood pressure has been explained by the following theory. A decrease in Na^+-K^+-ATPase pump activity enhances intracellular Na^+ concentration with a concomitant reduced calcium efflux. The result is an increased intracellular calcium ion concentration that, in turn, increases arteriolar smooth muscle tone and vascular resistance [55]. Some investigators have found intracellular Na^+ and Ca^+ elevated only in obese hypertensive patients or with a familial predisposition for hypertension [56], suggesting that this mechanism may be critical to the understanding of obesity hypertension.

1.5 *Insulin resistance and hyperinsulinemia.* Some workers believe that the hyperinsulinemia and insulin resistance found in the upper-body obesity type result from a large accumulation of lipolytic hyperactive abdominal cells that release large amounts of free fatty acids into the portal vein, leading to excess hepatic synthesis of triglycerides, inhibition of insulin intake, hyperinsulinemia, and insulin resistance [57, 58]. As already stated, the upper-body, but not the lower-body, type of obesity may be associated with increased risk of hypertension, impaired glucose tolerance, and hyperinsulinemia. This frequent association suggests a common pathogenetic mechanism [14–17]. In this regard, DeFronzo et al. [59] have shown that insulin increases sodium absorption in the diluting segment of the distal nephron; and these workers have related these findings to the development of hypertension and obesity among genetically predisposed patients. Other investigators have explained the link between obesity and hypertension as follows: (a) tissue insulin resistance alters transmembrane ionic sodium and potassium distribution that causes vascular resistance to increase, (b) the hyperglycemia that accompanies hyperinsulinemia may increase vascular resistance by increasing intracellular osmolality through enhanced positive diffusion of glucose, and (c) insulin has a stim-

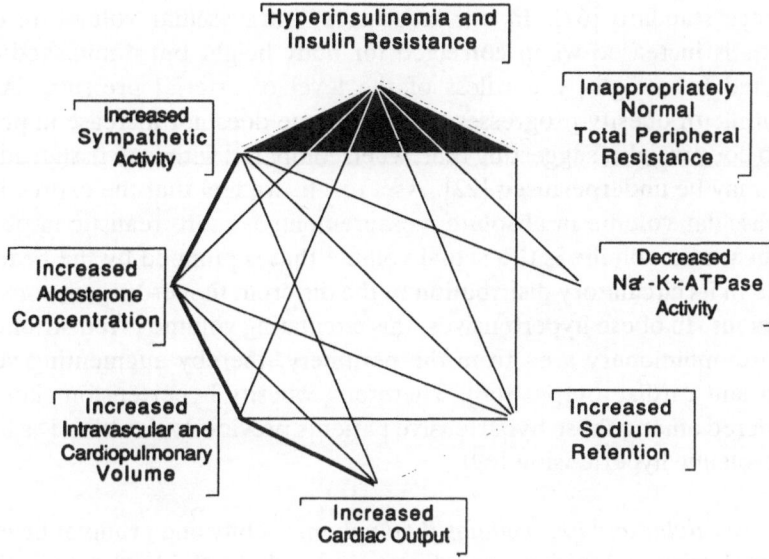

Figure 1. Mosaic concept including pathophysiological mechanisms suggested thus far for obesity-hypertension. Adapted from Page [104].

ulatory effect on the sympathetic nervous system that promotes hypertension [16, 60–63].

Thus, the link between insulin resistance-hyperinsulinemia and blood pressure does not prove cause and effect, but it supports the concept that hypertension and obesity may be controlled, in part, by the tendency of patients with upper-body obesity to have greater insulin resistance with consequent increased levels of plasma insulin that in some fashion seems to elevate arterial pressure.

2 *Fluid compartmental distribution and systemic hemodynamics in obesity hypertension*

2.1 *Intravascular volume.* In earlier studies, obese hypertensive patients demonstrated an absolute increase in plasma and total blood volume [64–66]. In each of those studies the increased total blood volume was well correlated with the degree of excess in body weight. In contrast, intravascular volume may be normal or reduced when calculated by deviation from desirable weight or expressed with reference to the body surface area [64–66]. Some, however, have raised several objections to the use of ideal or desirable weight as a reference standard [67]. In our laboratory, intravascular volume in obese patients is increased when corrected for body height but diminished when corrected for weight, regardless of the level of arterial pressure. As the magnitude of obesity progresses, blood volume does not increase in proportion to body weight, suggesting that, when compared with lean tissue, adipose tissue may be underperfused [22]. As a result, we feel that the expression of intravascular volume in absolute measurements is more realistic in obesity. The measured volume is the actual volume that is pumped by the heart and altered in its circulatory distribution to the different tissues, organs, or vascular regions. In obese hypertensives, this circulating volume is redistributed to the cardiopulmonary area from the periphery, thereby augmenting venous return and cardiac output [68]. Therefore, obesity hypertension should be considered among those hypertensive patients previously described as having hypervolemic hypertension [69].

2.2 *Extracellular and intracellular fluid volumes.* Only one group of investigators has determined the extracellular and intracellular fluid volumes in obesity hypertension as measured with inulin and antypirin, respectively [70, 71]. They concluded that, for the same degree of obesity, hypertensive patients had a greater extracellular and interstitial fluid volume than did normotensives subjects, although the total body water and intracellular fluid volumes were similar.

Considering the difficulty of expressing fluid volume based on reference frame indices, these authors analyzed only the indexes of partition of fluid volume, plasma volume/interstitial fluid volume (PV/IF), and the intracellular fluid volume/interstitial fluid volume (ICV/IF) [70]. They reported an altered partition of body water between the intracellular and extracellular spaces in obese hypertensive patients, explaining the increased ICV/IF ratio on the basis of an intracellular body water that is too great for the level of interstitial fluid volume (or an interstitial fluid volume that is too low for the level of intracellular fluid volume) [70]. Until now, no study has addressed the differences in fluid compartmental distribution between patients with upper- and lower-body obesity.

3 *Hemodynamics in obesity-hypertension*

3.1 *Systemic hemodynamics.* Early hemodynamic studies have shown that oxygen consumption and heart rate was increased slightly in obese hypertensive patients [64–65, 72]. Other reports have shown that in normotensive and hypertensive obese subjects the expanded intravascular volume was associated with an increased cardiac output, stroke volume, and left ventricular work [66]. In our studies, we have compared three groups of patients: normotensive, borderline hypertensive, and established hypertensive – each further classified as lean, mildly obese, and obese [22]. We found that intra-arterial pressure tended to rise progressively from the lean subgroup to the mildly obese to the obese.

The lean borderline hypertensive patients had an increased heart rate, cardiac output, and cardiac index, but the lean established hypertensive patients had a faster heart rate but their cardiac output and index were normal. In contrast, the mildly obese and obese patients demonstrated an elevated cardiac output in both borderline and established hypertensive patients. The elevated cardiac output in the obese hypertensive patients was related to an expanded intravascular volume that was redistributed to the cardiopulmonary area. The cardiac index, however, was normal, a finding that most likely relates to the lack of appropriate indices to express blood flow for patients groups having differences in body masses [73]. The calculated total peripheral resistance was normal in obese hypertensive patients when compared with lean patients having essential hypertension; however, in the face of an augmented cardiac output this normal total peripheral resistance must be considered 'inappropriately normal' [22]. The pulse-wave velocity, which is directly related to the stiffness and the thickness of large arteries, was found to be greater in obese than in nonobese hypertensive patients [74].

Thus whether obese patients are hypertensive or not, they have an increased cardiac output and stroke volume, and an inappropriately normal total peripheral resistance that is associated with an expanded intravascular volume [22]. However, other investigators have reported that the cardiac output of obese hypertensive patients was significantly higher than that of the nonobese hypertensive but not of obese normotensive controls [75]. When the cardiac output was expressed in relation to body surface area this difference disappeared. Thus, the total peripheral resistance, was significantly higher in both hypertensive groups, whether of normal weight or obese. They, therefore, concluded that hemodynamic characteristics do not separate obese from nonobese hypertensives when the functions are expressed in relation to body weight. In an analysis of obese hypertensives who were studied by means of cross-sectional sampling, Dustan concluded that the hypertension was not always related to obesity, and that more conclusive data would be obtained from a longitudinal study that examined hemodynamic functions as body weight was gained and lost [70]. To follow the same line of thinking these data would be all the more meaningful if the differences in hemodynamic variables considered differences between upper- and lower-body obesity in these patients.

3.2 *Other cardiac factors*. In obese hypertensive patients the increased arterial pressure and absolute increase in cardiac output and blood volume were associated with an increased oxygen consumption, left ventricular stroke volume, and stroke work [72]. As we already indicated, the heart adapts to increasing arterial pressure, total peripheral resistance, stroke work, and left ventricular overload in lean patients with hypertension by increasing its mass through concentric hypertrophy [73, 77, 78]. However, in the obese hypertensive patient this adaptation is complicated by the factor of volume overload that serves to reduce an eccentric component to the ventricular hypertrophy. Echocardiographic studies showed increases in diastolic and systolic volumes and aortic root diameters, as well as increases in septal wall thickness and left ventricular mass [78]. Thus, both pathological disorders – hypertension and obesity – affect the heart functionally and structurally through different mechanisms. Arterial hypertension promotes a concentric left ventricular hypertrophy (increased afterload), and obesity promotes, ventricular dilatation and eccentric hypertrophy (increased preload) [78].

3.3 *Peripheral circulation.* Studies of obese patients have shown that blood distribution to the brain and kidneys was normal, but the flow distribution to the spleen was slightly elevated [65]. Recently, we have reported that, when compared with lean normotensivees or hypertensive patients, whose pressures were matched with normotensive and hypertensive obese subjects, those who were obese had increased renal blood flow and a decreased renal vascular resistance [79]. We concluded that in obesity body weight correlated directly with renal blood flow and that the elevated cardiac output and intravascular volume expansion in obese patients was associated with the increased renal perfusion, and we suggested that these findings might explain the recent observation that overweight hypertensive patients had a better prognosis than did those who were lean [80].

Part Two: Effect of weight reduction

Several reports have demonstrated that, in obese hypertensive patients arterial pressure decreases as weight decreases and that this effect was independent of sodium restriction [18–21, 70, 71, 81–84]. These findings are in conflict with earlier findings that attributed the fall in pressure to sodium, rather than caloric, restriction [45]. This fall in arterial pressure with reduction in body weight has been explained on the basis of the adrenergic, hormonal, and metabolic factors [20, 23, 25, 34–40, 85–90] and the altered fluid volume partition [70, 91–95] and hemodynamic changes [70, 84, 91–94] (Figure 2). However, it is worthy to note that these studies were not always able to differentiate the independent effect of caloric restriction or weight reduction and did not specify those patients with upper-body distribution of obesity.

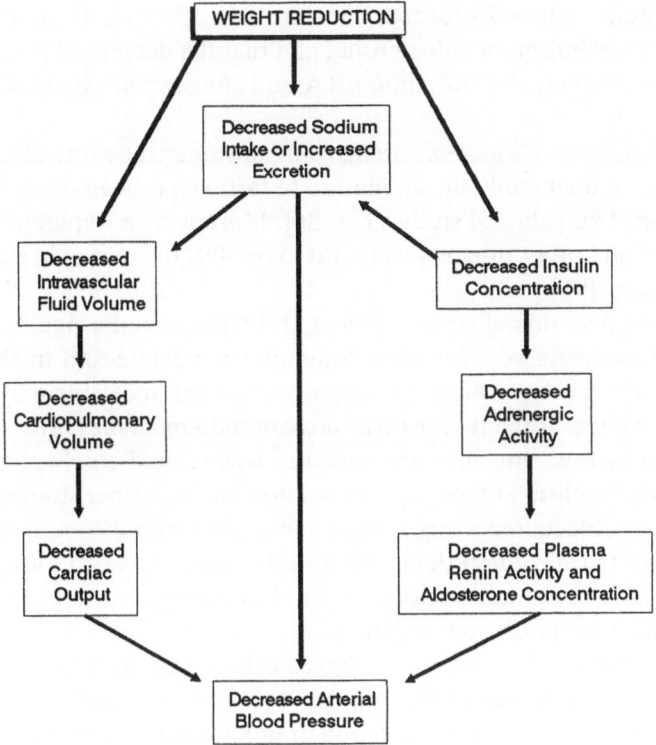

Figure 2. Pathophysiological changes produced by weight reduction.

4 *Metabolic-endocrinic changes following weight reduction*

4.1 *Plasma renin activity and aldosterone levels.* In an earlier study from our laboratory plasma renin acitivity (PRA) did not decrease in a group of obese hypertensive patients after weight reduction despite a significant decrease in blood pressure [91]. Other investigators, however, did find changes in the renin-aldosterone system that were associated with starvation and body weight reduction [20, 85, 88–99]. Thus, Sowers and co-workers [85] found that plasma renin activity and aldosterone levels declined significantly during weight reduction in obese hypertensives, and that the decrease in PRA in those patients correlated with the reduction in blood pressure. A PRA decrease was also reported [20] during the natriuresis of fasting that occurs early (6th day on diet); but, this decrease was also observed ten months after a fifteen percent weight reduction (achieved with a 800 caloric and 150 mEq per day diet) [89].

Marks and co-workers reported a significant decrease in urinary aldosterone level and PRA following weight reduction [80]. They postulated that the decrease in tetrahydroaldosterone-3 glucuronide was an indication of a lowered rate of metabolism of aldosterone, and that the decreased pressure after weight reduction may depend upon PRA and aldosterone changes.

4.2 Sympathetic nervous system and thyroid hormones. The role of the sympathetic system in the metabolic adaptation to fasting has been described previously in animal and clinical studies [35, 36]. Moreover, norepinephrine turnover in heart and other organs was found to be 40% decreased in rats after 48 hours of fasting [96].

Confirming that animal study, Jung et al. [97] reported a significant fall in the urinary excretion of 4-hydroxy-3-methoxymandelate and in the plasma norepinephrine levels in obese normotensive women receiving a hypocaloric diet (low carbohydrate content with a constant sodium intake). This significant reduction in systolic and diastolic pressure was related to changes in catecholamine metabolism independent of sodium intake. Other studies on obese hypertensive subjects receiving a hypocaloric diet with different sodium intakes (40 and 120 mEq/day) demonstrated that weight loss was accompanied by a progressive reduction in blood pressure and decreases in plasma norepinephrine and epinephrine levels [20].

Some investigators have indicated that catecholamines may interact with the thyroid hormone not only at the cellular level, where triiodothyronine (T3) may modulate the thermogenesis action of noadrenaline, but also by modifying peripheral thyroid metabolism or a decreased conversion of T4 to T3 in peripheral tissue [37]. In a group of subjects receiving a low caloric diet (9.2 cal/kg of desirable weight), the reduced resting metabolic rate was associated with a decline in T3 and norepinephrine [37].

Thus, as we have reported previously [91], it seems reasonable that the lower norepinephrine levels associated with the fall in arterial pressure accompanied by weight reduction could reflect a state of diminished adrenergic input to the cardiovascular system. This suppressed adrenergic activity also suggests a means for conservation of calories – by diminishing metabolism and heat production [92].

4.3 Sodium and Na^+-K^+-ATPase. Dahl and co-workers attributed the reduction of blood pressure in obese hypertensive patients after weight reduction to a concomitant decrease in sodium intake [45]. A moderate sodium intake has been reported to reduce arterial pressure of essential hypertensive patients [98].

This relationship between sodium and arterial pressure clearly is a complex one (as well as controversial). Some investigators, however, have shown that the natriuresis of fasting was associated with a drastic decrease in sympathetic activity and consequent impairment of renal tubular sodium reabsorption [88].

Others [86] have attributed the natriuresis of fasting to the decreased insulin secretion associated with starvation. Only two studies were concerned with the effect of weight reduction on the erythrocyte Na^+-K^+ transport in obese subjects [87, 99]. In a group of obese hypertensive adults receiving a 12-week regimen of caloric and sodium restriction, the Na^+-K^+-ATPase activity was shown to increase with a considerable decrease in intracellular sodium concentration [87]. No relationship was found, however, between erythrocyte sodium pump activity and changes in blood pressure in these patients. According to other authors [99] the previously mentioned findings were produced by sodium restriction and not by the caloric reduction in the diet. These workers have shown in normotensive obese young subjects, after a 6-month hypocaloric diet with normal sodium intake, that erythrocytic sodium concentration was significantly increased as mean arterial pressure was reduced [99].

In consequence (and considering these contradictory results), we must conclude that more data are necessary to evaluate the changes of Na^+-K^+-ATPase and intracellular sodium changes in obese hypertensive patients before and after weight reduction.

4.4 *Insulin resistance and insulin concentration levels.* One group of investigators [100] has studied the changes in insulin resistance in obese normotensive patients with type II non-insulin-dependent diabetes. After weight reduction, standing blood pressures fell significantly. In those patients fat mass, and insulin concentration decreased significantly whereas hepatic sensitivity to insulin increased significantly. The changes were explained on the basis of a decreased basal endogenous glucose production and an increased hepatic sensitivity to insulin.

Other workers have shown [101] that caloric restriction in obese hypertensives reduced plasma insulin concentration within a day, and this fall was attributed to an increased in the number and affinity of insulin receptors. However, the effect of weight reduction independent of caloric restriction on insulin levels has not been reported.

5 *Fluid compartmental distribution and systemic hemodynamics following weight reduction*

5.1 *Intravascular, extracellular, and intracellular fluid volumes.* After weight reduction in obese hypertensive patients, intravascular volume decreased significantly [43, 94]. In 1983, we reported [91] that a moderate weight reduction (± 10 kg) in obese hypertensives resulted in a decrease in intravascular and central cardiopulmonary blood volumes.

Raison et al. [70] have studied the effect of a 10% to 15% reduction of body weight on the fluid compartmental distribution in a group of obese hypertensive patients obtained after one month using a low caloric diet, with a moderate sodium intake (90 mEq/day). They found that the plasma volume/interstitial fluid volume and the intracellular fluid volume/total body water ratios significantly increased after weight reduction, changes that they believed expressed a shift of fluid volume from the intracellular to the interstitial space.

5.2 *Systemic hemodynamics.* Earlier studies have shown that total body oxygen consumption (by arteriovenous-oxygen difference) decreased after a 50% weight reduction [93]. Another investigation involving patients having jejunoileostomy with ensuing weight loss (50 kg) showed reduced oxygen consumption, cardiac output, and left ventricular stroke work without changes in total peripheral resistance [94].

In our study of obese hypertensive patients with a moderate weight reduction (± 10 kg) but without sodium restriction (± 173 mEq/day), a significant decrease in cardiac output was directly related to a contracted total blood volume and a decreased cardiopulmonary blood volume [91]. This reduction in cardiac output was associated with improved cardiac function, as reflected by reduced left ventricular stroke work; total peripheral resistance remained unchanged. These studies have been confirmed by others [70] who also have shown in addition an improvement of arterial distensibility and compliance after weight reduction [74].

5.3 *Other cardiac factors.* Only one study [102] has shown the effect of weight reduction (± 8 kg) with low caloric diet (sodium content was not mentioned) on M-mode echocardiographic measurements of the thickness and mass of the left ventricular wall on a group of obese hypertensive patients. In that study interventricular septal and posterior wall thicknesses decreased by 14% and 11%, respectively, and left ventricular mass also was decreased by 20%.

The changes in body weight were directly related to the diminished left ventricular mass, independent of fall in arterial pressure (and this decrease was also significant when adjusted to body surface area). These findings strongly suggest that weight reduction of the obese hypertensive is not only beneficial for the control of arterial pressure but also for the prevention or correction of left ventricular hypertrophy. This work confirms an earlier report that showed that heart size, as confirmed by roentgenkymograms, was significantly decreased in all dimensions after a drastic caloric restriction and loss of weight [103].

Summary and conclusions

An association between increased body mass and hypertension is a consistent epidemiological finding irrespective of age, sex, or social origin. Those patients who show a preponderance of fat in the abdominal region (upper-body obesity), however, are associated with increased risk of hypertension, impaired glucose tolerance, and hypersulinemia. Obesity in hypertensive subjects induces some metabolic, hormonal, and hemodynamic characteristics; some of these metabolic-hormonal characteristics have been specifically studied in obese hypertensives classified as having upper-body obesity. Levels of plasma renin activity were inversely correlated with the increase of relative body weight, and the level of serum aldosterone was elevated in young and adult obese hypertensives. The decreased Na^+-K^+-ATPase activity, found by many but not all investigators, in obese hypertensives could enhance the intracellular sodium concentration. These changes could decrease intracellular calcium efflux, thereby increasing intracellular calcium concentration, smooth muscle tone, and vascular resistance. The increased insulin level associated with higher insulin resistance in obese hypertensives having upper-body obesity could have a stimulatory effect on the sympathetic nervous system (as measured by higher supine plasma norpinephrine, epinephrine, and norepinephrine response to upright posture).

The hemodynamic characteristics described above as studied in the obese population without differentiation with respect to body fat distribution were: an increased circulating plasma volume that is associated with a high ratio of intracellular body water to interstitial fluid volume. The increased circulating volume is redistributed to the cardiopulmonary area, thereby increasing venous return, ventricular preload, and cardiac output. The ventricles adapt structurally to this augmented volume load and to the increased arterial pressure with a dimorphic (concentric-eccentric) type of hypertrophy.

Weight reduction, independent of sodium and caloric restriction, reduces arterial pressure in the obese hypertensive patient. With weight reduction, plasma renin activity and aldosterone and norepinephrine levels may become reduced, and the lower adrenergic levels could reflect a state of diminished adrenergic input to the cardiovascular system. Studies showing changes in the Na^+-K^+-ATPase activity or in insulin levels after weight reduction in obese hypertensives are lacking.

The hyperdynamic circulatory state, described in the obese hypertensive patients, is reversed with weight reduction, but the total peripheral resistance remains unchanged. Fluid volume then is apparently shifted from the intracellular to the interstitial space, and the changes in body weight are directly associated with reduction in cardiac mass and wall thicknesses.

References

1. Kannel W, Brand N, Skinner J, Dawber J, MacNamera P (1976): Relation of adiposity of blood pressure and development of hypertension: The Framingham Study. *Ann Intern Med* 68: 48–59.
2. Stamler R, Stamler J, Riedlinger WE, Algera G, Roberts RH (1978): Weight and blood pressure findings in hypertension screening of a million Americans. *J Am Med Assoc* 240: 1607–1610.
3. Epstein FM (1965): Prevalence of chronic disease and distribution of selected physiological variables in a total community of Tecumseh, Michigan. *Am J Epidemiol* 81: 307–322.
4. Levi RL, White PD, Stroud WD (1946): Overweight: A prognostic significance in relation to hypertension and cardiovascular-renal diseases. *J Am Med Assoc* 131: 951–953.
5. Hsu PH, Mathewson FAL, Rabkin SW (1977): Blood pressure and body mass index patterns a longitudinal study. *J Chronic Dis* 30: 93–113.
6. Rabkin SW, Mathewson FAL, Hsu PH (1977): Relation of body weight to development of ischemic heart disease in a cohort of young North American mean after a 26 year observation period: The Manitoba Study. *Am J Cardiol* 39: 452–458.
7. Goldring D, Londe S, Sivakoff M (1977): Blood pressure in a high school population standards for blood pressure and the relation of age, sex, weight, height and race to blood pressure in children 14 to 18 years of age. *J Pediatr* 91: 884–889.
8. Garn SM (1969): Relative fat patterning: An individual characteristic. *Hum Biol* 26: 75–89.
9. Edwards DAW (1950): Observations on the distribution of subcutaneous fat. *Clin Sci* 9: 259–270.
10. Vogue J (1956): The degree of masculine differentiation of obesities: A factor determining predisposition to diabetes, atherosclerosis, gout and uric calculus disease. *Am J Clin Nutr* 4: 20–34.
11. Albrink MJ, Meigs JW (1965): The relationship between serum triglycerides and skinfold thickness in obese subjects. *Ann NY Acad Sci* 131: 673–683.
12. Hartz AJ, Rupley D, Kalkhoff RK, Rimm AA (1983): Relationships of obesity to diabetes: Influence of obesity level and body fat distribution. *Prev Med* 12: 351–357.
13. Ashwell M, Cole TJ, Dixon AK (1985): Obesity new insight into the antropometric classification of fat distribution shown by computed tomography. *BMJ* 290: 1692–1694.
14. Berglund G, Ljungman S, Hartford M, Wilhemsen L, Bjorntorp P (1982): Type of obesity and blood pressure. *Hypertension* 4: 692–696.
15. Seidell JC, Bokx JC, Deboer R, Deurerberg P, Heutvast JGAJ (1985): Fat distribution of overweight persons in relation to morbidity and subjective health. *Int J Obesity* 9: 363–374.
16. Jarret RJ, Keen H, McCartney J, Fuller JH: Hamilton PJS, Reid DD, Rose G (1978): Glucose tolerance and blood pressure in two populations sample their relation to diabetes mellitus and hypertension. *J Epidemiol* 7: 15–34.
17. Butler WJ, Ostrander LD, Jr, Carmen WJ, Lamphlear DE, (1982): Diabetes mellitus in Tecumseh, Michigan: Prevalence in incidence and associated conditions. *Am J Epidemiol* 7: 116, 971–980.
18. Reisin E, Abel R, Modan M, Silverberg DS, Eliahou HE, Modan B (1978): Effects of weight loss without salt restriction on the reduction of blood pressure. *New Engl J Med* 298: 1–5.
19. Gillum RF, Prineas RJ, Jeffery RW, Jacobs DR, Elmer PJ, Gomez O, Blackburn H (1983): Nonpharmacological therapy of hypertension: The independent effect of weight reduction and sodium restriction in overweight borderline hypertensive patients. *Am Heart J* 105: 128–133.
20. Tuck MJ, Sowers J, Dornfeld L, Kledzik G, Maxwell MH (1981): The effect of weight

reduction on blood pressure, plasma renin activity and plasma aldosterone levels in obese patients. *New Engl J Med* 304: 12–13.

21. Reisin E, Frohlich ED (1982): Effects of weight reduction on arterial pressure. *J Chronic Dis* 35: 887–891.

22. Messerli FH, Christie B, DeCarvalho GR, Aristimuno GG, Suarez DH, Dreslinski GR, Frohlich ED (1981): Obesity and essential hypertension, intravascular volume, sodium excretion and plasma renin activity. *Arch Intern Med* 141: 81–85.

23. Hiramatzu K, Yamada T, Ichikawa K, Izumiyama T, Nagata H (1981): Changes in endocrine activities relative to obesity in patients with essential hypertension. *J A Geriatr* 29: 25–30.

24. Bull MB, Hillman RS, Cannon PJ, Laragh JH (1970): Renin and aldosterone secretion in man as influenced by changes in electrolyte balance and blood volume. *Circ Res* 27: 953–960.

25. Rocchini AP, Katch VL, Grekin R, Moorehead C, Anderson J (1986): Role for aldosterone in blood pressure regulation of obese adolescents. *Am J Cardiol* 57: 613–617.

26. Scavo D, Borgia C, Isacobelli A (1968): Aspetti di funzione corticosurenalica nell obesita Nota VI, II: Comportamento della secrezione di aldosterone e della escrezione dei suoi metabolite nel corso di alcune prove dinamiche. *Folia Endocrinol* 21: 591–602.

27. Kalkroff RK, Hartz AH, Rupley D, Kissebah AH, Kelber S (1983): Relationship of body fat distribution to blood pressure, carbohydrate tolerance and plasma lipids in healthy obese women. *J Lab Clin Med* 621–627.

28. Migeon CJ, Green OC, Eckert JP (1963): Study of adrenocortical function in obesity. *Metabolism* 12: 718–739.

29. Prezio JA, Carreon G, Clerkin E, Meloni CR, Kyle LH, Canary JJ (1964): Influence of body composition on adrenal function in obesity. *J Clin Endocr Metab* 24: 481–485.

30. Modan M. Halkin H, Almog S, Lusky A, Eshkol A, Shefi M (1985): Hyperinsulinemia: A link between hypertension obesity and glucose intolerance. *J Clin Invest* 75: 809–817.

31. Lopez A, Kerhl WA (1967): A possible interrelation between glucose-6-phosphate dehydrogenose and dehydroepiondrosterone in obesity. *Lancet* 1967/2: 485–487.

32. Evans DJ, Hoffman RG, Kalkhoff RK, Kissebah AH (1983): Relationship of adrogenic activity to body fat topography, fat cell morphology, and metabolic aberrations in premenopausal women. *J Clin Endocr Metab* 57: 304–310.

33. Hediger ML, Katz SH (1986): Fat patterning, overweight, and adrenal androgen interactions in black adolescent females. *Hum Biol* 58: 985–600.

34. Landsberg L, Young JB (1978): Fasting, feeding and regulation of the sympathetic nervous system. *New Eng J Med* 298: 1295–1301.

35. Young JB, Landsberg L (1982): Diet induced changes in sympathetic nervous system activity, possible implication for obesity and hypertension. *J Chronic Dis* 35: 879–886.

36. Young JB, Landsberg L (1977): Catecholamines and intermediary metabolism. *J Clin Endocrinol Metabol* 6: 559–631.

37. Danforth JE, Horton ES, O'Connell M, Sims EAH, Burger AG, Ingbar SH, Braverman L, Vagenakis AG (1979): Dietary induced alterations in thyroid hormone metabolism during overnutrition. *J Clin Invest* 64: 136–1347.

38. Sims EAH (1982): Mechanisms of hypertension in the overweight. *Hypertension* 4 (Suppl III): III 43–49.

39. Sowers JR, Whitfield LA, Catania RA, Stern N, Tuck ML, Dornfeld L, Maxwell M (1982): Role of the sympathetic nervous system in blood pressure maintenance in obesity. *J Clin Endocrinol Metabol* 54: 1181–1186.

40. Boehringer K, Beretta Picoli C, Weidmann P, Meier A, Ziegler W (1982): Pressor factors and cardiovascular pressor responsiveness in lean and overweight normal or hypertensive subjects. *Hypertension* 4: 697–708.

41. Pickering G (1980): Salt intake and essential hypertension. *Circ Reviews & Reports* 1: 13–17.
42. Tobian L (1979): The relationship of salt to hypertension. *Am J Clin Nutr* 32: 2739–2748.
43. Page LB, Danion A, Moellerung Jr RC (1974): Antecedents of cardiovascular disease in six Solomon Island Societies. *Circulation* 49: 1132–1146.
44. Takahashi E, Sasaki N, Takeda J, Ito H (1957): The geographic distribution of cerebral hemorrhage and hypertension in Japan. *Hum Biol* 29: 130–166.
45. Dahl KK, Silver L, Christie RW (1958): Role of salt in the fall of blood pressure accompanying reduction of obesity. *New Engl J Med* 258: 1186–1192.
46. Tobian L (1978): Salt and hypertension. *Ann NY Acad Sci* 304: 178–202.
47. DeChamplain J (1977): The sympathetic system in hypertension. *J Clin Endocrinol Metabol* 6: 633–655.
48. Cole FE, Frohlich ED, MacPhee AA (1978): Angiotensin binding affinity and capacity in the midbrain area of spontaneously hypertensive and normotensive rats. *Brain Res* 154: 178–181.
49. Garay RP, Meyer P (1979): A new test showing abnormal net Na^+ and K^+ ATPase in erythrocytes of essential hypertensive patients. *Lancet* 1979/1: 349–353.
50. Avenell A, Leeds AR (1981): Sodium intake, inhibition of Na^+-K^+-ATPase and obesity. *Lancet* 1981/1: 836.
51. Whittman R, Blond DM (1965): Respiratory control by an adenosine triphosphatase involved in active transport in brain cortex. *Biochem J* 92: 117–158.
52. DeLuise M, Blackburn GL, Flier JS (1980): Reduced activity in the red cell sodium-potassium pump in human obesity. *New Engl J Med* 303: 1017–1022.
53. Klimes I, Nagulesparan M, Unger RH, Aronoff SL, Mott DM (1982): Decreased Na^+-K^+-ATPase activity in erythrocyte membranes and intact erythrocytes from obese men. *J Clin Endocrinol* 54: 721–724.
54. Mir MA, Charalambons BM, Morgan K, Evans PJ (1981): Erythrocyte sodium-potassium-ATPase and sodium transport in obesity. *New Engl J Med* 305: : 1264–1261.
55. Blaustein MP (1977): Sodium ions, calcium ions, blood pressure regulation and hypertension: A reassessment and a hypothesis. *Am J Physiol* 232: C-165–173.
56. Baumgart AV, Zidek W, Losse H, Karoff C, Wehling M, Vetter W, Vetter H (1983): Obesity, hypertension and intracellular electrolytes. *Klin Wochenschr* 6: 803–805.
57. Bjorntorp P (1986): Hypertension and other complications in human obesity. *J Clin Hypertension* 2: 163–165.
58. Krotkiewski M, Bjorntorp P, Sjostrom L, Smith V (1983): Impact of obesity on metabolism in men and women: Importance of regional adipose tissue distribution. *J Clin Invest* 72: 1150–1162.
59. DeFronzo RA, Cooke CR, Andres R, Faloona GR, Davis PJ (1975): The effect of insulin or renal handling of sodium, potassium, calcium and phosphate in man. *J Clin Invest* 55: 845–855.
60. Voors AW, Webber LS, Frerichs RR, Berenson GS (1981): Body height and body mass as determinants of basal blood pressure in children: The Bogalusa Heart Study. *Am J Epidemiol* 106: 101–108.
61. Winquist RJ, Webb RC, Bohr DF (1982): Vascular smooth muscle in hypertension. *Fed Proc Am Soc Exp Biol* 41: 2386–2393.
62. Christensen NJ (1983): Acute effects of insulin on cardiovascular function and noradrenaline uptake and release. *Diabetologio* 25: 377–381.
63. Friedman SM (1983): Monovalent and divalent ions in vascular tissue. *Ann Intern Med* 98: 753–758.
64. Alexander JK (1963): Obesity and the circulation. *Mod Cardiovasc Dis* 32: 799–803.
65. Alexander JK, Dennis EW, Smith WG, Amad KH, Austin RC (1963): Blood volume,

cardiac output and distribution of systemic blood flow in extreme obesity. *Cardiovasc Res Cent Bull*, Suppl II: 39–44.

66. Backman L, Freyschuss V, Hollberg D, Melcher A (1973): Cardiovascular function in extreme obesity. *Acta Med Scand* 193: 437–446.

67. Knopp TR (1983): A methodological critique of the 'ideal weight' concept. *J Am Med Assoc* 250: 506–510.

68. Reisin E, Frohlich ED (1986): Hemodynamics in obesity, in: Zanchetti A, Tarazi RC (eds), *Handbook of Hypertension*, Vol 7: *Pathophysiology of hypertension. Cardiovascular aspects*, p. 281. Amsterdam: Elsevier Science Publishers.

69. Tarazi RC, Dustan HP, Frohlich ED, Gifford Jr RW, Hoffman GC (1970): Plasma volume and chronic hypertension relationship to arterial pressure levels in different hypertensive diseases. *Arch Intern Med* 125: 835–842.

70. Raison J, Achimastos A, Bouthier, London G, Safar M (1983): Intravascular volume, extracellular fluid volume and total body water in obese and nonobese hypertensive patients. *Am J Cardiol* 51: 165–170.

71. Raison J, Achimastos A, Asmar R, Simon A, Safar M (1986): Extracellular and interstitial fluid volume in obesity with and without associated systemic hypertension. *Am J Cardiol* 57: 223–226.

72. Alexander JK, Amad KH, Cole VW (1962): Observations on some clinical features of extreme obesity, with particular reference to cardiorespiratory effects. *Am J Med* 32: 512–523.

73. Frohlich ED, Messerli FH, Reisin E, Dunn FG (1983): The problem of obesity and hypertension. *Hypertension* 5 (suppl III): III 71–78.

74. Toto-Moukouo JJ, Achimastos A, Asmar RG, Hughes CJ, Safar ME (1986): Pulse wave velocity in patients with obesity and hypertension. *Am Heart J* 21: 136–140.

75. Mujais SK, Tarazi RC, Dustan HP, Fouad FM, Bravo EL (1982): Hypertension in obese patients hemodynamic and volume studies. *Hypertension* 4: 84–92.

76. Dustan HP (1983): Mechanisms of hypertension associated with obesity. *Ann Intern Med* 98: 860–864.

77. Messerli FH, Sundgaard-Riise K, Reisin E, Dreslinski GR, Dunn FG, Frohlich ED (1983): Disparate cardiovascular effects of obesity and essential hypertension. *Am J Med* 74: 808–812.

78. Messerli FH, Sundgaard-Riise K, Reisin E, Dreslinski GR, Ventura HO, Oigman W, Frohlich ED, Dunn FG (1983): Dimorphic cardiac adaptation to obesity and arterial hypertension. *Ann Intern Med* 99: 757–761.

79. Reisin E, Messerli FH, Ventura HO, Frohlich ED (1987): Renal hemodynamic studies in obesity-hypertension. *J Hypertension* 5: 397–400.

80. Barret-Connor E, Kow KT (1985): Is hypertension more benign when associated with obesity? *Circulation* 72: 53–60.

81. MacMahon SW, Bernstein L, MacDonald GS, Andrew SG, Blacket RB (1985): Comparison of weight reduction with metoprolol in treatment of hypertension in young overweight patients. *Lancet* 1985/1: 1233–1250.

82. Cohen N, Flamenbaum W (1985): Obesity and hypertension. Demonstration of a 'floor effect'. *Am J Med* 80: 177–181.

83. Dornfeld LP, Maxwell MH, Waks AV, Schroth P, Tuck ML (1985): Obesity and hypertension: Long-term effect of weight reduction on blood pressure. *Int J Obesity* 9: 381–389.

84. Reisin E (1986): Weight reduction in the management of hypertension: Epidemiologic and mechanistic evidence. *Can J Physiol Pharmacol* 64: 818–824.

85. Sowers JA, Nyby M, Naftali BS, Beck F, Baron S, Catania R, Vlachis N (1983): Blood

pressure and hormone changes associated with weight reduction in the obese. *Hypertension* 4: 686–691.

86. Kolanowski J (1981): Influence of insulin and glucagon on sodium balance in obese subjects during fasting and refeeding. *Int J Obesity* 5: 5105–5114.

87. Weder AB, Toneti BA, Skatch VL, Rochini AP (1984): The antihypertensive effect of caloric restriction in obese adolescents: Dissociation of effect on erythrocyte countertransport and cotransport. *J Hypertension* 2: 507–514.

88. Boulter PR, Spark RF, Arky RA (1973): Dissociation of the renin aldosterone system and refractoriness to the sodium-retaining action of minerolocorticoid during starvation in man. *J Clin Exp Metab* 38: 248–254.

89. Marks P, Wilson B, Delasalle A (1985): Aldosterone studies in obese patients with hypertension. *Am J Med Sci* 289: 224–228.

90. Garnett ES, Cohen H, Nehmias C, Viol G (1973): The roles of carbohydrate, renin and aldosterone in sodium retention during and after total starvation. *Metabolism* 22: 867–874.

91. Reisin E, Frohlich ED, Messerli FH, Dreslinski GR, Dunn FG, Jones MM, Batson HM Jr (1983): Cardiovascular changes after weight reduction in obesity hypertension. *Ann Intern Med* 98: 315–319.

92. Shetty PS, Jung RT, James WPT (1979): Effect of catecholamine replacement with levodopa on the metabolic response to semistarvation. *The Lancet* 1979/1: 77–79.

93. Alexander JK, Peterson KL (1972): Cardiovascular effects of weight reduction. *Circulation* 69: 310–318.

94. Backman L, Freyschuss V, Hallberg D, Melcher A (1979): Reversibility of cardiovascular changes in extreme obesity: Effects of weight reduction through Yeyunoicleostomy. *Acta Med Scand* 205: 367–373.

95. Achimastos A, Raison J, Levenson J, Safar M (1984): Adipose tissue cellularity and hemodynamic indexes in obese patients with hypertension. *Arch Intern Med* 144: 265–268.

96. Young JB, Landsberg L (1977): Stimulation of the sympathetic nervous system during sucrose feeding. *Nature* 269: 615–617.

97. Jung RT, Shetty PS, Barrand M (1979): Role of catecholamine in hypotensive response to dieting. *Br Med J* 1: 12–13.

98. MacGregor GA, Best FE, Conn JM, Markandu ND, Elder DM, Sagnella GA, Squires M (1982): Double blind randomized crossover trial of moderate sodium restriction in essential hypertension. *Lancet* 1982/1: 351–354.

99. Sowers JR, Whitfield LA, Beck IWJ, Catania RA, Tuck ML, Donfeld L, Maxwell M (1982): Role of enhanced sympathetic nervous system activity and reduced Na-K dependent adenosine triphosphatose activity in maintenance of elevated blood pressure in obesity: Effect of weight loss. *Clin Sci* 63: 1215–1245.

100. Bogardus C, Ravussin E, Robbins DC, Wolfe RR, Horton ES, Sims EAH (1984): Effects of physical training and diet therapy on carbohydrate metabolism in patients with glucose intolerance and noninsulin dependent diabetes. *Mellitus Diabetes* 33: 311–318.

101. Grey N, Kipinis DM (1971): Effect of diet composition on the hyperinsulinemia of obesity. *New Engl J Med* 385: 827–831.

102. MacMahon SW, Wilcken DEL, MacDonald GJ (1986): The effect of weight reduction on left ventricular mass: A randomized controlled trial in young overweight hypertensive patients. *New Engl J Med* 314: 334–339.

103. Keys A, Henschel A, Taylor HL (1947): The size and function of the human heart at rest in semi-starvation and in subsequent rehabilitation. *Am J Physiol* 150: 153–169.

104. Page IH (1987): The Mosaic Theory, in: *Hypertension Mechanisms*, p. 914. Grune Stratton, Inc.

12. Atherosclerotic hypertension
Systolic hypertension and arterial compliance in patients
with arteriosclerosis obliterans of the lower limbs

MICHEL E. SAFAR

Arteriosclerosis obliterans usually denotes a degenerative arteriopathy of the aorta, and of the extremities and the aortic branches that go to them [1]. It is characterized by occlusive lesions, primarily atheromatous but often accompanied by fibrosis and calcification of the tunica media. They may be associated with a varying degree of thrombosis. In the past, arteriosclerosis obliterans has been considered to be an occlusive arterial disease, exclusively or predominantly affecting the lower limbs. However, recent studies have shown that lesions affecting a significant part of the large artery system, as observed in arteriosclerosis obliterans of the lower limbs (AOLL), may have general consequences for overall circulatory dynamics [2–3] for several reasons. First, large arteries act as a reservoir that stores blood during cardiac ejection and releases it during diastole, enabling the intermittent cardiac output to be converted to a steady flow through the capillaries [4] and thus participating to the general cardiovascular homeostasis. Second, an elevated incidence of systolic hypertension is observed in patients with arteriosclerosis obliterans of the lower limbs.

In the present review, the abnormalities of circulatory homeostasis in patients with AOLL are analyzed with particular reference to the modifications in systolic pressure and arterial compliance and distensibility. Consequences with regard to diseased limbs, and the relationship with cardiovascular morbidity and mortality, are also analyzed.

Systemic hemodynamics in patients with AOLL

For many years, the incidence of systolo-diastolic hypertension, assessed using indirect determinations of blood pressure, has been reported to be consistently higher in patients with AOLL than in age-matched control subjects [1]. How-

M.E. Safar & F. Fouad-Tarazi (eds.), The heart in hypertension.
© *1989 Kluwer Academic Publishers, Dordrecht –*

ever, this assumption may be discussed on the basis of methodological problems due to the blood pressure determination. Since the initial description by Osler [5], it has become well accepted that elderly patients with atherosclerotic disease may have inappropriately elevated cuff pressure when compared with intra-arterial pressure, due to excessive atheromatosis and/or medial hypertrophy of the arterial tree [6–7]. Recent studies in elderly patients with AOLL have indeed shown that cuff determinations overestimate diastolic pressure, whereas systolic pressure measurements are largely accurate [8]. Such findings strongly suggest that the incidence of hypertension in AOLL patients should be reviewed on the basis of intra-arterial measurements.

Intra-arterial determinations of brachial artery blood pressure have been performed after 3 days' hospitalization in patients with AOLL (aged between 30 and 70), compared with age and sex-matched normal subjects [2, 9]. While diastolic pressure was mostly maintained within the normal range, a significant and sustained increase in systolic pressure was observed, resulting in a substantial elevation of pulse pressure. This finding was observed even in AOLL patients with the same mean arterial pressure as normal subjects [2, 10]. In the latter case, it was even shown that not only systolic pressure was significantly increased but also that diastolic pressure was slightly reduced, contributing to the elevated pulse pressure [11]. However, it is important to note that these hemodynamic modifications were recorded at the brachial artery, a site where the pressure wave is usually of higher amplitude than in the central aorta [4]. Although there is some reduction in amplification of the pulse with age, the age-related increase in pulse pressure in the central aorta can be considered as probably greater than is apparent from recordings of brachial artery pressure [4]. Thus, it follows that an elevated incidence of increased systolic and pulse pressure does exist in patients with AOLL.

The finding of an increased pulse pressure with nearly normal values of mean arterial pressure in patients with AOLL is important with regard to analysis of the blood pressuree curve, as described by specialists in pulsatile arterial hemodynamics [4, 12–14]. As shown by the study of the arterial impedance spectrum, the pressure curve may be divided into two components: a steady component, i.e. mean arterial pressure, which reflects steady flow and a pulsatile component, i.e. pulse pressure – the difference between systolic and diastolic pressure – which reflects pulsatile flow. Whereas mean arterial pressure is influenced only by cardiac output and vascular resistance, pulse pressure is determined by independent hemodynamic mechanisms such as the pattern of ventricular ejection, the timing of reflected waves and the degree of reduction of arterial compliance and distensibility [4]. Taking this into account, it is important to notice that, in patients with AOLL, cardiac output and systemic vascular resistance remain largely within the normal range [2, 9]. On the other hand, ventricular ejection, assessed from the ratio between stroke volume and left ventricular ejection time [2, 9], is comparable to that of age-matched normal subjects. Finally, the increase in pulse pressure in patients with AOLL seems to be predominantly due to modifications in arterial compliance and distensibility, or to timing of reflected waves, or to a combination of both factors. In that regard, modifications in the status of large arteries seem to be particularly important to evaluate in patients with AOLL. Experimental studies have indeed shown that reduced elasticity of the arterial system is able to cause not only an increase in systolic pressure, but also to a reduction in diastolic pressure, as observed in AOLL patients [4, 12–14].

Arterial compliance and timing of reflected waves in patients with AOLL

It is well known that, physiologically speaking, large arteries have not only a conduit function, but also a buffering function [4, 12–13]. Because of their distensibility, they are able to dampen the pulsatile systolic output of the ventricle. Indeed, after left ventricular ejection has distended the aorta and its large branches, and the aortic valves have closed, the elastic aorta and its branches recoil, thereby sustaining the pressure head and rendering the blood flow to the periphery steadier than it would otherwise be. This buffering function is due to the visco-elastic properties of the arterial wall. Since arteries are tubular, it is usual to examine the visco-elastic properties of the wall by increasing the distending pressure inside the tube and measuring the change in radius (or in volume). The change in volume divided by the change in pressure (or arterial compliance) represents the slope of the pressure-volume relationship, and is used as a quantitative index to describe the elasticity of the system. Since the visco-elastic arterial wall gets stiffer as it is distended, the pressure-volume relationship is curvilinear. Thus, arterial compliance may be defined only for a given pressure.

Propagative and nonpropagative models have been proposed in man to determine arterial compliance. The latter conceives the arteries as a system of interconnected tubes with fluid storage capacity [4, 12–13]. The basic assumption of the model is that all pressure changes within the arterial tree occur simultaneously (i.e., pulse wave velocity is infinite), an approximation which has been validated for the systemic circulation [15] and may be accepted in particular systems such as the forearm [16]. However, pulse wave velocity has been shown to differ greatly according to the site of measurement, and the presence or absence of pharmacological agents [4, 12–13]. Thus in man, propagative models, which assume a finite value of pulse wave velocity, seem to be more suitable for the evaluation of arterial compliance, studied under different conditions of stimulation and treatment. Propagative models are all derived from the Moens-Korteweg equation, applied to the case of thin-wall elastic tubes [13]. Under such conditions, arterial compliance is equal to the product of arterial volume (or cross-sectional area per unit length) and distensibility. In man, it is possible to evaluate noninvasively the cross-sectional area and distensibility of intact superficial straight arteries, such as the brachial artery and the common carotid artery. Cross-sectional area is deduced from determination of the inner diameter, using a pulsed Doppler methodology with range-gated systems and double transducer probe, as previously validated in the literature [17]. Distensibility is derived from the determination of pulse wave velocity. Wave velocity is measured by displaying two pressure or flow pulses simultaneously [4]. The time difference between the feet of the two pulses, which contain the high frequency information, is measured. The distance between the two sites of measurement along the arterial system divided by this time difference gives the pulse wave velocity (PWV), as described elsewhere [13–14, 18–19]. According to the Bramwell and Hill formula, arterial distensibility is given by $(3.75/PWV)^2$ [18–19].

Several studies have shown that arterial distensibility, measured either in the aortic or in the forearm circulations, is reduced in elderly patients with untreated isolated systolic hypertension, when compared with age- and sex-matched controls [18–19]. Such results agree with data derived from experimental models of atherosclerosis [20–22], and may be extended to the problem of systolic hypertension in AOLL patients [8, 23]. Since arterial distensibility falls as the distending pressures rise, it is possible that the reduced distensibility of large arteries in systolic hypertension may be explicable solely on the basis of arterial distension, the applied load shifting with increasing pressure from the extensible elastin to the relatively inextensible collagen component of the wall. In order to resolve this problem, clinical studies were performed in order that the distending pressure of normal subjects and patients with systolic hypertension could be regulated by placing the right arm in an air-tight box, which was then subjected to various steady pressures [18–19]. When arterial distensibility was measured in subjects at identical arterial distending pressure, no difference was found between elderly subjects with isolated systolic hypertension and age- and sex-matched normal subjects [18–19]. From these observations, it was suggested that the low distensibility of large arteries in systolic hypertensives was a simple mechanical consequence of the elevated distending pressure. However, such an interpretation does not seem relevant in patients with AOLL. First, for the same mean arterial pressure as in controls, patients with AOLL undoubtedly have the same level of volume distensibility as controls, but at the same time different levels of pulse pressure [8]. This important parameter cannot be measured when using an airtight box around the forearm. Second, as confirmed experimentally [4, 12–14], arterial stiffening produces not only an elevation of systolic pressure, but also a significant lowering of diastolic pressure, a finding which is observed in patients with AOLL when intra-arterial blood pressure measurements [8] (and not cuff measurements [18–19]) are performed. Finally, volume distensibility represents the ratio between arterial compliance (dV/dP) and arterial volume (V), as noticed above. Therefore, any evaluation of the stiffness of the arterial wall must take into consideration independent determinations of arterial volume (V) and compliance (dV/dP) for the same mean arterial pressure in patients and controls. In patients with AOLL, simultaneous determination of inner brachial artery diameter and pulse wave velocity in the forearm showed clearly that the slope of the pressure-volume relationship (dV/dP) is reduced in comparison with controls matched for age, sex and mean arterial pressure [8]. Thus elderly patients with AOLL and systolic hypertension exhibit intrinsic alterations of the brachial artery wall, unrelated to the level of mean arterial pressure. Furthermore, such intrinsic alterations of the arterial wall may be observed in sites where clinical symptoms of arterial disease are absent [8, 23]. Thus the reduced arterial compliance in patients with AOLL does not simply reflect alterations in the lower limbs, but rather more generalized modifications of large vessels. Indeed, reduced compliance of the general arterial tree has also been recognized in patients with AOLL [2, 9], and may be responsible for the increase in systolic pressure.

For the mechanism of the increased systolic pressure in patients with AOLL, another factor may interfere. When arterial compliance is reduced, the propagation velocity of the pulse wave is greater. This has been shown in several experimental studies, particularly in arteriosclerotic monkeys [20–22]. Under these conditions, addition of forward and backward waves leads to amplification of the pressure curve during systole and thus produces a high systolic peak, as in isolated systolic hypertension [4]. However, the reflection time is also critical in the summation of forward and backward waves. This depends on the length of the vessel: the shorter the vessel, the sooner the reflection occurs [4, 12–13]. In normal human subjects, the region of the terminal abdominal aorta may potentially act as one important reflection site [4, 12–13]. In arteriosclerosis obliterans of the lower limbs, which involves gross arterial lesions of the lower part of the body, the terminal abdominal aorta may be a major site of reflection, the reflections occurring in the direction of the heart. The pressure waves thus traverse the arterial system more quickly because of their smaller dimensions. This causes superimposition of the forward and backward waves during systole, and leads to a marked increase in systolic pressure. Indirect evidence for this mechanism has been provided by the study of subjects over 50 years old with traumatic amputation of the lower limbs. Such subjects display a high incidence of systolic hypertension, resulting from the reduction of arterial compliance and the shorter length of the arterial system [24–25].

Structural and functional components of reduced arterial compliance in patients with AOLL

Since decreased arterial compliance in patients with AOLL reflects intrinsic alterations of the arterial wall, it seems likely that the increased rigidity could be due to structural modifications of the arterial wall secondary to atherosclerosis. Studies in non-human primate models of atherosclerosis have shown that aortic pulse wave velocity reaches 1.5 to 2.0 times the values seconded in control animals [20–22]. There was no difference in the incremental (Young's) modulus of elasticity between the two populations. In contrast, the in vitro pressure-strain elastic modulus of the atherosclerotic aorta was more than twice that of controls, indicating that the increased arterial stiffness was mainly due to the increased wall thickness caused by the atherosclerotic plaques rather than to material changes described by Young's modulus [20–22]. Such findings suggest that, in humans with atherosclerotic complications, such as occur in patients with AOLL, structural modifications of the arterial wall may induce arterial stiffening, with a resulting increase in systolic blood pressure.

For a long time, it was believed that structural changes of the arterial wall provided the exclusive explanation for increased systolic and pulse pressure in elderly patients with AOLL. More recently, the role of functional factors has been recognized, derived from studies of the effects of: (1) sodium intake, (2) administration of nitrates, and finally (3) abnormalities in the functioning of the sympathetic nervous system.

Isotonic saline infusion causes a higher increase in systolic pressure in patients with AOLL and systolic hypertension than in age matched controls [23]. The increase in systolic pressure is mainly due to a reduction in arterial compliance following salt administration, whereas diastolic pressure is only marginally modified. The findings suggest that sodium may act on the arterial wall either directly, or through associated modifications of the autonomic nervous system, or by a combination of both factors [23]. In the literature [26–27], the observation in elderly subjects of an increase in pulse wave velocity with sodium intake, and a decrease with salt restriction, is consistent with the effects of saline infusion in patients with AOLL.

While sodium intake acts to increase systolic pressure in patients with AOLL, nitrate substances have, in contrast, a beneficial effect on systemic hemodynamics [28]. Following acute administration, nitroglycerine has been shown to decrease systolic pressure selectively in patients with AOLL and systolic hypertension [9]. This reduction in systolic pressure is related to an increase in arterial compliance. No significant change in ventricular ejection and vascular resistance is observed [28]. Similar effects on systolic blood pressure reduction have been observed in elderly subjects with isolated systolic hypertension, and confirm that nitrate compounds improve arterial compliance in such patients [25].

Several lines of evidence suggest that the autonomic nervous system may be affected in patients with AOLL. A slight but significant decrease in baseline heart rate has been reported [2, 9, 23]. Since age or previous treatment could not explain this relative bradycardia, two possibilities were explored: an alteration in the intrinsic pacing function of the heart and a baroreflex-mediated mechanism related to the observed arterial findings (reduced compliance and increased systolic pressure). To test the latter hypothesis, baroreflex mechanisms were evaluated according to the method of Smyth et al. [29]. The curve relating systolic pressure to the RR interval after phenylephrine was clearly reset, so that a higher stretch was required in patients with AOLL to obtain the same heart rate as in controls [23]. Furthermore, the expected enhancement of baroreflex sensitivity usually observed in normal subjects following administration of cardiotonic substances [30] was not found in patients with AOLL [23], a result which suggests a complex disturbance of the baroreflex mechanisms involving sodium pumps [31]. Finally, acute administration of propranolol in patients with AOLL showed that the abnormalities of the autonomic nervous system affected not only the heart but also blood vessels [2]. Following propranolol administration, arterial compliance was significantly reduced in the absence of blood pressure change. The acute effect of propranolol on the arterial wall could reflect an unopposed effect of alpha-receptors in the presence of decreased sensitivity of beta-receptors with age [2].

The abnormalities of the autonomic nervous system in patients with AOLL are difficult to interpret. They may be involved in the overall evolution of the atherosclerotic process, or take place within the context of disease of the lower limbs. In a previous study in patients with AOLL and unilateral intermittent claudication, Lorentsen [3] observed that both systemic systolic and diastolic pressure increased to significantly higher levels during exercise with the diseased limb than during exercise with the healthy limb. Furthermore, after the first minutes of recovery following exercise, the systemic systolic pressure (but not the diastolic pressure) in the diseased limb stayed higher than the pressure measured at rest immediately before exercise. Such findings suggested that active contraction of muscle cells under ischemic conditions might cause stimulation of local receptors involving generalized circulatory pressor reflexes, with a predominant influence on systolic pressure [32].

Relevance of systolic hypertension and systemic hemodynamics for the interpretation of intermittent claudication

The hemodynamic changes of the diseased lower limbs of patients with AOLL are usually analyzed in terms of a linear model resulting from the association of two major resistances coupled in series (the stenotic and the arteriolar resistances), rather than predominantly in terms of the downstream arteriolar resistance as is normally the case [33]. Under these conditions, mean blood flow is determined by the driving pressure across these two resistances, the mean systemic arterial pressure being an important component. However, studies of human atherosclerotic femoral arteries have shown that non linear models are more useful to describe the hemodynamic changes. In that condition, vascular impedance is a more reliable index of the severity of large vessel atherosclerotic stenosis than is resistance [34]. Therefore, the oscillatory component of blood flow and blood pressure is important to consider with regard to the mechanisms of the disease in the lower limbs. In clinical studies, both mean arterial pressure and pulse pressure should be considered separately in evaluating the role of systemic hemodynamics in the severity of intermittent claudication.

Under resting conditions, calf blood flow is known to remain within the normal range in patients with AOLL [35–36]. Furthermore, calf blood flow is positively correlated with blood pressure in patients with AOLL, but not in normal subjects [10]. This finding suggests that systemic arterial pressure in patients with AOLL acts to maintain adequate perfusion of the lower limbs. Interestingly, baseline calf blood flow is positively correlated with both mean arterial pressure and pulse pressure. Despite the interest of hemodynamic determinations at rest, it is clear that the limiting influence of the AOLL disease will occur rather at elevated flow rates, i.e. during exercise and post-occlusive reactive hyperemia. Indeed the pressure drop caused by the stenosis increases with increasing flow [34–37]. Under such conditions, it is interesting to observe that walking distance and post-occlusive reactive hyperemia are strongly correlated with pulse pressure, and not with mean arterial pressure: the higher the pulse pressure, the greater the reduction in walking distance and the greater the alteration in vascular reserve, as evaluated from post-occlusive reactive hyperemia [10]. Although such findings remain difficult to interpret, they clearly point to the role of the oscillatory component of blood pressure (i.e. pulse pressure) in the mechanism of the intermittent claudication. In that regard, it is important to note that exercise in man produces not only arteriolar vasodilatation, but also an increase in pulse wave velocity, and a decrease in arterial compliance and distensibility [38]. This observation may be important in patients with reduced baseline arterial compliance, as in AOLL, and emphasizes the point that compliance abnormalities may play a major role in the severity of intermittent claudication.

Concluding remarks

For the evaluation of the contribution of AOLL in the cardiovascular risk, several previous reports have drawn attention to the strong association between AOLL and stenosis of the internal carotid artery and coronary heart disease [39]. Given this association, the value of the symptomatic expression of AOLL, intermittent claudication, as a predictive factor of cardiovascular mortality has been widely discussed. It has been suggested that claudication is not an independent marker of mortality, once adjustments have been made for other risk factors, and signs and symptoms of coexisting coronary heart disease [40]. On the other hand, more recent studies using highly reliable non-invasive hemodynamic tests of large vessel disease have indicated a more than four-fold excess risk of subjects with AOLL, independent of other cardiovascular risk factors or disease [41]. In our opinion, discrepancies in assessment of the validity of intermittent claudication as a cardiovascular risk factor may be better understood in the light of the pathophysiological mechanisms of AOLL as described above. Indeed, systolic pressure is the most important cardiovascular risk factor in individuals of around 50 years of age [42], and increased systolic pressure is also an important feature in patients with AOLL, in whom it plays a significant part in the systemic hemodynamic modifications.

Accepting the hemodynamic changes observed in patients with AOLL, the possible links between AOLL and mortality due to coronary heart disease may be better understood. As far as the cardiac muscle is concerned, it is known that the metabolic needs of the left ventricle are greatly influenced by the level of systolic pressure, and therefore by the reduction in systemic arterial compliance and the modification of the timing of reflected waves produced by AOLL [4, 25]. On the other hand, the coronary circulation is primarily dependent on mean diastolic pressure, due to the predominant diastolic perfusion of coronary arteries. Since diastolic pressure tends to be reduced in patients with AOLL, the supply/demand ratio may be altered under various circumstances, such as the development of cardiac hypertrophy, or exercise, or both. For these reasons alone, the alterations of systemic hemodynamics which characterize patients with AOLL (i.e. increase systolic pressure and decrease diastolic pressure due to reduced arterial compliance) may by themselves be detrimental to the heart. Clearly these are important fields for further clinical research in patients with AOLL.

References

1. Juergens JL, Baker NW, Hines EA (1960): Arteriosclerosis obliterans: Review of 520 cases with special reference to pathogenic and prognostic factors. *Circulation* 21: 188–195.
2. Levenson JA, Simon AC, Fiessinger JN, Safar ME, London GM, Housset EM (1982): Systemic arterial compliance in patients with arteriosclerosis obliterans of the lower limbs: Observations on the effect of intravenous propranolol. *Arteriosclerosis* 2: 266–271.
3. Lorentsen E (1972): Systematic arterial blood pressure during exercise in patients with atherosclerosis obliterans of the lower limbs. *Circulation* 46: 257–263.
4. O'Rourke MF (1982): *Arterial Function in Health and Disease*, pp 68–71. Edinburgh-London-Melbourne-New York: Churchill Livingstone.
5. Osler W (1892): *The Principles and Practices of Medicine*. New York: D. Appleton.
6. Spence JD, Sibbald WJ, Cape RD (1978): Pseudohypertension in the elderly. *Clin Sci Molec Med* 55: 399s–402s.
7. Messerli FH, Ventura HO, Amodeo C (1985): Osler's maneuver and pseudohypertension. *New Engl J Med* 312: 1348–1351.
8. Safar ME, Laurent St, Asmar RE, Safavian A, London FM (1987): Systolic hypertension in patients with arteriosclerosis obliterans of the lower limbs. *Angiology* 38: 287–295.
9. Levenson JA, Simon ACh, Safar ME, Fiessinger JN, Housset EM (1982): Systolic hypertension in arteriosclerosis obliterans of the lower limbs. *Clin & Exper Hyper Theory & Practice* A4(7): 1059–1072.
10. Totomoukouo JJ, Safar ME, Asmar RA, Laurent St (1987): Increased pulse pressure in patients with arteriosclerosis obliterans of the lower limbs. *Arteriosclerosis* 7: 232–237.
11. Safar ME, Totomoukouo JJ, Bouthier JA, Asmar RE, Levenson JA, Simon ACh, Levenson JA, London GM (1987): Arterial dynamics, cardiac hypertrophy and antihypertensive treatment. *Circulation* 75 (suppl I): I 156–161.
12. Noordergraaf A (1978): The arterial tree, in: *Circulatory System Dynamics*, pp 137–139. New York: Academic Press.
13. Milnor WR (1982): *Hemodynamics*, pp 56–91. Baltimore-London: Williams and Wilkins.
14. O'Rourke MF (1976): Pulsatile arterial hemodynamics in hypertension. *Austral and New Zeal J Medicine* 6 (suppl 2): 40–46.
15. Simon AC, Safar ME, Levenson JA, London GM, Levy BI, Chau NP (1979): An evaluation of large arteries compliance in man. *Am J Physiol* 237: H550–H556.
16. Simon AC, Laurent S, Levenson JA, Bouthier JE, Safar ME (1983): Estimation of forearm arterial compliance in normal and hypertensive men from simultaneous pressure and flow measurements in the brachial artery, using a pulsed Doppler device and a first-order arterial model during diastole. *Cardiovasc Res* 17: 331–338.
17. Safar ME, Peronneau PA, Levenson JA, Totomoukouo JA, Simon AC (1981): Pulsed Doppler: Diameter, blood flow velocity and volumic flow of the brachial artery in sustained essential hypertension. *Circulation* 63: 393–400.
18. Smulyan H, Vardan S, Griffiths A, Gribbin B (1982): Forearm arterial distensibility in systolic hypertension. *JACC* 2: 387–393.
19. Gribbin B, Pickering TG, Sleight P (1979): Arterial distensibility in normal and hypertensive man. *Clin Sci* 56: 413–417.
20. Farrar DJ, Green HD, Bond MG, Wagner WD, Gobbee RA (1978): Aortic pulse wave velocity, elasticity, and composition in a nonhuman primate model of atherosclerosis. *Atherosclerosis* 43: 52–62.
21. Farrar DJ, Bond MG, Sawyer JK, Green HD (1984): Pulse wave velocity and morphological changes associated with early atherosclerosis progression in the aortas of cynomolgus monkeys. *Cardiovasc Res* 18: 107–118.

22. Farrar DJ, Green HD, Wagner WD, Bond MG (1980): Reduction in pulse wave velocity and improvement of aortic distensibility accompanying regression of atherosclerosis in the rhesus monkey. *Circ Res* 47: 425–432.

23. Levenson JA, Simon AC, Maarek BE, Gitelman RJ, Fiessinger JN, Safar ME (1985): Regional compliance of brachial artery and saline infusion in patients with arteriosclerosis obliterans. *Arteriosclerosis* 5: 80–97.

24. Labouret G, Achimastos A, Benetos A, Safar M, Housset E (1983): L'hypertension artérielle systolique des amputés traumatiques. *La Presse Médicale* 12: 1349–1350.

25. Safar ME, Simon ACh (1986): Hemodynamics in systolic hypertension, in: Zanchetti A, Tarazi RC (eds), *Handbook of Hypertension,* Vol 7: *Pathophysiology of Hypertension; Cardiovascular Aspects.* Amsterdam: Elsevier Science Publishers.

26. Avolio AP, Deng FQ, Li WQ, Luo YF, Huang ZD, Xing LF, O'Rourke MF (1985): Effects of aging on arterial distensibility in populations with high and low prevalence of hypertension: Comparison between urban and rural communities in China. *Circulation* 71: 202–210.

27. Avolio AP, Clyde CM, Beard TC, Cooke HM, Kenneth KL, O'Rourke MF (1986): Improved arterial distensibility in normotensive subjects on a low salt diet. *Arteriosclerosis* 6: 166–169.

28. Simon ACh, Levenson JA, Levy BI, Bouthier JE, Perroneau PP, Safar ME (1982): Effect of nitroglycerin on peripheral large arteries in hypertension. *Br J Clin Pharmacol* 14: 241–245.

29. Smith HS, Sleight P, Pickering GW (1969): The reflex regulation of arterial pressure during sleep in man: A quantitative method of assessing baroreflex sensitivity. *Circ Res* 24: 109–115.

30. Ferrari A, Gregorini L, Ferrari MC, Preti L, Mancia G (1981): Digitals and baroreceptor reflexes in man. *Circulation* 61: 279–285.

31. McGregor GA, De Wardener HE (1984): A circulating sodium transport inhibitor and essential hypertension. *J Cardiovasc Pharmacol* 6: S55–S60.

32. Rowell LB, Freund PR, Hobbs SF (1981): Cardiovascular responses to muscle ischemia in humans. *Circ Res* I 48: 37–47.

33. Young DF, Cholvin NR, Roth AC (1978): Pressure drop accross artificially induced stenosis in the femoral arteries of dogs. *Circ Res* 36: 735–743.

34. Farrar DJ, Malindzak GS, Johnson G (1977): Large vessel impedance in peripheral atherosclerosis. *Cardiovascular Surg* II–56: 170–178.

35. Strandness DE, Bell JW (1964): An evaluation of the hemodynamic response of the claudication extremity to exercise. *Surg Gynecol Obstet* 119: 1237–1245.

36. Yao VST, Hobbs JT, Irvine WI (1969): Ankle systolic pressure measurements in arterial disease affecting the lower extremities. *Br J Surg* 56: 676–687.

37. Skinner JS, Strandness DE (1964): Exercise and intermittent claudication, I: Effect of repetition and intensity of exercises. *Circulation* 36: 15–22.

38. Murgo JP, Westerhof N, Giolma JP, Altobelli SA (1981): Effects of exercise on aortic input: Impedance and pressure wave forms in normal humans. *Circ Res* 48: 334–343.

39. Friedman SA, Pandya M, Greif E (1973): Peripheral arterial occlusion in patients with acute coronary heart disease. *Am Heart J* 86: 415–421.

40. Reunanen A, Takkunen H, Aromaa A (1982): Prevalence of intermittent claudication and its effect on mortality. *Acta Med Scand* 211: 249–256.

41. Criqui MH, Coughlin SS, Fronek A (1985): Noninvasively diagnosed peripheral arterial disease as a predictor of mortality: Results from a prospective study. *Circulation* 72: 768–773.

42. Kannel WB, Gordon T, Schwartz MJ (1971): Systolic versus diastolic blood pressure and risk of coronary disease. *Am J Cardiol* 27: 335–346.

13. Postmyocardial revascularization hypertension
The role of the heart

F.G. ESTAFANOUS and F.M. FOUAD-TARAZI

Our initial description of post myocardial revascularization hypertension in 1973 [1] has been confirmed by other centers and is now recognized as a frequent complication of coronary bypass surgery [2–4]. It has been reported to occur in 30 to 50 percent of operated patients [1–3]. The rise in blood pressure can be quite serious [1, 5, 6], and the final outcome depends on the rapidity of diagnosis and early initiation of adequate therapy [1, 7].

Although hypertension associated with cardiac surgery is not limited to coronary bypass grafting or to the postoperative period [8, 9], we will focus this discussion on hypertension following myocardial revascularization.

Hypertension after cardiac surgery

Paroxysmal hypertension in the immediate postoperative period is a frequent and potentially dangerous condition. Many precipitating factors could be implicated: arousal from anesthesia, tracheal and nasopharyngeal manipulations, pain, hypothermia, shivering, poor ventilation and the use of pressor agents as well as the diminishing effects of preoperative antihypertensive medications. In addition, postoperative coronary insufficiency or myocardial infarction might increase blood pressure since signs of cardioadrenergic stimulation are particularly marked after coronary bypass in those patients who sustained a postoperative infarction [10]. Finally, hypervolemia is often cited as a possible cause of postoperative hypertension, although the relation of fluid overload to increased arterial pressure is well known to be more complex than the relation between container and content [11]. In this context, compensatory neural and renal mechanisms may adequately buffer sizable variations in blood volume [12]; so that it is only in the functional absence of such reflexes or of renal excretory function that arterial pressure was found to correlate

M.E. Safar & F. Fouad-Tarazi (eds.), The heart in hypertension.
© *1989 Kluwer Academic Publishers, Dordrecht –*

directly with hypervolemia [11, 13]. Moreover, at the other end of the spectrum, marked sympathetic reaction to hypovolemia may cause hypertension and impaired tissue perfusion [14].

Postcoronary bypass hypertension

Since its original description in 1973 [1], this type of hypertension has been recognized as possibly the most common complication of coronary bypass surgery [2–4]. It was found to occur in 30 to 50 percent of patients as opposed to an incidence rate of 8 to 10 percent after cardiac valve replacement [1, 15].

The frequency of the condition and its serious implications [1–3, 5] have stimulated a large number of studies. These studies have outlined a clinical syndrome with typical hemodynamic characteristics and have investigated the possible pathophysiologgic mechanism and lines of treatment [1, 16].

Clinical description. The increase in arterial pressure usually occurred during the first four hours after myocardial revascularization operations and ran a paroxysmal course [1–3, 17]. Whether patients were already awake or still anesthetized, and whether the patient was normotensive or hypertensive preoperatively, these hypertensive episodes were not related to pain, ventilatory difficulties, or obvious anxiety; also pressure elevations persisted despite adequate sedation and muscle relaxation [1, 5]. Indeed, clinical examination revealed no evidence of pallor, cyanosis or sweating, although the pressure may have occasionally exceeded preoperative levels by 60/35 mm Hg and caused increased oozing and blood loss from the chest tube [5]. Despite the increase in pressure, pulse rate was usually unchanged or, tended to be slightly more rapid than in those patients who did not develop hypertension and in the same patients prior to blood pressure rise [17]. Only occasional premature ventricular complexes were detected [1] and ventricular fibrillation was reported only in two of our initial series of patients [18]. Central venous and left atrial pressures usually remained within normal limits [17, 19].

Serious postoperative complications were observed initially. One patient who had a ventricular aneurysmectomy developed hemorrhage from a previously intact ventricular suture line during the hypertensive episode. In another patient, the hypertensive episode was associated with a sudden severe hemorrhage from the aorta at the insertion line of the saphenous vein graft. Although every effort, including immediate thoracotomy, was made to resuscitate these two patients, bleeding was massive and both eventually died. Subsequently, early and systematic efforts at reducing blood pressure were adopted with resultant notable decrease in the occurence and/or severity of complications.

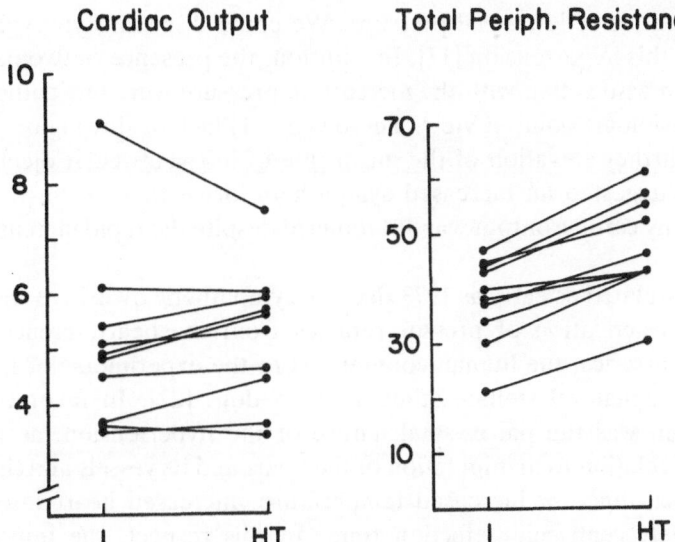

Figure 1. Changes in cardiac output (liter/minute) and total peripheral resistance (units · M²) in 10 patients who developed a hypertensive episode (HT) in the immediate period following coronary bypass surgery. I = Initial data, before development of the hypertensive episode.
Reproduced from Fouad et al. [16] by the courtesy of the *American Journal of Medicine*.

There remained, however, increased oozing from the site of incision as blood pressure rose in some patients.

Pathophysiology. A search for predisposing factors by several investigators did not produce any consistent results; findings were also mostly negative in our experience [1, 17]. By now, most authors agree that the type of anesthetic agent, the duration of cardiopulmonary bypass and the distribution of coronary arterial lesions do not significantly influence the incidence of postoperative hypertension. Our impression was that this hypertension occurred more frequently among patients with well preserved myocardial function. This impression was strengthened by our experience with early systemic hypertension after cardiac valve replacement [15]. Not only did hypertension develop more frequently after aortic valve replacement than after mitral valve replacement (12.1 vs. 5.9 percent), but also none of the 18 patients who had double valve replacement had postoperative hypertension. This difference in incidence was attributed to the difference in myocardial status among these groups.

Moreover, the increase in blood pressure after coronary bypass surgery was related in all published reports [2, 17, 16, 20] to an increase in total peripheral resistance with no significant change in either cardiac output (Figure 1) or central venous or left atrial pressure. We could discount hypervolemia as a cause for this hypertension [17]. In addition, the presence of two paradoxical findings in association with the increase in pressure were intriguing from the pathophysiologic point of view. These were (1) lack of slowing of heart rate, and (2) further elevation of the mean rate of left ventricular ejection. Both findings suggested an increased sympathetic drive that, in turn, helped to explain why cardiac output was not reduced despite the rapid increase in blood pressure.

We postulated as early as 1973 that the sympathetic overdrive was possibly related to activation of pressor reflexes from the heart, great vessels or coronary arteries, the human counterpart to the experiments of Liard et al. [21] with unilateral stellate stimulation in dogs [22]. In favor of a reflex mechanism was the paroxysmal nature of the hypertension, as well as its temporal relation to manipulation of the heart and its vessels and the simultaneous occurrence of increased temperature, increased heart rate, and decreased left ventricular ejection time. In this respect, the importance of pressor reflexes originating from the heart and great vessels was repeatedly demonstrated by many authors [23–28]. Such pressor reflexes were reported to be triggered from distension of coronary vessels [29, 30], myocardial ischemia [31] or specific chemoreceptors [32], as well as from rhythmic stretch of the aortic wall [28]. As pointed out by Brown [33], two prominent inputs originate from the heart and reach the central nervous system. One input is spinal and is mediated by afferent cardiac sympathetic nerve fibers; the other is medullary and mediated by afferent vagal fibers. The reflex effects produced by excitation of the two inputs were reported to be either pressor or depressor. The resulting picture can therefore, be quite complex: tachycardia with relatively little change in blood pressure [34], bradycardia and hypertension [35] or tachycardia and hypertension [36, 37]. Of particular importance in relation to these pressor reflexes is the unstable, potentially dangerous positive feedback state that they may induce [28]. Thus, vascular distension or distortion of myocardial receptors by increased pressure or increased cardiac action may initiate such pressor reflexes and lead to further rise in pressure and cardiac stimulation, generating a dangerous vicious circle.

Our previous experience with stellate ganglion stimulation [38], as well as the lack of any obvious predilection of postcoronary bypass hypertension for operations on any single coronary bed, suggested that of the various possible pressor reflexes, the more important in this context were those that involved sympathetic afferent fibers. We, therefore, elected to test the effect of unilateral stellate ganglion block in patients with hypertension after coronary bypass surgery. Both in our initial series of 27 patients [39] and in a subsequent larger group [17] an effective unilateral stellate ganglion blockade resulted in a rapid and definitive normalization of arterial pressure in the vast majority of

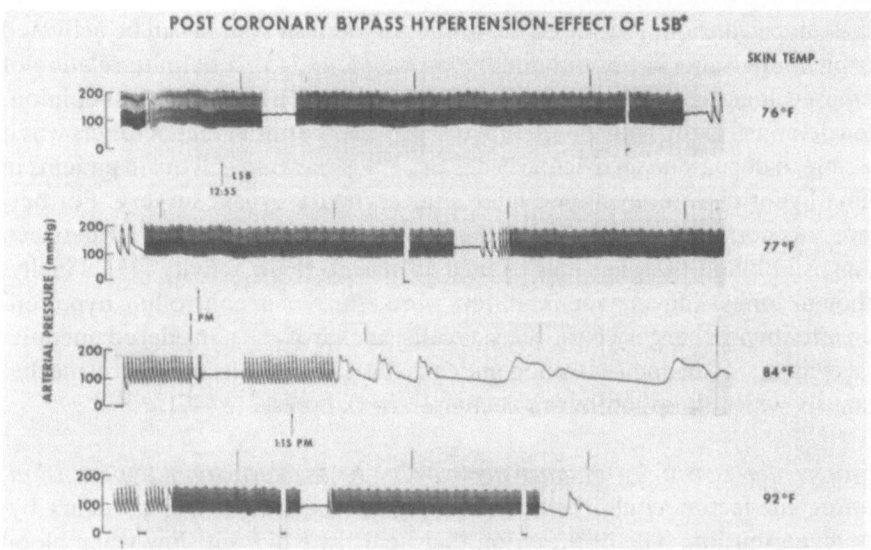

Figure 2. Continuous intra-arterial pressure recording before and after left Stellate Ganglion Blockade (LSB). The time elapsed from stellate blockade (12:55 pm) to normalization of blood pressure (1:19 pm) is marked. Skin temperature (Temp.) refers to the temperature recorded over the left index finger to determine the effectiveness of stellate blockade.
Reproduced from Tarazi et al. [39] by courtesy of the *American Journal of Medicine.*

cases (Figure 2). The reduction in blood pressure was rapid, smooth and related to a decrease in systemic resistance with no evidence of diminished cardiac performance [39]. These results were interpreted to indicate that the blood pressure response was probably due to interruption of afferent fibers coursing through or relaying in either stellate ganglion. If the blockade had acted mainly by interfering with efferent cardiac sympathetic drive, one would have expected a depression of cardiac output, an increase in total peripheral resistance and no change in blood pressure, similar to what happens with acute beta adrenergic blockade [40]. This pattern is obviously quite different from the immediate reduction in both arterial pressure and peripheral resistance produced by the unilateral stellate block. This widespread hemodynamic effect of a unilateral block suggested the interruption of a pressor reflex. Other possible causes of hypertension after cardiac surgery were not, however, ruled out. In particular the possible role for an activated renin-angiotensin system has to be considered at least in some cases [2] in view of the relationship between sympathetic stimulation and potentiation of renin release.

Renin-angiotensin system in post myocardial revascularization hypertension.
Reports by Roberts et al. [2] and other investigators [41–43] emphasized the pathogenic importance of increased plasma renin activity in postcoronary

bypass hypertension. Although the renin-angiotensin system can be activated during nonpulsatile cardiopulmonary bypass [4, 44, 45], a definite relation of increased angiotensin II to postoperative hypertension has not, in our opinion, been demonstrated. Thus, neither in our experience nor in that of others was it possible to document a particularly elevated plasma renin activity in patients in whom hypertension developed later after coronary bypass surgery. Furthermore, no correlation was found during the postoperative period between changes in blood pressure and change in plasma renin activity [17]. Finally, although converting enzyme inhibitors were effective in controlling hypertension after bypass surgery [46], these results can hardly be considered unequivocal evidence of an angiotensinogenic causation since there are several mechanisms by which these inhibitors decrease arterial pressure [47].

Baroreceptor sensitivity in post myocardial revascularization hypertension. Neurogenic factors could conceivably play another role in postcoronary bypass hypertension. The observation that heart rate did not slow when blood pressure increased might indicate a possible diminution in baroreceptor sensitivity, as happens in deafferentation hypertension. General anesthesia is known to suppress baroreceptor sensitivity [48]. This agrees with our findings of diminished baroreceptor sensitivity. However, this blunting of the reflex was observed in all patients, both those who remained normotensive and those who became hypertensive. There were only inconsistent changes in baroreceptor sensitivity in sequential determinations during the development of hypertension. It would seem, therefore, that this paroxysmal increase in blood pressure was not the result of reduced baroreceptor control. However, the reduction of baroreceptor sensitivity in the postoperative period might help set the stage for the development of hypertension from other causes.

In summary, hemodynamic findings and results of unilateral stellate ganglion blockade point out to a sympathetic reflex mechanism mediating postmyocardial revascularization hypertension in the immediate postoperative period. The reflex mechanism probably originates from the heart and/or great vessels. Although, unilaterate stellate ganglion blockade was generally effective in rapid and definitive normalization of postoperatively elevated arterial pressure, the routine use of prophylatic stellate block to avoid possible postoperative rise of arterial pressure in 30% of patients should be carefully evaluated against possible risks of the procedure.

References

1. Estafanous FG, Tarazi RC, Viljoen JF, et al. (1973): Systemic hypertension following myocardial revascularization. *Am Heart J* 85: 732–738.

2. Roberts AJ, Niarchos AP, Subramanian VA, et al. (1977): Systemic hypertension associated with coronary artery bypass surgery. *J Thorac Cardiovasc Surg* 74: 846–859.
3. Grolleau-Raoux PA, Chaptal R, Grolleau-Raoux F, et al. (1974): Le diazepam (valium) ans l'exploration et la chirurgie de l'insuffisance coronarienne. *Ann Anestheiol Fr* 15: 293–296.
4. Taylor KM, Morton IJ, Brown JJ, et al. (1977): Hypertension and the renin-angiotension system following open-heart surgery. *J Thorac Cardiovasc Surg* 74: 840–845.
5. Viljoen JF, Estafanous FG, Tarazi RC (1976): Acute hypertension immediately after coronary artery surgery. *J Thorac Cardiovasc Surg* 71: 548–550.
6. Buckberg GD, Archie JP, Fixler DE, et al. (1971): Experimental subendocardial ischemia during left ventricular hypertension. *Surg Forum* 22: 124–127.
7. Estafanous FG (1975): Management of systemic hypertension following myocardial revascularization, in: Arias A (ed): *Recent Progress in Anaesthesiology and Resuscitation*, pp 437–438. Amsterdam: Excerpta Medica.
8. Rastelli GC, Kirklin JW (1966): Hemodynamic state early after prosthetic replacement of mitral valve. *Circulation* 34: 448–461.
9. Taylor KM, Bain WH, Russell M, et al. (1979): Peripheral vascular resistance and angiotensin II levels during pulsatile and non-pulsatile cardiopulmonary bypass. *Thorax* 34: 594–598.
10. Boudoulas H, Lewis RP, Vasko JS, et al. (1976): Left ventricular function and adrenergic hyperactivity before and after saphenous vein bypass. *Circulation* 53: 802–806.
11. Tarazi RC (1976): Hemodynamic role of extracellular fluid in hypertension. *Circ Res* 38 (suppl II): II 72–83.
12. Leutscher JA, Boyers DG, Cuthberson JG, et al. (1983): A model of the human circulation. *Circ Res* 32–33 (suppl I): I 84–98.
13. Dustan HP, Tarazi RC, Bravo EL, et al. (1973): Plasma and extracellular fluid volumes in hypertension. *Circ Res* 32–33 (suppl I): I 73–83.
14. Cohn JN (1966): Paroxysmal hypertension and hypovolemia. *New Eng J Med* 275: 643–646.
15. Estafanous FG, Tarazi RC, Buckly S, et al. (1978): Arterial hypertension in immediate postoperative period after valve replacement. *Br Heart J* 40: 718–724.
16. Fouad FM, Estafanous FG, Tarazi RC (1978): Hemodynamics or postmyocardial revascularization hypertension. *Am J Cardiol* 41: 564–569.
17. Fouad FM, Estafanous FG, Bravo EL, et al. (1979): Possible role of cardioaortic reflexes in postcoronary bypass hypertension. *Am J Cardiol* 44: 866–872.
18. Chaptal PA, Grolleau-Raoux D, Millet F, et al. (1975): Les crises hypertensive dans la chirurgie de l'insuffisance coronarienne: Prevention par le diazepam. *Ann Chir Thorac Cardiovasc* 14: 255–261.
19. Price HL (1976): Circulatory actions of general anesthetic agents and the homeostatic roles of epinephrine and norepinephrine in man. *Clin Pharmacol Ther* 2: 163–176.
20. Hoar PF, Hickey RF, Ullyot DG (1976): Systemic hypertension following myocardial revascularization: A method of treatment using epidural anesthesia. *J Thorac Cardiovasc Surg* 71: 859–864.
21. Levinson GE, Pacifico AD, Frank MJ (1966): Studies of cardiopulmonary blood volume: Measurement of total cardiopulmonary blood volume in normal human subjects at rest and during exercise. *Circulation* 33: 347–356.
22. Liard JF, Tarazi RC, Ferrario CM, Manager WM (1975): Hemodynamic and humoral characteristics of hypertension induced by prolonged stellate stimulation in conscious dogs. *Circ Res* 36: 455–464.
23. James TN, Hageman FR, Urthaler F (1978): Anatomic and physiologic considerations of cardiogenic hypertensive chemoreflex. *Am J Cardiol* 42: 1013–1018.
24. Malliani A, Pagani M, Bergamaschi M (1979): Positive feedback sympathetic reflexes and hypertension. *Am J Cardiol* 44: 860–865.

25. Malliani A, Peterson DF, Bishop VS, et al. (1972): Spinal sympathetic cardiocardiac reflexes. *Circ Res* 30: 158–166.
26. Malliani A, Brown AM (1970): Reflexes arising from coronary receptors. *Brain Res* 24: 352–355.
27. Peterson F, Brown AM (1971): Pressor reflexes produced by stimulation of efferent fibers in the cardiac sympathetic nerves of the cat. *Circ Res* 28: 605–610.
28. Malliani A, Pagani M, Bergamashi M (1979): Positive feedback sympathetic reflexes and hypertension. *Am J Cardiol* 44: 860–865.
29. Brown AM (1967): Excitation of afferent cardiac sympathetic nerve fibers during myocardial ischemia. *J Physiol* (London) 190: 35–53.
30. Malliani A, Brown AM (1970): Reflexes arising from coronary receptors. *Brain Research* 24: 352–355.
31. Kent KM, Cooper T (1975): Editorial: Cardiovascular reflexes. *Circulation* 52: 177–178.
32. James TN, Isobe JH, Urthaler F (1975): Analyses of components in a cardiogenic hypertensive chemoreflex. *Circulation* 52: 179–182.
33. Brown AM (1974): Coronary pressor reflexes. *Am J Cardiol* 44: 849–851.
34. Liden RJ (1975): Reflexes from the heart. *Progress in Cardiovascular Diseases* 18: 201–221.
35. Oberg B, Thoren P (1973): Circulatory response to stimulation of left ventricular receptors in the cat. *Acta Physiol Scan* 88: 8–22.
36. James TN, Hageman GR, Urthaler F (1979): Anatomic and physiologic considerations of a cardiogenic hypertensive chemoreflex. *Am J Cardiol* 44: 852–859.
37. Fouad FM, Estafanous FG, Bravo EL, et al. (1979): Possible role of cardioaortic reflexes in postcoronary bypass hypertension. *Am J Cardiol* 41: 866–872.
38. Liard JF, Tarazi RC, Ferrario CM, et al. (1975): Hemodynamic and humoral characteristics of hypertension induced by prolonged stellate ganglion stimulation in conscious dogs. *Circ Res* 36: 455–464.
39. Tarazi RC, Estafanous FG, Fouad FM (1978): Unilateral stellate block in the treatment of hypertension after coronary bypass surgery. *Am J Cardiol* 42: 1013–1018.
40. Ulrych M, Frolich ED, Dustan HP, et al. (1968): Immediate hemodynamic effects of β-adrenergic blockade with propranolol in normotensive and hypertensive man. *Circulation* 37: 411–416.
41. Bailey DR, Miller ED, Kaplan JA, et al. (1975): The renin-angiotensin-aldosterone system during cardiac surgery with morphine-nitrous oxide anesthesia. *Anesthesiology* 42: 538–544.
42. Motlagh F, Alavi F, Najmabadi MH, et al. (1977): The relation of cardiopulmonary bypass induced hypertension and renin-angiotensin system (abstract). *Circulation* 56 (suppl III): III 142.
43. Wallach R, Karp RB, Reves JG, et al. (1977): Mechanism of hypertension after saphenous vein bypass surgery (abstract). *Circulation* 56 (suppl III): III 141.
44. Many M, Soroff HS, Birtwell WC, et al. (1968): Effects of bilateral renal artery depulsation on renin levels. *Surg Forum* 19: 387–391.
45. Taylor KM, Brannan JJ, Bain WH, et al. (1979): Vasoconstriction during cardiopulmonary bypass. *Cardiovasc Res* 13: 269–273.
46. Niarchos AP, Roberts AJ, Case DB (1979): Hemodynamic characteristics of hypertension after coronary bypass surgery and effects of converting enzyme inhibitor. *Am J Cardiol* 43: 586–593.
47. Bravo EL, Tarazi RC (1979): Converting enzyme inhibition with an orally active compound in hypertensive man. *Hypertension* 1: 39–46.
48. Bristow JD, Prys-Roberts C, Fisher A, et al. (1969): Effects of anesthesia on baroflex control of heart rate in man. *Anesthesiology* 31: 422–428.

PART TWO

Cardiac structure and function

14. Cardiac structure and function in animal models and in human hypertension
Basic concepts

P.I. KORNER

1. Introduction

The left ventricle (LV) in hypertension has to pump against a chronically increased workload, so that *a priori,* we would expect LV hypertrophy (LVH) to be an inevitable consequence of hypertension. Yet the reported prevalence of LVH in human hypertension is relatively low, much more so than in animal models. The first part of this chapter considers possible reasons for the apparent paradox. Similarly, if we regard LVH as a *physiological* response to hypertension, LV myocardial function would be expected to be either normal or enhanced. But here too there is no consensus, with divergent conclusions based on studies in humans and animals. The experimental conditions under which LV function has often been compared, probably contribute to the above differences. For example, the performance of the normal and LVH heart have often been assessed under different loading conditions, as discussed in the second part of the chapter. However, there are problems of oxygen delivery through the coronary circulation, which ultimately set limits on myocardial performance. The last part of the chapter considers regression of myocardial hypertrophy during anti-hypertensive drug therapy and whether this should be an explicit therapeutic target in management.

2. Prevalence of LVH

2.1 *Animal models*

In adult animals, cardiac hypertrophy is caused entirely by enlargement of individual cells. By contrast, when hypertrophy develops immediately after

M.E. Safar & F. Fouad-Tarazi (eds.), The heart in hypertension.
© *1989 Kluwer Academic Publishers, Dordrecht –*

birth and for a number of weeks thereafter, it is due to increases in cell number and in cell size [1].

In animal models of secondary hypertension, the time of onset of the rise in blood pressure is much more clearly defined than in human hypertension and can be accurately related to the time course of development of LVH. Increased protein synthesis occurs within the hour of a rise in blood pressure in a range of hypertrophy models [2–4]. In rats with experimental renovascular hypertension a gross increase in LV mass can be detected within 2–3 days and the process of hypertrophy is complete within about 3 weeks after 'square-wave' elevation of blood pressure (BP) [5]. Similarly in renal hypertensive dogs, rabbits and rats, the ratio of LV weight to body weight (LV/BW) is increased by about 50–100% after 4–6 weeks of hypertension [5–9]. As expected, the rise affects virtually all the experimental animals.

In primary hypertension in the spontaneously hypertensive rat (SHR), a significant increase in LV weight has been found by several investigators soon after birth [10, 11], when there is little, if any, elevation in blood pressure. However, in a recent study of the time course of the development of LVH, from 4 to 50 weeks of age, we found little difference in LV mass/BW ratio at 4 weeks between carefully age- and weight-matched SHR and Wistar-Kyoto (WKY) normotensive controls [12]. In this series, there was no obvious difference in systolic or in mean arterial BP between the strains at 4 weeks and the LV/BW ratio was only about 6–8% higher (n.s.) in SHR than in WKY [12]. The main rise in LV mass occurred between 4 and 14 weeks and was associated with the main rise in BP during the rapid growth phase. At the end of this time, LV/BW ratio in SHR exceeded that of WKY by about 25%, which rose by a further 10% by 20 weeks to the final young 'adult' difference between the strains [12].

2.2 Human primary hypertension

In the earlier literature assessment of LVH was based largely on X-Ray and electrocardiographic (EKG) findings, which are relatively insensitive to minor changes in LV mass. Hence, it is likely that many patients diagnosed as having LV *hypertrophy,* may have had some degree of LV *dilatation.* The latter may have contributed to the strikingly poor prognosis of LVH in the earlier epidemiological surveys, such as the Framingham study [see ref. 13].

The development of M-mode and of 2-dimensional echocardiography and the associated Doppler methods for determining transmitral blood flow velocity have allowed more precise assessment of human LV dimensions and function. There are now well validated formulae for assessing LV mass from measurements of wall thickness and other dimensions [14], which permit diagnosis of milder degrees of LVH. However, despite these more sensitive techniques, the reported prevalence of human LVH is still surprisingly low [e.g. 15, 16], when compared to the almost 100% prevalence in animal models.

In patients with established hypertension, estimates of the prevalence range from 20–60%, with the findings of most series closer to the lower end of this range [15–17]. Possible reasons for the discrepancy between human and experimental hypertension include: (1) a greater severity of hypertension in experimental models, (2) prior treatment with antihypertensive drugs in many studies in human hypertension, which could reduce the apparent prevalence by causing regression of LVH, and (3) use of inbred strains in animal experiments, with a smaller normal range of variation of LV mass than in the human population. The latter is genetically more heterogenous as regards the factors likely to influence LV mass; for example, there is a much greater variation in body build in the human population than in WKY and SHR.

A high variance of LV mass in the normal population makes it more difficult to establish realistic criteria which take adequately into account the numerous biological factors that influence the 'normal' variation. The conventional yardstick is to define as 'abnormal' a value that lies more than 2 standard deviations (SD) above the mean of the normal population. This criterion is rather severe with a variable like LV mass where the range of normal variation is large, and will result in categorizing as 'abnormal' only those with gross degrees of LVH. With other criteria of congruence, such as matching individuals for the same body build or lean body mass, we could probably detect hypertensive individual with smaller degrees of LVH. Such an approach for providing the best 'index' of LV mass has been suggested [e.g. ref. 17]. An alternative way is to use anatomical variables with a smaller range of variation in the normal population that provided similar information about LVH. With a low variance, the categorization of 'abnormality' will be less ambiguous when considering as our yardstick, values that lie 2 SD's above the mean of the normal population.

A recent echocardiographic study by Laufer et al. [18], suggests that it is indeed the high variance of LV mass index (LVMI) in the normal human population, that contributes to the low estimate of prevalence of LVH in hypertension. The study population included normal subjects and hypertensive patients with mild (borderline) and established hypertension. None of the patients had previously received anti-hypertensive drug treatment. However, despite this, only 30% of patients with established hypertension, and only 12% of those with mild hypertension, had values of LVMI that were at least 2 SD's above the mean of the normal group (Figure 1). This, accords exactly with the low level of prevalence reported in the earlier literature and suggests that prior drug treatment was not the major determinant of the estimated low prevalence of LVH in some of the earlier series. With anatomical variables, including wall thickness corrected for body surface area (WT*) and the ratio of wall thickness/internal radius (WT/R) in which the variance in the normal population was lower, a greater proportion of hypertensives were categorized as having LVH. With either of the latter variables about 60–65% of patients with established hypertension and about 30% with mild hypertension were classified as having 'abnormal' LV structure on the basis of values 2 SD's above the mean of the normal group (e.g. Figure 1).

Another approach, that allows maximum separation between hypertensive and normotensive individuals is the use of multivariate discriminant function analysis [19]. In the study of Laufer et al. [18] when two predictor variables were used to categorize the groups, [LVMI (or WT*) and LV internal diameter (LVID) 72% of normal subjects and 70% of patients with *established* hypertension were classified correctly, but those classified as having *mild* hypertension were only marginally greater than could be ascribed to chance. With the multivariate technique of the estimates of prevalence of LVH in hypertension were identical whether LVMI or WT* was used, suggesting that the multivariate technique makes some allowance for more congruent matching of individuals in the two populations. Thus, with the multivariate technique, the estimates of prevalence of LVH are thus no longer inversely related to the magnitude of the variance in the normal population, as is the case with single variables.

Still greater improvement in discriminating capacity was obtained, when in addition to anatomical variables, functional predictor variables were added to the discriminant function [18]. The most important of these was the ratio of transmitral flow velocities in early (E) and late (A wave-related) diastole (E/A velocity ratio). In mild and established hypertension, the E/A ratio falls progressively, when compared with corresponding normal values. The E/A ratio deals with diastolic events which, in the context of hypertension, are largely a reflection of decreased in LV compliance. The latter is an early abnormality in hypertension, so that the E/A ratio can be regarded as a quasi-anatomical variable. Fractional systolic shortening (FS; the ratio of end-systolic/end-diastolic LV diameter) was also used in the analysis. FS was slightly elevated in mild hypertension, but in established hypertension, there was an almost complete overlap with the normal range. In the multivariate analysis, the use of FS greatly helped in the correct classification of patients with *mild* hypertension. Using three predictor variables (WT*, E/A and FS), there was correct classification of 81% of normal male subjects, 72% of those with established hypertension and 60% of those with mild hypertension (Figure 2).

Thus, because of the relatively high variance of LVMI in the normal population, the latter turns out to be one of the least discriminating anatomical variables and the criterion of abnormality above 2 SD's above the mean of the

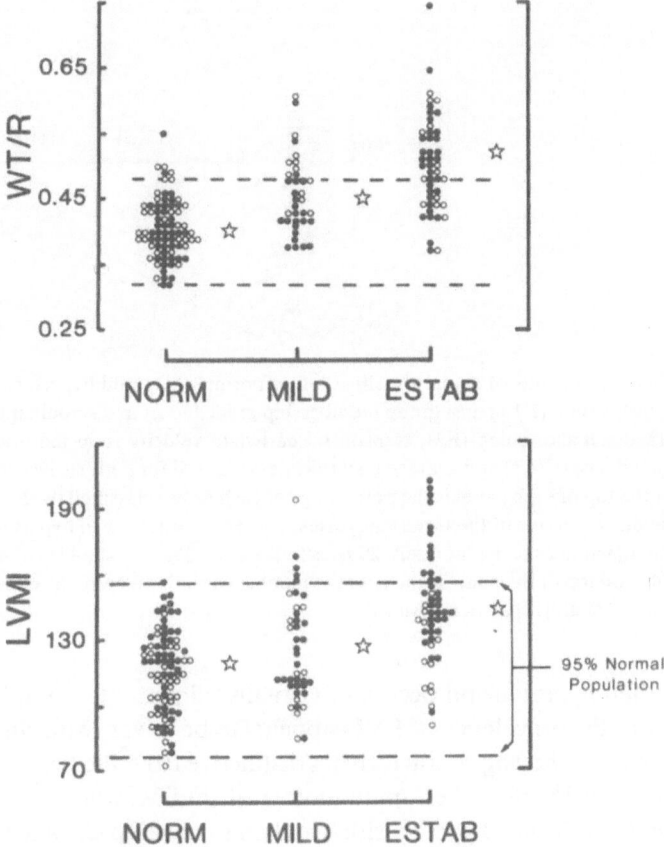

Figure 1. Individual data points of LV mass index (LVMI) and average wall thickness/internal radius (WT/R) ratio in 54 normal subjects (norm), 24 mild hypertensives (mild) and 57 patients with established hypertension (estab). Males = solid circles; females = open circles; stars are the mean values of each group; the dashed lines are the upper and lower 2 SD limits from the data of the normal group. (Based on data of Laufer et al. [18] by permission)

normal population appears to be too severe. Of the univariate variables that we have studied the estimated prevalence of LVH is greatest with WT* or WT/R (Figure 1). But the use of multivariate analysis with combined anatomical and functional variables, provides the highest estimate of prevalence of LVH.

Even with multivariate analysis it is unlikely that we can achieve 'perfect' matching of individuals in the normal and hypertensive populations. However, with this technique, the prevalence of LVH is very high and is not very far from the almost universal prevalence in animal models of hypertension. The results of Laufer et al. [18] suggest that, if some allowance is made for problems of matching of hypertensive and normal individuals, LVH in estab-

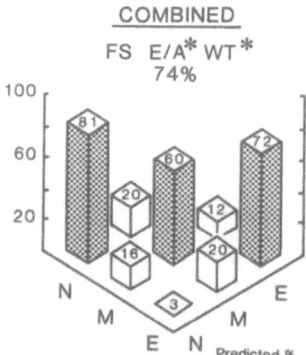

Figure 2. Results of actual classification as normal (N), mild hypertension (M) and established hypertension (E) against group membership predicted from discriminant function analysis, using fractional shortening (FS), transmitral early/late velocity ratio indexed for age by analysis of covariance (E/A*) and average wall thickness indexed for body surface area (WT*). The number at the top of each panel is the percentage of each group classified by the discriminant function as belonging to one of the three categories, e.g. 3% of established hypertensives were classified by the function as being 'normal', 20% as 'mild' and 72% as 'established' hypertension. The figure 74% on top of the panel is the average number of subjects correctly classified. (Based on data of Laufer et al. [18] by permission)

lished hypertension occurs in virtually all patients. In mild human hypertension, the prevalence of LVH appears to be lower, with slightly more than half the group having characteristics distinctive from the normal population. This is in accord with earlier epidemiological studies, where about half the subjects with borderline hypertension went on to develop chronic hypertension, whilst the blood pressure returned to normal in the others [13].

3. Myocardial function in LVH

3.1 *Methods of assessing myocardial function*

The indices of contractility which have been employed to assess LV myocardial function, include several 'isovolumic' indices of developed LV tension or force: (1) peak LV systolic tension, which is assessed in animal experiments from the peak LV pressure (LVP), following brief occlusion of the ascending aorta for 1–2 beats, and (2) measurement of time derivatives of LVP, including dP/dt_{max}, dP/dt_{DP40} and $([dP/dt]/TP)_{max}$, where dP/dt = instantaneous rate of change of LVP during isovolumic systole; dP/dt_{DP40} = instantaneous dP/dt at a developed LVP of 40 mmHg above LV end-diastolic pressure; TP = the instantaneous total LVP above atmospheric pressure [20–22].

   The index $([dP/dt]/TP)_{max}$ has been considered to estimate the peak velocity of myocardial contractile elements [23]. Its use is based on the assumption, that the force-velocity relationship of cardiac muscle closely resembles that of skeletal muscle, allowing assessment at least in principle of cardiac muscle 'active' state [23]. The validity of this assumption seems doubtful [24] and it is safer to consider all the indices to be *empirical* measures of contractile state.

Both dP/dt_{DP40} and $([dP/dt]/TP)_{max}$ occur early in isovolumic systole in contrast to dP/dt_{max}, which occurs just before the opening of the aortic valve. Indeed, dP/dt_{DP40} was introduced by Mason et al. [25], to avoid the ambiguity associated with having dP/dt_{max} below its 'true' maximum, when the aortic valve opened prematurely. Unfortunately, the timing in the cardiac cycle of dP/dt_{DP40} and $([dP/dt]/TP)_{max}$ occurs well before tension has developed throughout the ventricle and they are less responsive to the registration of changes in inotropic state, than dP/dt_{max} [20, 28]. The latter remains one of the best measures of isovolumic force development, provided loading conditions are carefully controlled and provided the aortic valve has not opened prematurely.

Several techniques are now available for assessing pump performance, including (1) measurement of cardiac output (stroke volume) responses during rapid volume loading (2) assessment of cardiac output (stroke volume) responses during alterations in afterload, (3) determining LV pressure-volume and LV-wall dimension loops and associated parameters such as E_{max} (the slope of the end-systolic pressure/volume ratio introduced by Sagawa and colleagues, 26), which are valuable in assessing systolic and diastolic myocardial properties, and (4) measurements of ejection fraction [see 20 for references], fractional systolic shortening and transmitral blood flow velocities during early (E) and late (A = atrial) LV diastole [14].

The main reasons for the divergent assessment of myocardial contractile and pumping performance in LVH probably include, (1) an inadequate control of loading conditions, and (2) reflex compensation through the autonomic nervous system in the *in situ* heart during the pressure changes associated with altered loading conditions. For example, an increase in dP/dt_{max} is completely masked during elevation in left atrial pressure [9, 20]. Thus, if it is *intrinsic* myocardial function that we wish to assess in the *in situ* heart it is necessary to rigidly control LV preload and afterload in the presence of autonomic blockade. Clearly, in the intact patient, the autonomic nervous system is of the greatest importance in providing inotropic support in chronic LVH; recent measurements indicate that in established hypertension cardiac sympathetic activity is preferentially enhanced and this becomes even greater in cardiac failure [27]. However, the high tonic sympathetic activity masks any deterioration of *intrinsic* myocardial function, which can only be assessed during autonomic blockade.

3.2 *Intrinsic LV properties in chronic hypertension*

Our group has studied myocardial properties in the *in situ* LV in open-chest dogs, in which loading conditions were controlled, autonomic effects were blocked and heart rate was held constant [28]. We compared the performance of the *in situ* LV in dogs with 2–4 months of experimental renovascular hypertension, with that of a group of well-matched control dogs of similar body weight and build [8, 29]. The hypertensive dogs had concentric LVH and significantly higher LV mass/BW ratio and greater LV wall thickness, than the normal group.

In one series of experiments, the mean arterial pressure (MAP) was held constant at 100 mmHg and left atrial pressure (LAP) was varied between 6 and 30 mmHg:– dP/dt_{max} at any LAP was higher in the LVH dogs than in the normal animals (Figure 3, upper left). We also measured cardiac index (CI ≡ stroke volume index, since heart rate remained constant). In the LVH dogs, CI was also higher at any given LAP than in the normal dogs (Figure 4). For example, at an LAP of 15 mmHg, the CI was 15% higher in LVH than in normal dogs, whilst the mean LV pressure (MLVP) was about 4 mmHg lower [29]. Since filling pressure (and probably end-diastolic volume) were the same in both groups, these results indicate that in LVH the ventricle *empties* more completely than in the normal heart. This is to be expected because of the increased WT/R ratio that is associated with concentric LVH. It makes the hypertrophied ventricle into a hemodynamic 'amplifier' of cardiac output and stroke volume in a manner that is analogous to the amplification of total peripheral resistance (Figure 5). The latter is one of the well known properties of the resistance vessels and is due to medial hypertrophy and narrowing of the lumen of the small arteries in hypertension (Figure 5) [30–32].

Hallbäck-Nordlander et al. [33] reached a similar conclusion, that intrinsic LV pump performance was somewhat enhanced in LVH. They compared LV volume loading curves in the *isolated hearts* of SHR and WKY. In each set of comparisons LV pumping was performed against the same arterial pressure load. By contrast, in numerous other studies, the heart has been allowed to pump against each group's resting MAP, which makes it impossible to validly compare pump performance. This may have been the reason why Averill et al. [34] and Ferrario et al. [35] considered that LV pump function was depressed in renal hypertensive rats and in SHR.

Broughton and Korner [8] studied the effects of altering afterload on dP/dt_{max} with LAP held at 15 mmHg. Under these conditions dP/dt_{max} remained constant in each group at aortic diastolic pressures above 100 mmHg in LVH, and above 80–90 mmHg in normal dogs (Figures 3 and 6). On average, at the plateaus dP/dt_{max} in LVH dogs was 1.28 times the value observed in normal animals, which was similar to the increase in wall thickness. This indicated that

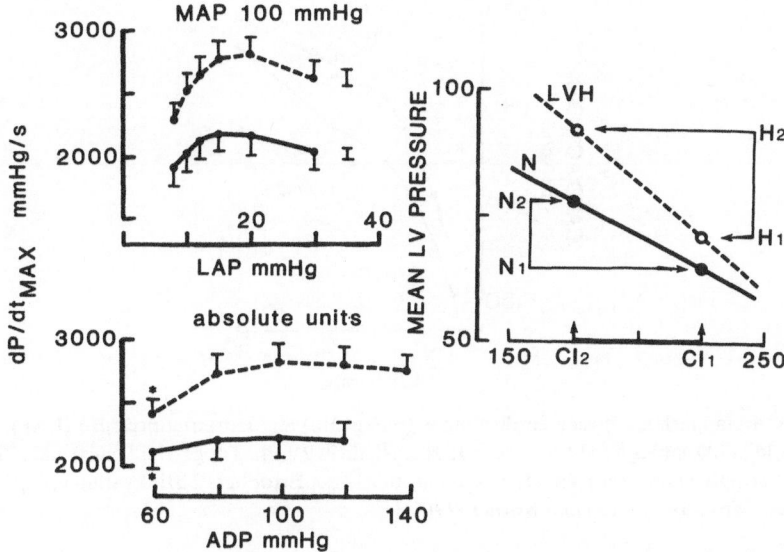

Figure 3. (Left). Top graph shows average effects and SE of mean of altering left atrial pressure (LAP) on dP/dt$_{max}$ in open-chest normal dogs (solid lines) and in dogs with LV hypertrophy; mean arterial pressure (MAP) and heart rate were held constant. *Lower graph* shows the relationship of aortic diastolic pressure (ADP) to dP/dt$_{max}$, with LAP and heart rate constant. *(Right)* Relationship of cardiac index (CI) to mean LV pressure (MLVP) in normal (N) and hypertensive dogs with LVH. A given change in CI is associated with a greater MLVP change in the hypertensive dogs than in the normal dogs, so that $(H_2 - H_1) = 1.92 (N_2 - N_1)$. All dogs were autonomically blocked. (Based on Broughton and Korner [9, 29] by permission)

LV wall stress was closely similar in both groups. However, at aortic diastolic pressures below the pressures referred to above, dP/dt$_{max}$ declined in both groups (Figure 3, lower left). The decline in normal dogs was due to premature opening of the aortic valve, but in LVH dogs the decline was much greater and represented a 'true' decline in contractile function [8].

We also studied the cardiac output-'afterload' relationship, using an approach first introduced by Elzinga & Westerhof [36]. With LAP held at 15 mmHg, MAP was varied and the resultant alterations in cardiac output were determined (Figure 6). Elzinga & Westerhof [36] have pointed out that the mean LVP (MLVP) provides a better measure of LV load than MAP, because it is independent of the rectification properties of the aortic valve. However, the MLVP-cardiac index (CI) relationship in this preparation was very similar to the MAP-CI relationship [29]. In both groups there was an inverse relationship between MAP and CI, but for a given rise in MAP, the reduction in CI was significantly smaller in LVH dogs than in the normal group (Figure 6).

Figure 3 (right) shows the data from the above experiments plotted as the

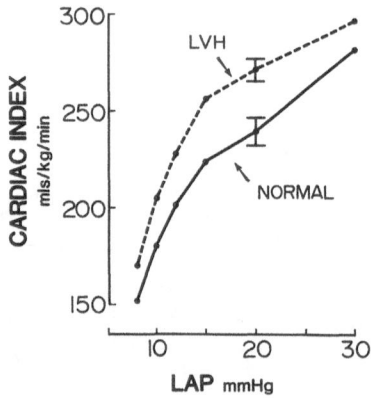

Figure 4. Relationship between cardiac index (ml/kg/min) and left atrial pressure (LAP), with MAP held at 100 mmHg and heart rate at 150 beats/min in 9 normal dogs (solid lines) and 13 LVH dogs (interrupted lines) subjected to autonomic blockade. Error bars 2 SEM within groups from ANOVA. (From Broughton and Korner [29])

CI-MLVP relationship [cf. ref. 36]. For a given change in CI the change in MLVP in the LVH group was 1.92 times the corresponding change in the normal group. This degree of amplification by the cyclically ejecting LV is much greater than the 1.28 amplification factor of dP/dt_{max} during the isovolumic phase of the cardiac cycle [29]. It should be noted that MLVP divided by WT/R also provides a measure of the average systolic wall stress, provided LAP remains constant. Hence the difference in the above two amplification factors suggests that the difference in wall/lumen ratio between normal and LVH hearts plays a greater role during LV ejection than during isovolumic systole. This is to be expected from the greater encroachment on the ventricular cavity during shortening of the hypertrophied LV than is possible during isovolumic systole (Figure 5). This is, of course, consistent with the results of the volume loading experiments in the same dogs (Figure 4).

The slope of the MLVP-CI relationship assesses the load-induced changes in LV end-systolic volume [29], thus providing somewhat similar information to the parameter E_{max} (the slope of the end-systolic pressure/LV volume ratio), introduced by Sagawa and colleagues [26].

In summary, the intrinsic LV pump function in LVH is enhanced when compared to that of a normal heart. This enhancement permits better maintenance of cardiac output (= stroke volume) against the increased arterial pressure load in chronic hypertension. The enhanced pump function appears predominantly to be due to (1) the presence of additional muscle units, each with normal contractile function, and (2) more complete systolic emptying due to the increased wall/lumen ratio. Of course, once LV dilatation supervenes, this will lead to progressive impairment of intrinsic pump function [20, 37].

HEART & VESSEL AMPLIFIERS

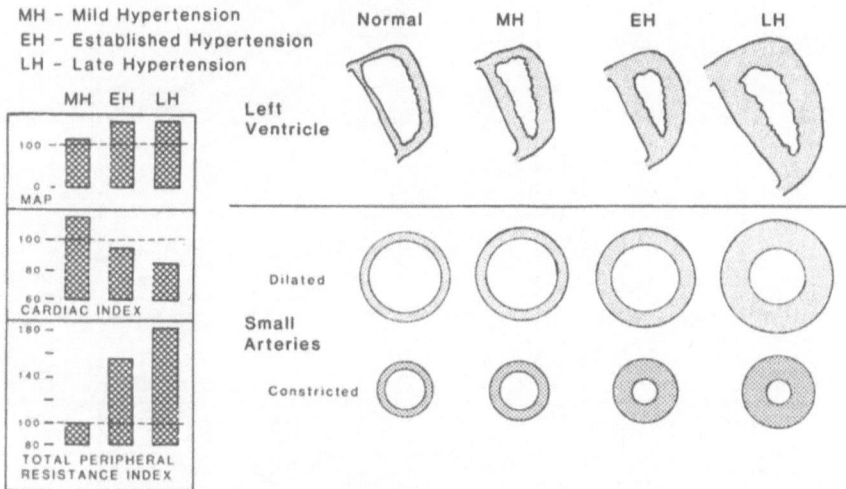

Figure 5. Schema showing progressive increase in the degree of muscle hypertrophy of the LV (top) in mild hypertension (MH), established uncomplicated hypertension (EH) and late hypertension (LH), where hypertrophy is associated with dilatation of the LV. The lower part shows muscle hypertrophy of the resistance vessels when fully dilated, showing progressive luminal narrowing. It is the latter which is responsible for the amplification of total peripheral resistance when the vessels constrict. A similar amplifier action of the concentrically hypertrophied LV accounts for the greater stroke volume at a given LAP, due to greater systolic emptying (see Figure 4 and text). The difference in cardiac index (CI) and stroke volume between normal and hypertrophied LV is accentuated, within limits, at high arterial pressure (see Figure 6). *(Insert)* Average hemodynamic profiles (mean arterial pressure – MAP) in mild, established and late hypertension expressed as percentages of control value of the normal population (interrupted line). The patterns can be explained on the basis of the structural changes without the need to postulate volume load, as discussed in Korner [31]).

3.3 *Myocardial blood flow*

Normally the LV blood flow per 100 gm is greater in the endocardium than in the epicardium [38]. This distribution pattern is preserved by autoregulatory vasodilatation when coronary perfusion pressure is reduced, whilst maintaining LV load constant, i.e. MAP. However, when both coronary pressure and MAP are reduced *simultaneously,* as in the experiments in Figure 6 for studying LV pump function, there is not only a decrease in perfusion pressure, but also a *decrease in the LV workload.*

Smolich et al. [39] recently investigated normal dogs and found that when aortic pressure was lowered, average LV myocardial blood flow declined, with the change most pronounced in the endocardium (Figure 7). The transmural redistribution of blood flow was not associated with an increased oxygen

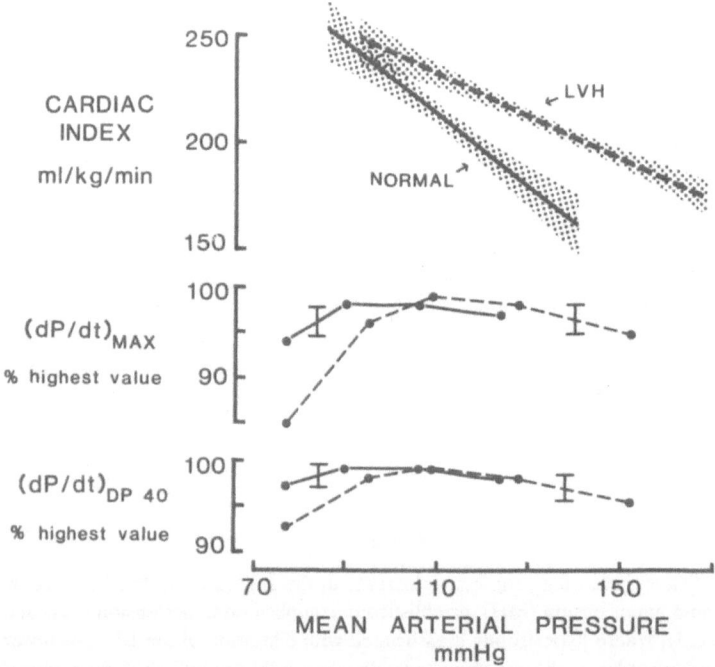

Figure 6. Mean results obtained in 13 LVH and 9 normal dogs, showing relationship of mean arterial pressure to cardiac index (top), isovolumic (dP/dt$_{max}$) expressed as percent of maximum of each group (middle) and isovolumic (dP/dt)$_{DP40}$ as percent of each group's maximum (bottom). LAP held at 15 mmHg and heart rate at 150 beats/min, in autonomically blocked dogs. (From Broughton and Korner [29], by permission).

extraction, or with depression of LV contractility or with electrical dysfunction. Moreover, the changes occurred when there was still a considerable coronary blood flow reserve to further vasodilatation. Electrical evidence of subendocardial ischemia appeared only when aortic diastolic pressure had been lowered to 32 mmHg. In contrast to the changes in LV flow and flow distribution, there were no corresponding changes in right ventricular blood flow or blood flow distribution, since in this preparation right ventricular load remains constant [40]. Absence of change of right ventricular blood flow during substantial reduction in coronary perfusion pressure, is presumably mediated by autoregulatory mechanisms.

By contrast, in 7 dogs with LVH, the decline in average myocardial blood flow during reduction in aortic pressure was more pronounced and the decline in endocardial blood flow was greater than in normal dogs [Smolich, Weissberg & Korner, unpublished data]. At aortic diastolic pressures below 90 mmHg myocardial contractile function declined in LHV dogs and this deterioration had become very pronounced at diastolic pressures of 60 mmHg.

LEFT VENTRICLE

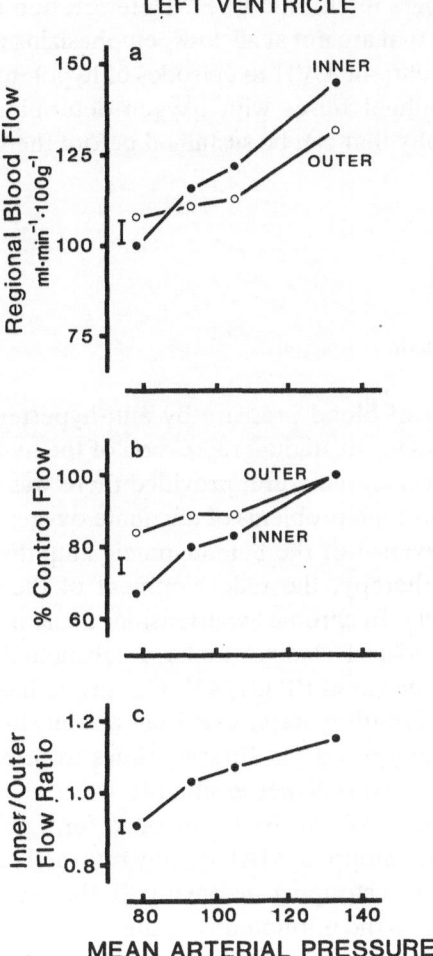

Figure 7. Regional LV blood flow during arterial pressure reduction. *Panel a:* flow to inner and outer halves. *Panel b:* inner and outer blood flow as a percentage of control flow. *Panel c:* inner-to-outer flow ratio.
Error bars = 1 SE of the difference between any 2 means within animals. (From Smolich et al. [40], by permission)

Altering aortic diastolic pressure from similar resting values in normal and LVH dogs to a level of 60 mmHg reduced average LV myocardial blood flow by 20% in normal dogs and by about 40% in LVH dogs; endocardial/epicardial blood flow ratio changed from 1.20 to 0.84 in normal dogs, and from 1.24 to 0.68 in LVH.

Thus, during reduction in the coronary perfusion pressure, there are limits in supplying adequate amounts of oxygen and other nutrients to the hypertrophied muscle fibers in chronic LVH. Deterioration of function occurs at perfusion pressures that are not at all 'low', emphasizing just how vulnerable is the myocardium in chronic LVH to episodes of hypotension. The problem of supplying hypertrophied fibres with oxygen determines that limits to the *degree* of hypertrophy that can be sustained before the fibres are irreversibly damaged.

4. Reversal of LVH

4.1 *Human hypertension*

Satisfactory control of blood pressure by anti-hypertensive drug treatment should, *a priori*, lead to substantial regression of the hypertrophy of both LV and resistance vessels musculature, provided there was no pre-existing damage to the muscle through problems of adequate oxygen supply. With regression, we will get reversal of the hemodynamic amplifier properties, so that upon cessation of therapy, the redevelopment of the hypertension should proceed rather slowly. In chronic hypertension, the amplifier properties associated with the structural changes make a substantial contribution to the maintenance of the elevated BP [31, 44]. Our group has, to date, performed three studies in which anti-hypertensive drugs (mainly β-blockers and thiazide diuretics) were administered for differing times to previously untreated patients with moderate/severe hypertension [41–44].

In the first group, MAP was well controlled for a period of 4 weeks [44]. When medication was stopped, MAP rapidly returned to pretreatment values within a few days after stopping treatment. In the second group, MAP was carefully maintained in the normotensive range for 1 year [41]. Hemodynamic measurements were made before treatment and soon after cessation of drug therapy [see ref. 41]. After 1 year CI was significantly greater than before treatment (Figure 8) and total peripheral resistance index (TPRI) had fallen to the normal range. Both these hemodynamic changes were also present when the measurements were made during autonomic blockade [1, 20, 41]. Thus, the observed pattern after prolonged therapy was independent of the activity of the autonomic nervous system. The hemodynamic pattern is strikingly similar to that observed in the heart during LVH, where CI is higher at any LAP than in the normal heart when both are pumping against the same MAP (Figure 4 and ref. 29). The pattern of high CI-normal TPRI is also found in about half the patients with mild (borderline) hypertension (see Figure 5 and ref. 31). On stopping treatment, the redevelopment of hypertension was slower than in the first group, but over the next 4–16 weeks, MAP had returned to the initial pretreatment values [31, 43].

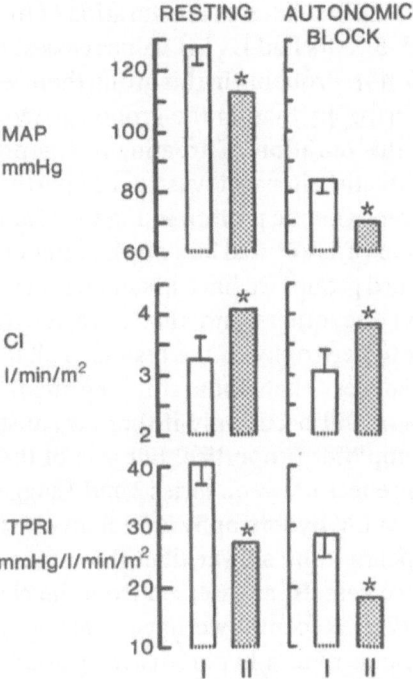

Figure 8. Results obtained in 13 patients with essential hypertension showing mean arterial pressure (MAP), cardiac index (CI) and total peripheral resistance index (TPRI). Study I (I) before the start of treatment, study II (II) a few days after ceasing all therapy after 1 year's excellent control of blood pressure. Open rectangles show resting supine data with functioning autonomic effectors; stippled rectangles during autonomic blockade. Bar = 1 SE of the difference within subjects; * p < 0.05. (Based on Jennings et al. [41] by permission)

In the third group the period of drug treatment was longer, from 15 months to 5 years, and the reduction in MAP during treatment was somewhat greater than in the second series [42–44]. After withdrawal of the diuretics 4 weeks before final drug withdrawal [42], 2 out of 13 patients rapidly redeveloped hypertension, requiring immediate reinstitution of medication. In the other 11, after all medication had stopped, the rate of redevelopment of hypertension was markedly slower than in the second group [42–44]. On average, after 12 weeks without drugs, supine MAP had risen by only one-quarter of the way towards the pretreatment value. Over the first 20 weeks systolic pressure rose, on average, by 0.9 mmHg per week, whilst diastolic pressure showed a small rise in the first week after treatment with little further rise subsequently. CI was only measured during the first 10 weeks after treatment and did not change.

This last group was the only group in which echocardiographic data was available but, unfortunately, only after the end of treatment [44]. Post-therapy

LV mass index was inversely related to the duration of treatment. Patients who had been treated for 3–5 years had LVMI values closest to the range observed in normal subjects [43, 44]. Probably in this group there was a greater degree of regression of LV hypertrophy than in the group treated only for 1 year.

In the first study, the duration of treatment was probably too short for causing substantial reduction in cardiovascular hypertrophy. The most likely explanation of the hemodynamic pattern in Figure 8, at the end of the second study, is that regression of LVH was less marked than regression of vascular hypertrophy. In the third group, we have assumed that regression of LVH was more marked than in the others and that here too there was substantial regression of vascular hypertrophy. If the results of all three series are considered together, they suggest that upon stopping medication, slow redevelopment of hypertension will occur only if there is substantial regression not only of the vascular amplifier properties, but also of the amplifier properties due to LVH. The differences between series 2 and 3 suggest that therapeutically-induced regression of LV hypertrophy is a relatively slow process in human hypertension and appears to be slower than the regression of medial hypertrophy of the resistance vessels, as assessed from the changes in non-autonomic component of TPRI. Recently we have again found that regression of LVH is slow, using a range of anti-hypertensive agents under conditions when BP was well controlled. The drugs include calcium channel antagonists and converting enzyme inhibitors, where little change in LVMI was observed within patients, though there was reduction in WT/R ratios, suggestive of structural remodelling [Jennings, personal communication].

4.2 *Animal models*

Sen et al. [45] first showed in SHR, that different anti-hypertensive drugs produced different degrees of regression of LVH. For example, with α-methyl dopa there was substantial lowering of LV mass, but the same lowering of blood pressure produced by minoxidil did not cause regression of LVH. In addition, propranolol produced substantial reversal of LVH in doses that did not lower blood pressure. By contrast, Motz & Strauer [46] found that hydralazine, another vasodilator agent, did produce regression of LVH. However, there was further reduction in LV mass when metoprolol was added to hydralazine, for only slight additional lowering of blood pressure. In this study, there was substantial reduction in LV mass/volume ratio with therapy, indicating structural remodelling similar to the findings in humans. In SHR, lowering MAP is associated with substantial reduction in LV mass, though the values reached remain usually somewhat above those of WKY [46, 47]. This was also observed by Fletcher [48] after normalizing BP after reversing renal cellophane wrap hypertension in rabbits, by removing the fibrous capsule encasing the kidney: in untreated renal hypertensive rabbits, LV mass/BW was 2 g/kg, compared with a mean value of 1.3 g/kg in normal rabbits. Six weeks after unwrapping the kidneys, LV mass/BW was 1.5 g/kg, indicating substantial regression of LVH.

In SHR, the development of LVH parallels the rise of blood pressure from 4–20 weeks [12]. We have recently examined to what degree hypertension could be aborted by brief periods of therapy. Three groups of SHR were treated with the ACE inhibitor enalapril, in a dose that normalized BP; treatment was given from (a) 4 to 10 weeks, (b) 4–14 weeks, which corresponds to the major phase of development of hypertension, and (c) 14–20 weeks, when 'adult' levels of blood pressure have been reached [Adams, Bobik & Korner, unpublished data]. In all three groups, LVH had been reversed completely by the end of treatment, with LV mass/BW ratios the same as those of WKY. When treatment was stopped, BP remained stable and at significantly lower values than in untreated SHR. In SHR treated from 4–14 weeks, BP rose by only a small amount till the end of the study, when the rats were 3–40 weeks of age and this was associated with a corresponding slight redevelopment in LVH. In the other two groups, 15–20 weeks after treatment, BP had stabilized about half-way between the levels obtained in untreated SHR and WKY, with corresponding redevelopment of a modest degree of LVH, which was somewhat greater than in SHR treated from 4–14 weeks.

These findings indicate that during anti-hypertensive therapy, LVH can be completely reversed in young animals, and that its subsequent redevelopment is in proportion to the elevation in BP. In older animals, regression of LVH, though substantial, appears to be less complete. We do not know whether this relates to the development of irreversible structural changes, such as the deposition of collagen, owing to damage associated with poor perfusion of the hypertrophied muscle fibres.

Conclusion

The prevalence of LVH in established hypertension appears to have been underestimated. With multivariate discriminant function analysis, a prevalence figure of about 80% is obtained in established hypertension, which suggests that LVH is present in almost all patients, similar to the high prevalence in animal models.

Analysis of intrinsic isovolumic contractile function and pump performance in LVH suggests that, provided coronary perfusion is adquate, the contractile function of the additional muscle units is normal, so that contractile and pump function of the *whole* LV is somewhat enhanced. In concentric LVH, there is greater systolic emptying, whilst during isovolumic systole, the enhancement of contractile function is less marked and is proportional to the increase in wall thickness. In the intact patient, the *intrinsic* enhancement of pump function is reinforced substantially through increased cardiac sympathetic activity, that appears to be a regular accompaniment of uncomplicated hypertension [27]. Although contractile and pump performance is greater in LVH than in the normal circulation, the LVH heart is much more vulnerable to moderate reduction in perfusion pressure at pressure levels that make ultimate depression of function almost inevitable.

It follows that therapy aimed at producing regression of LVH is a desirable target in management of hypertension. In humans, a period of prolonged therapy appears necessary to bring this about. We do not yet know what choice of drugs produces most rapid and pronounced regression of hypertrophy. Clearly, if irreversible damage to the heart is to be avoided, improved detection of early LVH in mild hypertension holds the key to earlier therapeutic intervention in the future.

Acknowledgements

Work from the Baker Institute was supported by the Australian National Health & Medical Research Council, and by the National Heart Foundation of Australia. I am grateful to Judith Segal and Tessa Morton for their help in the preparation of the manuscript.

References

1. Bugaisky L, Zak R (1986): Biological mechanisms of hypertrophy, in: Fozzard HA, Jennings RB, Haber H, Katz AM (eds), *The Heart and Cardiovascular System,* pp 1491–1506. New York, Raven Press.
2. Wikman Coffelt J, Parmley WW, Mason DT (1979): The cardiac hypertrophy process: Analyses of factors determining pathological vs. physiological development. *Circ Res* 45: 697–707.
3. Tarazi RC, Sen S (1979): Catecholamines and cardiac hypertrophy, in: *Catecholamines and the Heart,* No 8 (Royal Society of Medicine International Congress and Symposium Series). Academic Press and Royal Society of Medicine, London.
4. Schreiber SS, Evans CD, Oratz M, Rothschild MA (1981): Protein synthesis and degradation in cardiac stress. *Circ Res* 48: 601–611.
5. Lundgren Y, Hallbäck M, Weiss L, Folkow B (1974): Rate and extent of adaptive cardiovascular changes during experimental renal hypertension. *Acta Physiol Scand* 91: 103–115.
6. Folkow B, Hallbäck M (1977): Physiopathology of hypertension in rats, in: Genest J, Koiw E, Kuchel O (eds), *Hypertension,* pp 507–529. New York: McGraw Hill.
7. Fletcher PJ, Korner PI, Angus JA, Oliver JR (1976): Changes in cardiac output and total

peripheral resistance during development of renal hypertension in the rabbit: Lack of conformity with the autoregulation theory. *Circ Res* 39: 633–639.

8. Korner PI, Oliver JR, Casley DJ (1980): Effect of dietary salt on hemodynamic of established renal hypertension in the rabbit: Implications for the autoregulation theory of hypertension. *Hypertension* 2: 794–801.

9. Broughton A, Korner PI (1983): Basal and maximal inotropic state in renal hypertensive dogs with cardiac hypertrophy. *Am J Physiol* 245: H33–41.

10. Sen S, Tarazi RC, Khairallah PA, Bumpus FM (1974): Cardiac hypertrophy in spontaneously hypertensive rats. *Circ Res* 35: 775–781.

11. Pfeffer MA, Frohlich ED (1972): Hemodynamic and myocardial function in young and old normotensive and spontaneously hypertensive rats. *Circ Res* 32 (suppl. I): I 28–35.

12. Adams MA, Bobik A, Korner PI (1988): Differential development of vascular and cardiac hypertrophy in the spontaneously hypertensive rat: Relationship to regional sympathetic function. *Hypertension* (in press).

13. Pickering GW (1968): *High Blood Pressure,* 2nd ed. London: J. & A. Churchill.

14. Levine RA, Gillam LD, Weyman A (1986): Echocardiography in cardiac research, in: Fozzard HA, Jennings RB, Haber H, Katz AM (eds), *The Heart and Cardiovascular System,* pp 369–452. New York: Raven Press.

15. Ali-Sambra F, Fouad FM, Tarazi RC (1983): Determinants of left ventricular hypertrophy and function in hypertensive patients. *Am J Med* 75 (Suppl 3A): 26–43.

16. Hammond IW, Devereux RB, Alderman MH, Lutas EM, Spitzer MC, Crowley JS, Laragh JH (1986): The prevalence and correlates of echocardiographic left ventricular hypertrophy among employed patients with uncomplicated hypertension. *J Am Coll Cardiol* 7: 639–650.

17. Devereux RB, Casale PN, Hammond IW, Savage DD, Alderman MH, Campo E, Alonso DR, Laragh JH (1987): Echocardiographic detection of pressure overload left ventricular hypertrophy: Effect of criteria and patient population. *J Clin Hypertens* 3: 66–78.

18. Laufer E, Jennings GL, Korner PI, Dewar E (1989): Prevalence of cardiac structural and functional abnormalities in untreated primary hypertension. *Hypertension* 13: 151–162.

19. Fisher RA (1946): *Statistical Methods for Research Workers,* pp 285–298. Edinburgh: Oliver and Boyd.

20. Korner PI (1983): The role of the heart in hypertension, in: Robertson JIS (ed), *Handbook of Hypertension,* Vol 1: *Clinical Aspects of Essential Hypertension,* pp 97–132. Amsterdam: Elsevier.

21. Weber KT, Janicki JS, Shroff SG (1986): Measurement of ventricular function in the experimental laboratory, in: Fozzard HA, Jennings RB, Haber H, Katz AM (eds), *The Heart and Cardiovascular System,* pp 865–886. New York: Raven Press.

22. Smith V-E, Weisfeldt ML, Katz AM (1986): Relaxation and diastolic properties of the heart, in: Fozzard HA, Jennings RB, Haber H, Katz AM (eds), *The Heart and Cardiovascular System,* pp 803–818. New York: Raven Press.

23. Brutsaert DL, Paulus WJ (1979): Contraction and relaxation of the heart as a muscle and pump. *Int Rev Physiol* 18: 1–31.

24. Brady AJ (1968): Active state in cardiac muscle. *Physiol Rev* 48: 570–600.

25. Mason DT, Braunwald E, Covell JW, Sonnenblick EH, Ross J Jr (1971): Assessment of cardiac contractility: The relation between the rate of pressure rise and ventricular pressure during isovolumic systole. *Circulation* 44: 47–58.

26. Sagawa K (1978): The ventricular pressure volume diagram revisited. *Circ Res* 43: 677–687.

27. Esler M, Jennings G, Korner P, Willett I, Dudley F, Hasking G, Anderson W, Lambert G (1988): Assessent of human sympathetic nervous system activity from measurements of norepinephrine turnover. *Hypertension* 11: 3–20.

28. Broughton A, Korner PI (1981): Estimation of maximum inotropic responses from changes in isovolumic indices of contractility in the dog. *Cardiovasc Res* 15: 382–389.
29. Broughton A, Korner PI (1986): Left ventricular pump function in renal hypertensive dogs with cardiac hypertrophy. *Am J Physiol* 251: H 1260–1266.
30. Folkow B (1982): Physiological aspects of primary hypertension. *Physiol Rev* 62: 347–504.
31. Korner PI (1982): Causal and homeostatic factors in hypertension. *Clin Sci* 63 (suppl 8): 5s–26s.
32. Mulvany MJ (1987): The structure of the resistance vasculature in essential hypertension. *J Hypertension* 5: 129–136.
33. Hallbäck-Nordlander M, Noresson E, Thoren P (1979): Hemodynamic consequences of left ventricular hypertrophy in spontaneously hypertensive rats. *Am J Cardiol* 44: 986–993.
34. Averill DB, Ferrario CM, Tarazi RC, Sen S, Bajbus R (1976): Cardiac performance in rats with renal hypertension. *Circ Res* 38: 280–288.
35. Ferrario CM, Spech MM, Tarazi RC, Doi Y (1979): Cardiac pumping ability in rats with experimental renal and genetic hypertension. *Am J Cardiol* 44: 979–985.
36. Elzinga G, Westerhof N (1976): The pumping ability of the left heart and the effect of coronary occlusion. *Circ Res* 38: 297–302.
37. Strauer BE (1981): *The Heart in Hypertension,* pp 251–284. Berlin: Springer Verlag.
38. Feigl E (1983): Coronary physiology. *Physiol Rev* 63: 1–205.
39. Smolich JJ, Weissberg PL, Broughton A, Korner PI (1988): Aortic pressure reduction redistributes transmural blood flow in dog left ventricle. *Am J Physiol* 254: H 361–368.
40. Smolich JJ, Weissberg PL, Broughton A, Korner PI (1988): Comparison of left and right ventricular blood flow responses during arterial pressure reduction in the autonomically blocked dog: Evidence for right ventricular autoregulation. *Cardiovasc Res* 22: 17–24.
41. Jennings GL, Esler MD, Korner PI (1980): Effect of prolonged treatment on haemodynamics of essential hypertension before and after autonomic block. *Lancet* 1980/2: 166–169.
42. Jennings G, Korner P, Esler M, Restall R (1984): Redevelopment of essential hypertension after cessation of longterm therapy: Preliminary findings. *Clin Exp Hypertens* A6: 493–505.
43. Korner PI, Jennings GL, Esler MD, Bobik A, Adams M (1987): The role of cardiovascular hypertrophy in hypertension: Basis for a new therapeutic strategy. *J Cardiovasc Pharmacol* 10 (suppl 5): S72–78.
44. Korner PI, Jennings GL, Esler MD, Anderson WP, Bobik A, Adams M, Angus JA (1987): The cardiovascular amplifiers in human primary hypertension and their role in a strategy for detecting the underlying causes. *Can J Physiol Pharmacol* 65: 1730–1738.
45. Sen S, Tarazi RC, Bumpus FM (1977): Cardiac hypertrophy and antihypertensive therapy. *Cardiovasc Res* 11: 427–431.
46. Motz W, Strauer B (1984): Regression of structural cardiovascular changes by antihypertensive therapy. *Hypertension* 6 (suppl III): III 133–139.
47. Tarazi RC, Fouad FM (1984): Reversal of cardiac hypertrophy in humans. *Hypertension* 6 (suppl III): III 140–146.
48. Fletcher PJ (1984): Baroreceptor heart rate reflex in rabbits after reversal of renal hypertension. *Am J Physiol* 246: H 261–266.

15. Volume and cardiac factors in the genesis of mineralocorticoid hypertension in the conscious dog

KAORU ONOYAMA

Steroid induced hypertension is well known to be salt and water dependent. In both the clinical and experimental forms of this disorder, salt loading increases while salt deprivation decreases arterial blood pressure [1, 2]. We have previously reported our experience in conscious dogs [3] in which we performed serial quantitative assessment of hemodynamic and volume alterations during sodium deprivation and during gradual replenishment of total body sodium; the aim of the study was to dissociate between the role of sodium and the role of changes of blood and extracellular fluid volumes in the genesis of steroid induced hypertension. The sequence of changes in metyrapone treated dogs (100 mg/kg/day) was compared with untreated controls submitted to the same protocol. Restoration of sodium stores failed to alter arterial blood pressure in untreated dogs while, in contrast, it led to significant hypertension in metyrapone treated dogs. Changes in cardiac output and fluid volumes were virtually identical at every stage in the normotensive and hypertensive dogs. These findings suggested that changes in flow, which occurred in all dogs following salt and water administration, were not responsible for the subsequent rise in arterial pressure. The increased arterial pressure in metyrapone treated dogs was clearly due to a rise in total peripheral resistance when these dogs attained a critical amount of cumulative sodium intake. In fact, these studies have followed a quantitative evaluation of the relationship between sodium intake and total peripheral resistance changes in the presence of excess electrolyte active steroids; increases in cardiac output by as much as 20% were not associated with increased total peripheral resistance or blood pressure when cumulative sodium intake was limited to 140 mEq. In contrast, equivalent increases in cardiac output and in extracellular fluid volumes were associated with a rise in total peripheral resistance and blood pressure only at much higher cumulative sodium intakes. Of additional considerable importance was the demonstration that the rise in blood pressure was not time-dependent, but

M.E. Safar & F. Fouad-Tarazi (eds.), The heart in hypertension.
© *1989 Kluwer Academic Publishers, Dordrecht –*

was related entirely to the amount of sodium given. Thus, infusion of 10 mEq sodium for 14 days (total cumulative sodium = 140 mEq) failed to modify blood pressure although both volume and cardiac output were elevated, while the administration of 60 mEq sodium for 7 days (total cumulative sodium = 420 mEq) produced significant increases in blood pressure at levels of extracellular fluid volume and cardiac output not significantly different from those produced by 140 mEq cumulative sodium intake.

The mechanism underlying the increase in peripheral vascular resistance in mineralocorticoid hypertension is still unclear. It may be speculated that (1) total body vascular autoregulation occurs in response to increased cardiac output and tissue perfusion [4], (2) there is enhancement of activity of the peripheral sympathetic nervous system [5, 6] during steroid induced hypertensive responses, (3) electrolyte active steroids have direct or indirect myogenic effects [7, 8], and (4) steroids alter ion distribution in the vascular smooth muscles cell [9–12]. As regard the first possibility, results from several studies have supported the concept that an initial phase of high cardiac output is not always essential for the development of hypertension induced by electrolyte active steroids; the pig, for example, treated with deoxycorticosterone acetate (DOCA) develops hypertension within 3–5 days without any demonstrable increases in cardiac output [13]. Also in both the DOCA-saline [14] and metyrapone-treated hypertensive dogs [2], the rise in arterial pressure was not uniformly associated with increases in cardiac output nor did prevention of rises in cardiac output by beta blockade inhibit the development of hypertension. Neither did the sympathetic nervous system appear to be essential in the development of this type of hypertension in the dog. Thus, it was previously shown that in this model, plasma norepinephrine concentrations were decreased rather than increased [2]. In addition, the prior administration of either centrally or peripherally acting adrenergic blocking drugs could not prevent the development of hypertension, although the values of plasma norepinephrine concentrations were reduced further. On the other hand, enhanced sensitivity of vascular smooth muscle to vasoconstrictor substances during administration of electrolyte-active steroids has been demonstrated in a number of studies. In this respect, Schmid et al. [7, 8] showed that constriction of resistance and capacitance vessels in response to norepinephrine is potentiated by treatment with 9 alpha-fluoro-hydrocortisone. Berecek and Bohr [15] found a distinct lowering of threshold doses of both angiotensin II and norepinephrine during the early stages of the development of hypertension in the DOCA-hypertensive pig. Hinke [16] demonstrated hyperresponsiveness to exogenous vasopressin in DOCA-hypertension of rats while Mohring et al. [17] recently reported some observations suggesting a vasopressor role of antidiuretic hormone in the pathogenesis of malignant but not benign DOCA-hypertension of rats. This increased vascular reactivity could theoretically be

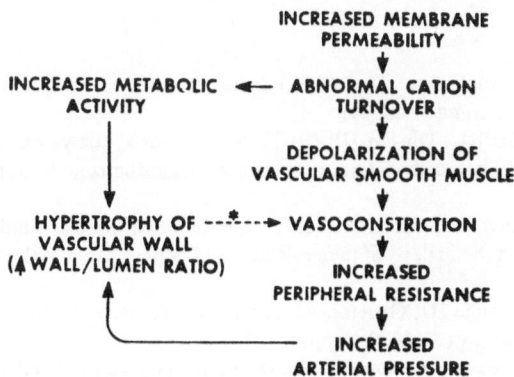

Figure 1. The possible sequence of events leading to hypertension induced by electrolyte-active steroids. * Increased reactivity.

related to changes in potassium since decreases in plasma potassium (less than 3 mEq/l) were found to increase vascular resistance [18]. However, in our studies plasma potassium in metyrapone treated hypertensive dogs averaged 3.9 mEg/l. In addition, other studies have shown that the local vascular changes encountered in the DOCA-saline hypertensive rat were independent of potassium balance [11]. Providing supplemental potassium in these rats did not influence the progress of vascular changes and hypertension.

We have hypothesized that primary changes in vascular smooth muscle could account entirely for increased total peripheral resistance and the eventual rise in arterial blood pressure in steroid-dependent hypertension in the dog model (Figure 1). This was based on previous work published by Jones and Hart [11], Friedman and Friedman [10, 12] and Berecek and Bohr [15]. Thus, changes in cell membrane permeability may lead to abnormal cation turnover which in turn could lead to vasoconstriction and increased peripheral vascular resistance. Also increased cation turnover would be expected to increase metabolic activity [19] and may provide an early signal for vascular and smooth muscle hypertrophy. The combined effects of increased blood pressure and these stimuli could lead to thickening of the media and increased wall to lumen ratio with enhancement of vascular reactivity [20].

Therefore, based on various studies including ours [2, 3], it could be concluded that steroid-induced hypertension is 'resistance mediated' from its early stages. Also, in the presence of mineralocorticoid excess, sodium repletion rather than volume expansion, plays a more important role in the initiation of hypertension. Furthermore, it is quite possible that sodium itself interacts with electrolyte active steroids on vascular smooth muscle to alter ion transport resulting in increased vascular resistance and hence arterial blood pressure.

References

1. Bravo EL, Dustan HP, Tarazi RC (1973): Spironolactone as nonspecific therapy for primary aldosteronism. *Circulation* 48: 491.
2. Bravo EL, Tarazi RC, Dustan HP (1977): Multifactorial analysis of chronic hypertension induced by electrolyte-active steroids in trained unanesthetized dogs. *Circ Res* 40 (suppl I): I-140.
3. Onoyama K, Bravo EL, Tarazi RC (1979): Sodium, extracellular fluid volume, and cardiac output changes in the genesis of mineralocorticoid hypertension in the intact dog. *Hypertension* 1: 331.
4. Coleman TG, Grange HJ, Gruyton AC (1971): Whole-body circulatory autoregulation and hypertension. *Circ Res* 28 & 29 (suppl II): II-76.
5. deChamplain J, Farley L, Cousineayu D, Van Amerigen MR (1976): Circulating catecholamine levels in human and experimental hypertension. *Circ Res* 38: 109.
6. Reid JL, Zivin JA, Kopin IJ (1975): Central and peripheral adrenergic mechanisms in the development of deoxycorticosterone-saline hypertension in rats. *Circ Res* 37: 569.
7. Schmid PG, Eckstein JW, Abboud FM (1965): Effects of 9-alpha-fluorohydrocortisone on forearm vascular responses to norepinephrine. *Circulation* 34: 620.
8. Schmid PH, Eckstein JW, Abboud FM (1967): Effect of 9-alpha-fluorohydrocortisone on forearm venous responses to norepinephrine and tyramine. *J Appl Physiol* 23: 571.
9. Overbeck HW, Pamnani MB, Akera T, Brody TM, Haddy FJ (1976): Depressed function of ouabain-sensitive sodium-potassium pump in blood vessels from renal hypertensive dogs. *Circ Res* 38 (suppl II): II-48.
10. Friedman SM (1974): An ion exchange approach to the problem of intracellular sodium in the hypertensive process. *Circ Res* 34 & 35 (suppl I): I-123.
11. Jones AW, Hart RG (1975): Altered ion transport in aortic smooth muscle during deoxycorticosterone acetate hypertension in the rat. *Circ Res* 37: 333.
12. Friedman SM, Friedman CL (1976): Cell permeability, sodium transport and the hypertensive process in the rat. *Circ Res* 39: 433.
13. Terris JM, Berecek KH, Cohen EL, Stanley JC, Whitehouse WM Jr, Bohr DF (1976): Deoxycorticosterone hypertension in the pig. *Clin Sci Mol Med* 51 (suppl III): 303.
14. Conway J, Hatton R (1978): Development of deoxycorticosterone acetate hypertension in the dog. *Circ Res* 43 (suppl I): I-82.
15. Berecek KH, Bohr DF (1978): Whole body vascular reactivity during the development of deoxycorticosterone acetate hypertension in the pig. *Circ Res* 42: 764.
16. Hinke JAM (1965): In vitro demonstration of vascular hyperresponsiveness in experimental hypertension. *Circ Res* 17: 359.
17. Mohring J, Mohring B, Petri M, Haack D (1963): Vasopressor role of ADH in the pathogenesis of malignant DOC hypertension. *Am J Physiol* 232: F260.
18. Haddy FJ, Scott JB, Florio MA, Daugherty RM Jr, Huizinga JN (1963): Local vascular effects of hypokalemia, alkalosis, hypercalcemia and hypomagnesemia. *Am J Physiol* 204: 202.
19. Whittam R (1964): Interdependence of metabolism and active transport, in: Hoffman JF (ed), *Cellular Functions of Membrane Transport,* Section 3, p 139. Englewood Cliffs, N.J.: Prentice-Hall.
20. Folkow B, Oberg B (1959): The effect of functionally induced changes of wall/lumen ratio on the vasoconstrictor response to standard amounts of vasoactive agents. *Acta Physiol Scand* 47: 131.

16. Heart and hypertension: The magnitude of the problem
Electrocardiographic and echocardiographic aspects

EDWARD D. FROHLICH and MARC A. PFEFFER

Introduction

A close association has been demonstrated across many animal species between the mass of the heart and external work of the ventricle [1]. Thus, within any single species of animals, any prolonged augmentation in the hemodynamic overload imposed on the ventricle will result in hypertrophy of that chamber sustaining that load. Systemic arterial hypertension is the most common condition leading to left ventricular hypertrophy since it is this chamber which is the source for the augmented energy needed to overcome the chronic burden of the pressure overload.

The first association made between hypertension and this augmentation of left ventricular mass is usually attributed to Richard Bright. However, it is well to recognize that Bright's observations proceeded indirect measurements of arterial pressure by many years. Nevertheless, Bright related the increased left ventricular mass to a 'hardness of the pulse' [2]. In 1868, however, George Johnson utilized sphygmographic evidence of increased arterial pressure to make the true association between arterial hypertension and left ventricular hypertrophy [2]. It wasn't until 1933 that Chanutin and Barksdale actually demonstrated left ventricular hypertrophy to be produced by inducing experimental hypertension [3]. These investigators used a renoprival model of arterial hypertension to show that left ventricular mass increased with the development of experimental hypertension [3]. This pioneering work also indicated clearly that this increased mass of the left ventricle could be attributed to ventricular hypertrophy since they demonstrated that left ventricular myocyte fiber diameter was increased in direct proportion to the height of the arterial pressure.

M.E. Safar & F. Fouad-Tarazi (eds.), The heart in hypertension.
© *1989 Kluwer Academic Publishers, Dordrecht –*

Electrocardiographic left ventricular hypertrophy (ECG-LVH)

Until only recently, clinical premorbid diagnosis of left ventricular hypertrophy was confined mainly to alterations in the electrocardiographic criteria
of LVH. These various criteria of ECG-LVH were based upon increased
electromotive precardial voltage forces plus repolarization changes on the
standard electrocardiogram. At present, there are over 30 different criteria
that have been developed by various investigators to relate electrocardiographic measurements to more direct evidence of increased anatomic ventricular mass. In general, these electrocardiographic criteria of LVH are rather
consistently insensitive, yet they are fairly specific for detecting increased left
ventricular mass [4]. These electrocardiographic criteria by definition provide
only a categorial variable for the continuous variable of left ventricular mass;
and therefore, the direct correlation to the actual LVH mass to the ECG
changes has been disappointing [5]. It follows, then, that the clinical premorbid diagnosis of LVH has generally referred to the ECG pattern rather than
actual mass of the left ventricle.

Prognostic significance of ECG-LVH

Electrocardiographic recognition of left ventricular hypertrophy has retained
an important role in the overall cardiovascular assessment of the patient, no
doubt as a result of the prognostic information it provides rather than the
relatively crude and imprecise measure of actual left ventricular mass. Thus,
the important dire implications of ECG-LVH as a risk factor of future cardiovascular morbidity and death has stood the test of time. It has been a consistent
finding of both large population studies as well as interventional clinical trials,
and thus, ECG-LVH continues to be an integral component of cardiovascular
assessment.

The existence of ECG-LVH markedly increases the relative risk for that
patient to develop an adverse cardiovascular event or death [6]. In the pros-
pectively conducted Fraingham study, development of ECG-LVH was documented in individuals having had previously normal ECG's. Thus, in this study
35 percent of all men that first manifested ECG-LVH died within five years of
the appearance of this adverse marker. Furthermore, men and women between 35 and 64 years of age had a 10 to 19-fold increased risk of cardiovascular
mortality when ECG-LVH was present as compared to age- and gender-
matched individuals without these ECG abnormalities [7]. Moreover, risk of
sudden death is particularly increased in patients with ECG-LVH [8]; and left
ventricular ectopy appears to be more prevalent on ambulatory monitoring in
individuals with ECG-LVH [9, 10].

Prognostic implications of ECG-LVH is also demonstrable in other forms of adverse cardiovascular events. Risk of later development of angina pectoris, myocardial infarction, stroke, symptomatic peripheral vascular disease, and overt congestive heart failure are all significantly increased in patients with ECG-LVH [7]. Indeed, the greatest risk of developing overt congestive heart failure could be predicted from the presence of ECG-LVH. In the Framingham study, asymptomatic men and women with ECG-LVH had more than a 17-fold chance of ultimately developing congestive heart failure than age- and gender-matched cohorts without evidence of ECG-LVH [7].

ECG-LVH and hypertension

The Framingham study also demonstrated a clear-cut increase in the prevalence of ECG-LVH in proportion to advancing age and increasing arterial pressure levels; and systemic arterial hypertension emerged as the major predicting factor for the later deveelopment of ECG-LVH in the general population. Fewer than six percent of men with systolic pressures of 139 mmHg or less exhibited ECG-LVH, whereas, the proportion of individuals manifesting ECG-LVH increased steeply as a function of baseline blood pressure (Table 1). Prevalence of ECG-LVH was increased by 15 percent in men with systolic pressures between 140 and 159 mmHg; and this increased to fully one-third of all men in the general population whose systolic pressures exceeded 159 mmHg. A similar steep arterial pressure related increase in the prevalence of ECG-LVH was observed in women [7].

The Framingham Heart study also demonstrated the incidence for development of ECG-LVH in individuals whose baseline electrocardiogram did not manifest the pattern of LVH. Based on the 30 year follow-up data provided by the Framingham Heart study, ultimate development of ECG-LVH was closely related to the blood pressure level of the individual patient at the time of baseline study. Those with mild hypertension (140/90 to 160/95 mmHg) had double the risk for ultimately developing ECG-LVH; and persons with higher levels of arterial pressure had more than a 10-fold chance of manifesting

Table 1. Risk of adverse cardiovascular event with respect to echocardiographic left ventricular mass. From Casale et al., *Ann Int Med,* 1986 [24].

ECHO LV mass index (gm/m²)	(n)	CV event rate (per 100 pt yrs)
<95	(53)	0.8
95–124	(58)	1.6
125+	(29)	4.6

ECG-LVH than other individuals in the general population with normal
baseline blood pressures [7].

Antihypertensive drug trials have consistently supported the information
generated from these logitudinal population studies. Two recurring themes
from every large clinical trial involving patients with hypertension are: (1) the
prevalence of ECG-LVH increases in relation to entry level arterial pressure,
and (2) the risk of sudden or other cardiovascular deaths is adversely influenced by the presence of ECG-LVH. In the initial Veterans Administration
Cooperative Study of antihypertensive agents, in which the inclusion criteria
was a diastolic pressure between 115 and 129 mmHg, 143 individuals were
randomized. Of these 143 patients, 46 (or 32 percent) had ECG-LVH at
baseline evaluation [11]. In the subsequent report from this Veterans Administration Coopeerative Study (in which entry diastolic pressure levels were less
severe – 90 to 114 mmHg) 16 percent of the enrolled patients had ECG-LVH at
baseline [12]. In the Hypertension Detection and Follow-up Program (HDFP)
over 150,000 individuals were screened in order to identify 10,940 patients with
increased diastolic pressure to permit inclusion into the multicenter trial. Of
these patients, 5 percent demonstrated ECG-LVH criteria at baseline. As in
the general population and in other antihypertensive drug trials, there was a
direct relationship of blood pressure level to the occurrence of ECG-LVH. In
HDFP, of the 7,825 individuals with entry diastolic pressure between 90 and
104 mmHg, only 256 (or 3 percent) demonstrated ECG-LVH at baseline. In
this same study, the prevalence of ECG-LVH was increased three-fold in
persons entering the trial with higher diastolic pressures (105 mmHg or
greater), with 285 of 3115 (or 9 percent) having ECG-LVH at baseline [13].

This valuable information coming from these longitudinal population studies has been consistently supported by clinical experience. Sokolow and Perloff were among the first to describe the adverse affects of ECG-LVH on
long-term survival of hypertensive patients. This was especially evident when
repolarization abnormalities were included in the definition of ECG-LVH
[14]. The more recent HDFP study confirmed this experience demonstrating
the five year mortality rate for those patients with ECG-LVH was 17.4
percent. This high rate was more than two and one-half times the five year
mortality rate (6.5 percent) of individuals without ECG-LVH at baseline [15].

Another interesting observation emanating from the Framingham Heart
Study concerns the temporal reduction in the prevalence of ECG-LVH in the
general population coinciding with the period when more attention was directed towards the detection and treatment of hypertension [16]. A considerable
decrease in the age-gender specific prevalence of ECG-LVH in the Framingham population from the 1950's to the 1970's was observed. Thus, in the
1950's, 5 percent of all men evaluated between ages 50 to 54 years demonstrated ECG-LVH. The prevalence of ECG-LVH was only 3 percent in

comparable age- and gender-matched sample 14 years later. Similar results of a reduction in the prevalence of ECG-LVH were obtained in other age groups [16]. These observations of the temporal decline in prevalence of ECG-LVH in the general population have been supported by other information from recent large clinical trials. Indeed, it is currently estimated that less than 5 percent of the hypertension population will exhibit ECG-LVH [17]. However, although this lower prevalence of ECG-LVH in the general and even hypertensive populations have been documented, the prognostic importance of ECG-LVH has not diminished. Thus, once ECG-LVH is established the risk does not diminish.

Although the MRFIT Study raised the question of a possible adverse effect of antihypertensive diuretic therapy of individuals with baseline ECG abnormalities, this observation was not confirmed by the HDFP Study. In both trials, overall prognosis of those patients with ECG abnormalities was worse than individuals with normal baseline electrocardiograms. However, in the HDFP trial, patients with baseline ECG-LVH randomized to the more aggressive antihypertensive therapy group (Stepped Care) resulted in a lower five year mortality rate than in those patients with baseline evidence of ECG-LVH who were randomized to the less stringently controlled (Referred Care) group.

Echocardiographic-LVH (ECHO-LVH)

Clinical trials and epidemiologic studies, therefore, have clearly provided, consistent and convincing evidence that ECG-LVH is an important indicator of adverse cardiovascular events. Yet, as has been apparent over these many years, the ECG has provided a relatively poor assessment of actual left ventricular mass. The consistent lack of sensitivity of the myriad of ECG criteria for LVH only underscores the point that anatomical evidence of LVH can certainly be present without being detected by the ECG. In more recent years, it has become apparent that the echocardiogram provides an excellent noninvasive means for more accurately assessing the presence of increased left ventricular mass. In expert hands, pre-mortem echocardiographic measurements of left ventricular mass has correlated very closely with actual anatomic measurements made from patients with a wide range of ventricular weights who died as a result of a wide variety of cardiovascular disorders [18].

Since mass clearly is a continuous variable, and the echocardiographic technique provides a reliable measure of left ventricular mass, it follows that for this non-invasive diagnostic measurement to be applied to general populations it must address more directly the question of the true prevalence of increased left ventricular mass. Levy and co-wworkers performed echocardiographic evaluations on almost 5,000 participants of the Framingham Heart Study. This important study demonstrated left ventricular hypertrophy (by the echocardiographic criteria) was not uncommon in the general population, being present in 16 percent of the men and 19 percent of the women evaluated [19]. Moreover, an important age affect was demonstrated as well as a significant association between blood pressure levels and the presence of ehocardiographic evidence of left ventricular hypertrophy. Another finding of this population based study was the influence of exogenous obesity as an independent risk for the occurrence of echocardiographic left ventricular hypertrophy. The importance of both age and the level of systolic arterial pressure on the prevalence of echocardiographically demonstrable LVH support the concept that the height of arterial pressure, as well as duration of hypertension, are important determinants of actual LVH.

ECHO-LVH hypertension

In one of the first applications of echocardiographic techniques to hypertensive individuals, Dunn et al., demonstrated that a graded increase in left ventricular mass was present in relation to the severity of the hemodynamic hypertensive process [20]. Of interest, this evidence of ECHO-LVH was observed, for the most part, in hypertensive patients who did not demonstrate ECG-LVH. In a larger series, this observation of a 7 to 10-fold higher prevalence of ECHO-LVH compared to ECG-LVH has been a consistent finding [21, 22]. Although ECG-LVH has been found in 3 to 5 percent of all hypertensive patients, ECHO-LVH was present in 20 to 50 percent of these same individuals [21, 22].

Since such a great disparity between the prevalence of ECG- and ECHO-LVH exists in the overall hypertensive population, it is difficult to conclude that the prognostic information that has accumulated over the decades with respect to ECG-LVH can be generally applied to ECHO-LVH. Only over the past few years the relevance of echocardiographic LVH in the hypertensive patient population has been addressed. At the outset it must be qualified that unlike ECG-LVH, large population numbers have not been followed for sufficiently protracted time periods. The epidemiologic variables with the lowest event rates therefore have the sparsest numbers. The crucial question as to whether echocardiographic-LVH is associated with increased risk for premature morbidity and mortality has yet to be answered. Thus, at the present time only preliminary information is available to indicate that the two-year mortality rate is actually increased in patients in the general population with echocardiographic evidence of LVH [23]. However, more information is clearly necessary before establishing ECHO-LVH as a risk factor for premature cardiovascular mortality in a large hypertensive population.

With respect to cardiovascular morbidity, one recent study has provided important first information as to the prognostic significance of ECHO-LVH in the hypertensive population [24]. Of 140 patients followed by a large hypertensive clinic, 29 (or 21 percent) had echocardiographic evidence of increased left ventricular mass. Although electrocardiograms were obtained from all patients, too few had electrocardiographic evidence of LVH for determination of the long-term consequences of ECG-LVH. The sample size and event rate was also too limited for a pure mortality analysis. Therefore, the predictive value of echocardiographic LVH was analyzed using combined endpoints of death, myocardial infarction, development of congestive heart failure, stroke, and angina pectoris requiring coronary artery bypass surgery. The follow-up period was approximately 5 years and during that time there were a total of 14 adverse cardiovascular events in the overall population. Of the 29 patients with echocardiographic evidence of left ventricular hypertrophy, 7 (or 24 percent) experienced an untoward cardiovascular event. In contrast, only 6 percent of patients without the echocardiographic evidence of LVH had developed cardiovascular events [24]. The difference between these groups was significant statistically at the 0.01 alpha level using a Chi square analysis.

In that same study, the concept that echocardiographic increase in left ventricular mass was associated with an increase in adverse effects was further supported by an analysis of risk of morbid events versus quartiles of left ventricular mass. A clear relationship was established: the greater the left ventricular mass the greater the chance of developing a morbid cardiovascular event during the follow-up period (Table 1). As acknowledged in this very important study, further work certainly is necessary involving larger patient populations in order to find the full prognostic importance of echocardiographic evidence of left ventricular hypertrophy in patients with hypertension. However, these recent data provide the first indication that the presence of increased left ventricular mass by echocardiographic criteria (rather than by ECG) does influence the overall prognosis after development of increased cardiovascular morbidity and mortality.

The presence of echocardiographically-detected LVH in the hypertensive population therefore strongly seems to be associated with an increased rate of ventricular ectopy including complex and paroxysmal runs of ventricular ectopic activity [10, 25, 26]. Although the association between ECHO-LVH and ambulatory arrhythmias has been documented, it must be underscored that the long-term significance of the presence of ambulatory arrhythmias in the hypertensive population has yet to be determined.

Summary

Hypertension is the major cause of left ventricular hypertrophy. While the electrocardiogram is an extremely insensitive measure of anatomic left ventricular hypertrophy, it provides a time-tested important marker of an adverse cardiovascular outcome. There has been a recent temporal decrease in the incidence of electrocardiographic evidence of LVH even within the hypertensive population; no doubt this is the result of large antihypertensive treatment experts. Anatomical evidence of left ventricular hypertrophy is best documented pre-morbidly using echocardiographic techniques. It therefore appears that between 20 and 50 percent of the hypertensive population has left ventricular hypertrophy by echocardiographic techniques. The prognostic significance of the echocardiographically determined increase in left ventricular mass is just beginning to be evaluated. Early information suggests that there is an increased rate of cardiovascular morbidity in patients with echocardiographic evidence of increased left ventricular mass. However, this information is only preliminary, and as yet only a limited number of events have been reported. Far more supporting information will be required before the full impact of echocardiographically-detected left ventricular hypertrophy can be determined. Nevertheless, it must be stated that the electrocardiogram still has the greatest predictive value of cardiovascular morbid and mortal events when the pattern of left ventricular hypertrophy plus repolarization abnormalities are present. It is quite possible that these repolarization abnormalities are indicative of a combination of increased left ventricular mass plus relative myocardial ischemia [27] that is not able to be detected by the echocardiogram. Larger population-based clinical trials are necessary to determine the prognostic significance of the more common finding of ECHO-LVH in hypertensive patients.

References

1. Holt JP, Rhode EA, Kines H (1968): Ventricular volumes and body weight in mammals. *Am J Physiol* 215: 705–715.
2. Pickering G (1982): Systemic arterial hypertension, in: Fishman AP, Richards DW (eds): *Circulation of the Blood: Men and Ideas*, pp 487–541. American Physiol Society.
3. Chanutin A, Barksdale EE (1933): Experimental renal insufficiency produced by partial nephrectomy. *Arch Intern Med* 52: 739–751.
4. Casale PN, Devereux RB, Alonso DR, Campo E, Kligfield P (1987): Improved sex-specific criteria of left ventricular hypertrophy for clinical and computer interpretation of electrocardiograms: Validation with autopsy findings. *Circulation* 75: 565–572.
5. Reichek N, Devereux RB (1981): Left ventricular hypertrophy: Relationship of anatomic, echocardiographic and electrocardiographic findings. *Circulation* 63: 1391–1398.

6. Frohlich ED (1986): Left ventricular hypertrophy as a risk factor, in: Messerli FH, Amodeo C (ed): *Cardiology Clinics,* Vol 4, pp 137–144. Philadelphia: W.B. Saunders.
7. Kannel WB, Dannenberg AL, Levy D (1987): Population implications of electrocardiographic left ventricular hypertrophy. *Am J Cardiol* 60: I 85–93.
8. Kannel WB, Doyle JT, McNamara PM, Quickenton P, Gordon T (1975): Precursors of sudden coronary death: Factors related to the incidence of sudden death. *Circulation* 51: 606–613.
9. Messerli FH, Ventura HO, Elizardi DJ, Dunn FG, Frohlich ED (1984): Hypertension and sudden death: Increased ventricular ectopic activity in left ventricular hypertrophy. *Am J Med* 77: 18–22.
10. McLenachan JM, Henderson E, Morris KI, Dargie HJ (1987): Ventricular arrhythmias in patients with hypertensive left ventricular hypertrophy. *New Engl J Med* 317: 787–792.
11. Veterans Administration Cooperative Study Group on Antihypertensive Agents (1967): Effects of treatment on morbidity in hypertension, I: Results in patients with diastolic blood pressures averaging 115 through 129 mmHg. *JAMA* 202: 116–1034.
12. Veterans Administration Cooperative Study Group on Antihypertensive Agents (1970): Effects of treatment on morbidity in hypertension, II: Results in patients with diastolic pressure averaging 90 through 114 mmHg. *JAMA* 213: 1143–1152.
13. Hypertension Detection and Follow-up Program Cooperative Group (1979): Five-year findings of the hypertension detection and follow-up program, I: Reduction in mortality of persons with high blood pressure, including mild hypertension. *JAMA* 242: 2562–2571.
14. Sokolow M, Perloff D (1961): The prognosis of essential hypertension treated conservatively. *Circulation* 23: 697–713.
15. Langford HG, Stamler J, Wassertheil-Smoller S, Prineas RJ (1986): All-cause mortality in the Hypertension Detection and Follow-up Program: Findings for the whole cohort and for persons with less severe hypertension, with and without other traits related to risk of mortality. *Prog Cardiovasc Disease* 29: 29–54.
16. Kannel WB, Sorlie P (1981): Left ventricular hypertrophy in hypertension: prognostic and pathogenetic implications (the Framingham study), in: Strauer BE (ed): *The Heart in Hypertension,* pp 223–242. Berlin: Springer Verlag. (Boehringer-Mannheim Symposium Series).
17. Devereux RB, Casale PN, Wallerson DC, Kligfield P, Hammond IW, Liebson PR, Campo E, Alonso DR, Laragh JH (1987): Cost-effectiveness of echocardiography and electrocardiography for detection of left ventricular hypertrophy in patients with systemic hypertension. *Hypertension* 9 (suppl II): II 69–76.
18. Devereux RB, Reichek N (1977): Echocardiographic determination of left ventricular mass in man: Anatomic validation of the method. *Circulation* 55: 613–618.
19. Levy D, Anderson KM, Savage DD, Kannel WB, Christiansen JC, Castelli WP (1988): Echocardiographically detected left ventricular hypertrophy: Prevalence and risk factors (The Framingham Heart Study). *Ann Intern Med* 108: 7–13.
20. Dunn FG, Chandraratna P, de Carvalho JGR, Basta LL, Frohlich ED (1977): Pathophysiologic assessment of hypertensive heart disease with echocardiography. *Am J Cardiol* 39: 789–795.
21. Savage DD, Drayer JIM, Henry WL, Mathews EC, Ware JH, Gardin JM, Cohen ER, Epstein SE, Laragh JH (1979): *Circulation* 59: 623–632.
22. Hammond IW, Devereux RB, Alderman MH, Lutas EM, Spitzer MC, Crowley JS, Laragh JT (1986): The prevalence and correlates of echocardiographic left ventricular hypertrophy among employed patients with uncomplicated hypertension. *J Am Coll Cardiol* 7: 639–650.
23. Savage DD, Garrison RJ, Castelli WP, Kannel WB, Anderson SJ, Feinleib M (1985): Echocardiographic left ventricular hypertrophy in the general population is associated with

increased 2-year mortality, independent of standard coronary risk factors (The Framingham Heart Study). *AHA Council Cardiovasc Epidemiol Newsletter* 37: 33.

24. Casale PN, Devereux RB, Milner M, Zullo G, Harshfield GA, Pickering TG, Laragh JH (1986): Value of echocardiographic measurement of left ventricular mass in predicting cardiovascular morbid events in hypertensive men. *Ann Intern Med* 105: 173–178.

25. Aronow WS, Epstein S, Schwartz KS, Koenigsberg M (1987): Correlation of complex ventricular arrhythmias detected by ambulatory electrocardiographic monitoring with echocardiographic left ventricular hypertrophy in persons older than 62 years in a long-term health care facility. *Am J Cardiol* 60: 730–732.

26. Levy D, Anderson KM, Savage DD, Balkus SA, Kannel WB, Castelli WP (1987): Risk of ventricular arrhythmias in left ventricular hypertrophy (The Framingham Heart Study). *Am J Cardiol* 60: 560–565.

27. Dunn FG, Pringle SD (1987): Left ventricular hypertrophy and myocardial ischemia in systemic hypertension. *Am J Cardiol* 60: I 19–22.

17. Acute volume expansion and pumping function of the heart in sustained essential hypertension

GÉRARD M. LONDON and MICHEL E. SAFAR

Introduction

The adequacy of the circulation depends on its filling pressure [1]. This, in turn, depends on intravascular blood volume, the capacity of the vascular compartment and their interrelationship, i.e. vascular compliance [2]. There are numerous control mechanisms involved in the regulation of cardiovascular function. There are called into play under abnormal conditions of capacitance and/or blood volume. An integrated response to acute hypervolemia involves a network of cardiovascular reflexes and hormonal changes and adjustments. These include the Frank-Starling relationship and stress-relaxation of the peripheral vessels [1, 3]. Such mechanisms have been extensively studied in isolated hearts and in animals. Hypervolemia secondary to infusion of intravenous fluids has also been induced in man, in attempt to stimulate venous return and to test the applicability of the Frank-Starling relationship to the intact human heart. For this purpose, a variety of fluids has been utilized, including saline [4, 5, 6], human serum albumin [4, 7], blood [8] and dextrans [9–18].

Limited data are available regarding the effects of blood volume expansion in patients with sustained essential hypertension [17–21]. Indeed, essential hypertension is a hemodynamically complex abnormality, involving derangements of several neurohumoral circulatory control mechanisms [22–26]. Furthermore, the cardiac hypertrophy which frequently complicates arterial hypertension may potentially modify the Frank-Starling relationship in man. The purpose of this review is to assess the effect of blood volume expansion on function of the heart in men with sustained essential hypertension.

M.E. Safar & F. Fouad-Tarazi (eds.), The heart in hypertension.
© *1989 Kluwer Academic Publishers, Dordrecht –*

Basic methodological concepts

In humans, conflicting results have been reported concerning the effects of volume loading on cardiac output and filling pressure. The differences are related principally to the nature of the substance infused and, more importantly, to the rate of perfusion. Substances that induce hemodilution and decrease blood viscosity are, by reducing the resistance to venous return, more likely to produce changes in central hemodynamics than those that induce blood volume expansion without hemodilutional 'anemia' [27]. For example dextran perfusion leads to a rise in cardiac output and cardiac filling pressure [9, 10, 12–15, 17, 18], whereas blood infusion does not affect these parameters [8]. As shown in a previous report, the most important factor in the cardiac output response is the rate of infusion. Flow-rates greater than 25 ml/minute are necessary to induce changes in cardiac output [5, 10, 12, 13]. As previously discussed, the central circulation is protected against vascular engorgement by several mechanisms, including reflex changes in venous tone [8, 28], pulmonary vessels [12, 13], stress relaxation and extracellular fluid volume partition. When perfusion rates are slow, the blood volume changes are progressive and the control mechanisms are capable of buffering the pressure and volume changes almost completely. When the rate of infusion is high, the mechanisms preventing the rise in central blood volume and pressures are temporarily overcome and measurable changes in filling pressure and cardiac output occur [12]. The present review, in line with previous reports [14, 15, 17], assesses the validity of the Frank-Starling relationship in the intact human heart using isoonkotic Dextran in normal and hypertensive subjects.

Dextran is a polysaccharide with no direct cardiac or vascular effect [14]. Nevertheless, intravenous perfusion of 750 ml (150 ml/min within 5 minutes using a Sogreath MP.6 pump) has a small dilutional effect, with a fall in systemic hematocrit and a reduction in the viscosity of whole blood at all shear rates (Figure 1). The changes of viscosity are minute or small for high shear rates, corresponding to blood flow velocity in arteries and arterioles [29]. At low shear rates, the reduction of blood viscosity is more pronounced, and therefore the decrease in resistance to flow is more marked in postcapillary venules and veins [29]. These rheologic changes induce a reduction in resistance to venous return, which therefore increases [30]. Anemia resulting from hemodilution could change the oxygen carrying capacity of the blood, but the fall in hematocrit is comparable (6 to 7%) in controls and in hypertensives, and it is unlikely that this factor would be important in the hemodynamic response. Furthermore, it has been shown that dextran displaces the oxygen dissociation curve to the right [31]. As shown in Figure 1, the changes in the rheologic properties of blood induced by dextran perfusion are quite similar in normotensive subjects and hypertensive patients.

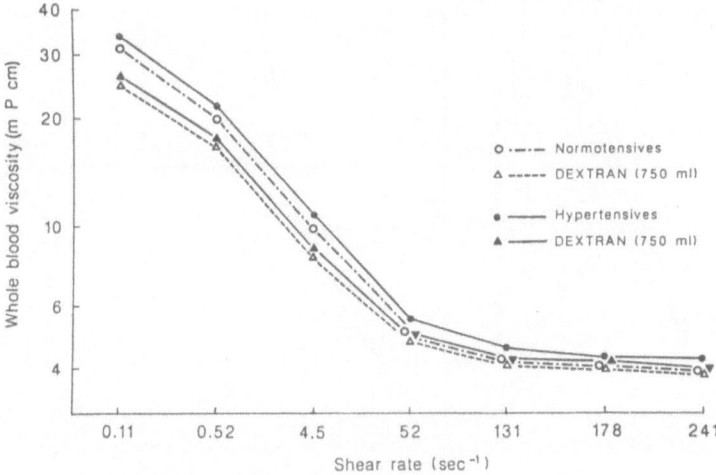

Figure 1. Whole blood viscosity before and after dextran infusion in normotensive (O △) and hypertensive (● ▲) subjects. [Personal data]

Since the pharmacological action of dextran does not seem to modify significantly cardio-circulatory parameters in normal subjects and hypertensives, this plasma expander has been widely used to evaluate the pumping function of the heart in hypertensives.

Changes in cardiac output following dextran infusion

Following dextran infusion, the filling pressure of the heart, cardiac output and the cardiac index are increased to a comparable extent in normal subjects and hypertensives (Figure 2). In most cases, the increase in cardiac output is moderate, rising by about $+34.7 \pm 8.6\%$ in normal subjects and by about $+42.8 \pm 18\%$ in hypertensives. The increase in cardiac output is related to an increase in stroke volume, and also to a slight acceleration of heart rate (Figure 3). A positive correlation is consistently observed between changes in pulmonary wedge pressure (PWP) and changes in cardiac output during dextran infusion. The curves obtained from pooled personal data are shown in Figure 4. A linear correlation is observed between PWP and cardiac index both in normal subjects and hypertensive patients. The slopes of these curves are similar. The pulmonary wedge pressure-stroke index relationship is curvilinear (Figure 4) and is of similar shape in both groups. The stroke work index increases in proportion to the PWP in both groups (Figure 4). In hypertensives, the plateau of the curves is at about $83.2 \pm 28 \, \text{gr} \cdot \text{min} \cdot \text{m}^{-2}$. However,

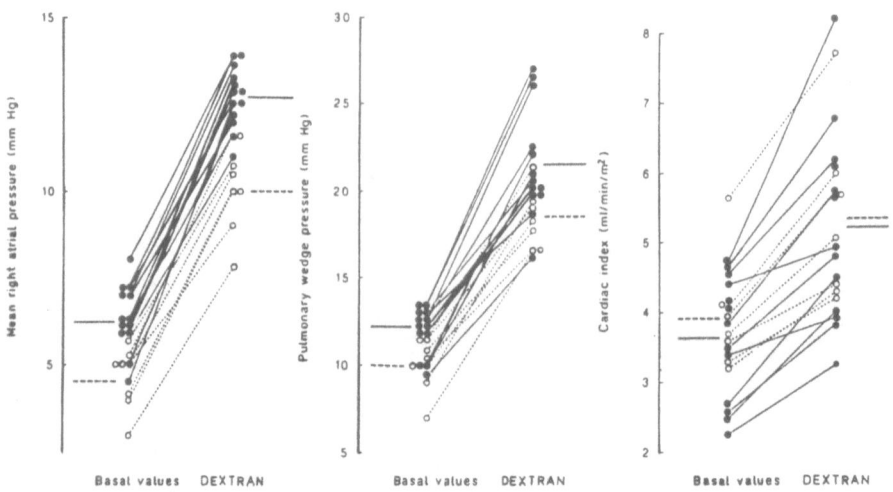

Figure 2. Changes in mean right atrial and pulmonary wedge pressures, and cardiac index, in normotensive (O) and hypertensive subjects (●). [Personal data]

ventricular function curves in human should be considered as 'effective ventricular curves' since the conditions under which the heart works during volume expansion are not constant, and reflex modifications of the peripheral circulation act to modify the curves. The shape of the ventricular function curve reflects the dependence of ventricular performance on preload, whereas shifts in the ventricular function curves can be produced by changes in contractile state, afterload or ventricular compliance.[32]. In essential hypertensive patients, the shape of the ventricular function curves is unchanged, but a

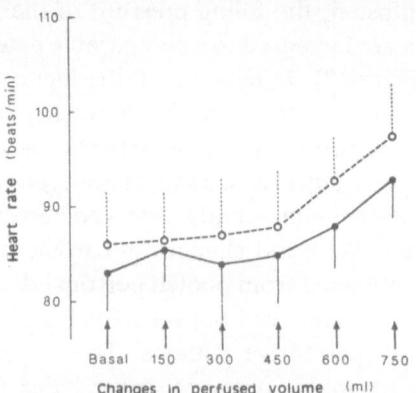

Figure 3. Changes in heart rate during blood volume expansion in normotensive (O) and hypertensive (●) subjects. [Personal data]

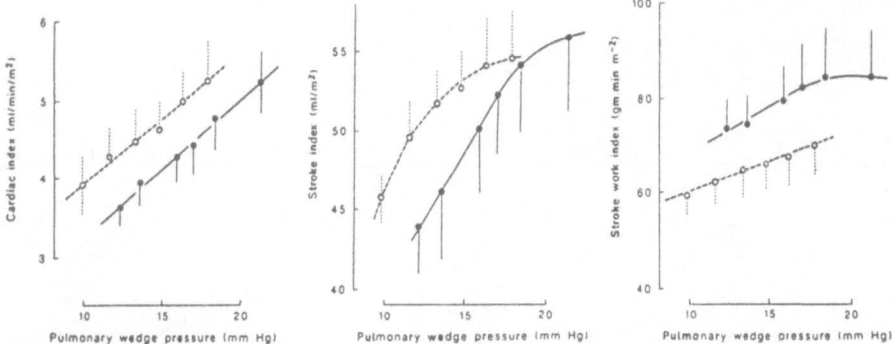

Figure 4. Relationship between pulmonary wedge pressure and cardiac index, and stroke index and stroke work index in normotensive (○) and hypertensive (●) subjects. [Personal data]

rightward shift in pressure/cardiac index or pressure/stroke index curves is observed. The initial linear part of these curves has the same slope in normotensives and hypertensives, and the plateau of the pressure/stroke index curves is similar in the two groups (Figure 4). Thus, the shift of the ventricular function curves is more likely to be related to the difference in afterload and/or in ventricular compliance than to changes in contractile state [33]. Finally, acute volume load seems to induce similar cardiac adjustments in normotensive controls and patients with sustained essential hypertension. Ventricular systolic performance must be considered as normal in uncomplicated essential hypertension in man.

Changes in blood pressure and vascular resistance following acute blood volume expansion

The responses of systemic arterial pressure and vascular resistance are quite different in essential hypertensive subjects and controls. Acute volume expansion has been shown to result in a small increase in arterial and/or pulse pressure in normal humans [4, 8, 9, 10, 12, 14, 15], or no change at all [11, 17], depending on the infusion rate and type of fluid used. Dextran infusion increases systolic and mean blood pressure in normotensive subjects but not in essential hypertensives (Figure 5). Furthermore, an inverse relationship is usually observed between the resting value of the blood pressure, and blood pressure response to volume load (Figure 6). Acute volume load has been shown to have no effect on arterial pressure in essential hypertensive patients [17, 18]. Experimental studies in animals have shown that when the baseline level of arterial pressure was relatively low, blood volume expansion tended to

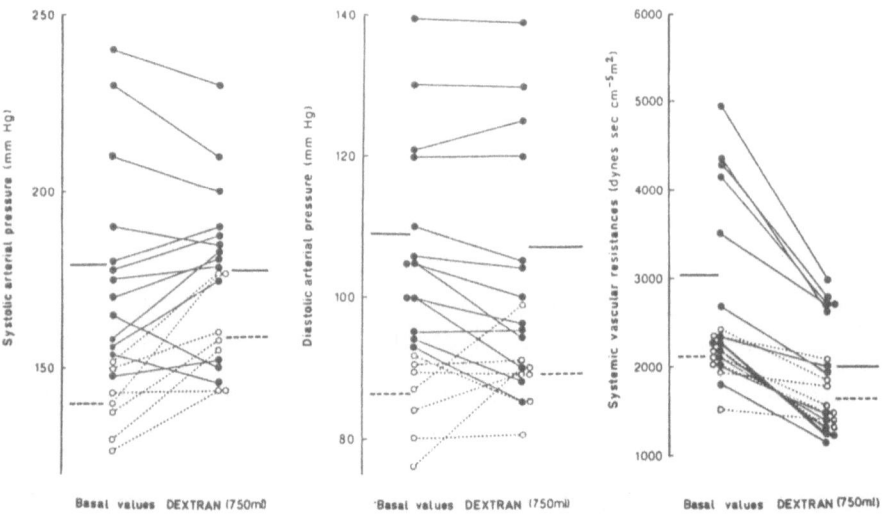

Figure 5. Changes in systemic arterial pressure and systemic vascular resistance during blood volume expansion with dextran in normotensive (O) and hypertensive subjects (●). [Personal data]

result in hypertension [34, 35, 36], whereas in anesthetised preparations with high blood pressure, arterial pressure remained unchanged [37] or actually fell [38].

As shown in Figure 6, the level of the prevailing arterial pressure prior to dextran infusion is a contributory factor in the different responses observed in controls and hypertensives. The mechanisms controlling the arterial pressure variations during blood volume load indicate progressively increased efficiency in hypertensives, the maximum value being achieved in patients with the highest basal blood pressure and highest initial systemic vascular resistance (Figure 6). This surprising result is difficult to explain. Studies in man have shown that the baroreceptor control of heart rate is reset in hypertension, and that its sensitivity is reduced [39, 40]. On the other hand, Mancia et al. [40] have shown that carotid baroreceptor influence on blood pressure control is unchanged in human hypertension. On the contrary, the depressor response to an increase in carotid transmural pressure was minimal in normotensive subjects, and increased progressively to achieve its maximal value in severe hypertension, as observed during blood volume load.

The unchanged or increased sensitivity of arterial pressure and vascular resistance control in hypertensive patients could be due to an increase in the inhibitory influence of low-pressure baroreflexes [24]. However, the similar changes in plasma renin activity and plasma catecholamine levels induced by alterations in central blood volume and/or pressure in normotensive subjects and patients with sustained essential hypertension do not support a major role

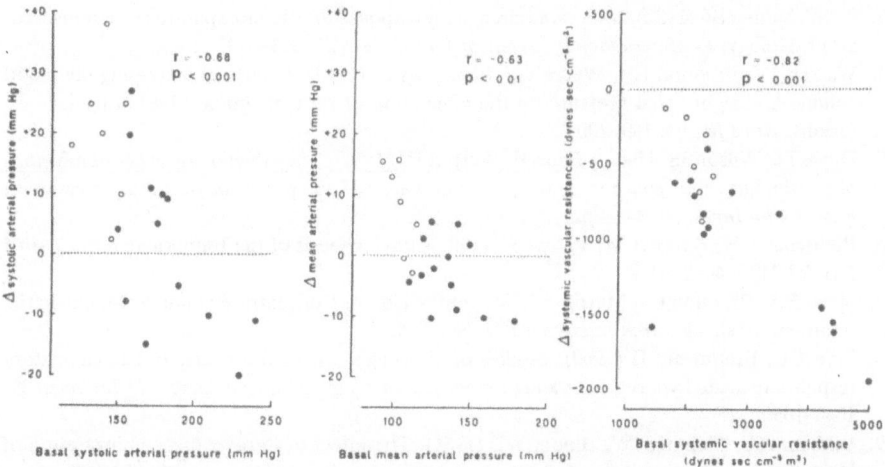

Figure 6. Correlation between arterial pressure and systemic vascular resistance changes during blood volume expansion, and between basal values of arterial pressure and systemic vascular resistance, in normotensive (O) and hypertensive subjects (●). [Personal data]

for this mechanism [25, 26, 41]. On the other hand, Folkow et al. [42] showed that in hypertension, the increase in systemic resistance is largely related to an increase in the arteriolar wall-to-lumen ratio, making the change in resistance in response to a given alteration in sympathetic outflow greater than that in normal subjects. Indeed, changes in peripheral resistance are amplified in hypertensive patients, and this 'amplification' is proportional to the initial value of vascular resistance (Figure 6). Such observations suggest that the preserved or increased vasodilatation observed in essential hypertensives could be related to a 'non-specific' amplification of reflex response, related to structural (or functional) changes of the vascular effector.

In conclusion, there is no basic difference in the integrated cardiovascular response to acute volume expansion in essential hypertensives, compared with normotensive subjects. The greater vasodilatatory response in essential hypertensives is related to a higher resting arterial tone. The pump function of the heart is normal, or even increased, in patients with sustained essential hypertension.

References

1. Guyton AC, Coleman TG, Granger HJ (1972): Circulation: Overall regulation. *Ann Rev Physiol* 34: 13–46.
2. Gauer OH, Henry JP (1976): Neurohumoral control of plasma volume in cardiovascular physiology, II. *International Review of Physiology.* 9: 145–190.

3. Sit SP, Vatner SF (1982): Integrated circulatory response to volume expansion in cardiovascular physiology, IV. *International Review of Physiology.* 26: 323–354.

4. Warren JV, Brannon EB, Weens HS, Stead EA Jr (1948): Effects of increasing the blood volume and right atrial pressure on the circulation of normal subjects by intravenous infusions. *Am J Med* 4: 193–200.

5. Doyle JT, Wilson JS, Harvey Estes E, Warren JV (1951): The effect of intravenous infusions of physiologic saline solution on the pulmonary arterial and pulmonary capillary pressure in man. *J Clin Invest* 30: 345–352.

6. Boettcher DH, Zimpfer M, Vatner SF (1982): Phylogenesis of the Bainbridge reflex. *Am J Physiol* 242: 244–246.

7. Stead EA, Brannon ES, Merrill AJ, Warren JV (1946): Concentrated human albumin in the treatment of shock. *Arch Intern Med* 77: 564–575.

8. Frye RL, Braunwald E (1960): Studies on Starling's law of the heart, I: The circulatory response to acute hypervolemia and its modification by ganglionic blockade. *J Clin Invest* 39: 1043–1050.

9. Witham AC, Fleming JW, Bloom WL (1951): The effect of intravenous administration of Dextran on cardiac output and other circulatory dynamics. *J Clin Invest* 30: 897–902.

10. Fleming JW, Bloom WL (1957): Further observations on the hemodynamic effect of plasma volume expansion by dextran. *J Clin Invest* 36: 1233–1238.

11. Schnabel TG, Eliash H, Thomasson B, Werko L (1959): The effect of experimentally induced hypervolemia on cardiac function in normal subjects and patients with mitral stenosis. *J Clin Invest* 38: 117–137.

12. Freitas FM, Faraco EZ, Azevedo DF, Zaduchliver J, Lewin I (1965): Behavior of normal pulmonary circulation during changes of total blood volume in man. *J Clin Invest* 44: 366–378.

13. Giuntini C, Maseri A, Bianchi R (1966): Pulmonary vascular distensibility and lung compliance as modified by Dextran infusion and subsequent atropine injection in normal subjects. *J Clin Invest* 45: 1770–1789.

14. Cohn JN, Luria MH, Daddario RC, Tristani FE (1967): Studies in clinical shock and hypotension, V: Hemodynamic effects of Dextran. *Circulation* 35: 316–326.

15. Sanghvi VR, Khaja F, Mark AL, Parker JD (1972): Effects of blood volume expansion on left ventricular hemodynamics in man. *Circulation* 46: 780–787.

16. Echt M, Duweling J, Gauer OH, lange L (1974): Effective compliance of the total vascular bed and the intrathoracic compartment derived from changes in central venous pressure induced by volume changes in man. *Circ Res* 34: 61–68.

17. London GM, Safar ME, Simon AC, Alexandre JM, Levenson JA (1978): Total effective compliance, cardiac output and fluid volumes in essential hypertension. *Circulation* 57: 995–1000.

18. Safar ME, London GM, Levenson JA, Simon AC, Chau NP (1979): Rapid Dextran infusion in essential hypertension. *Hypertension* 1: 615–623.

19. Ulrych M, Hofman J, Hejl Z (1964): Cardiac and renal hyperresponsiveness to acute plasma volume expansion in hypertension. *Am Heart J* 68: 193–198.

20. Lund-Johansen P (1967): Hemodynamics in early essential hypertension. *Acta Med Scand* 183 (suppl): 482.

21. Julius S, Pascual AV, Sannerstedt R, Mitchell C (1971): Relationship between cardiac output and peripheral resistance in borderline hypertension. *Circulation* 43: 382–389.

22. Bevegard BS, Castenfors J, Lindblad LE (1977): Effects of changes in blood volume distribution on circulatory variables and plasma renin activity in man. *Acta Physiol Scand* 99: 237–245.

23. Esler M, Zweifler A, Randall O, Julius S, De Quattro V (1978): The determinants of plasma renin activity in essential hypertension. *Ann Intern Med* 88: 746–752.

24. Mark AL, Kerber RE (1982): Augmentation of cardiopulmonary baroreflex control of forearm vascular resistance in borderline hypertension. *Hypertension* 4: 39–46.
25. London GM, Levenson JA, Safar ME, Simon AC, Guerin AP, Payen D (1983): Hemodynamic effects of head-down tilt in normal subjects and sustained hypertensive patients. *Am J Physiol* 245: H 194–202.
26. London GM, Guerin AP, Bouthier JD, London AM, Safar ME (1985): Cardiopulmonary blood volume and plasma renin activity in normal and hypertensive humans. *Am J Physiol* 249: H 807–813.
27. Fowler NO, Franch RH, Bloom WL (1956): Hemodynamic effects of anemia with and without plasma volume expansion. *Circ Res* 4: 319–324.
28. Bondurant S, Hickam JB, Isley JK (1957): Pulmonary and circulatory effects of acute pulmonary vascular engorgement in normal subjects. *J Clin Invest* 36: 59–66.
29. Messmer K, Sunder-Plasmann L (1974): Hemodilution. *Progr Surg* 13: 208–217.
30. Guyton AC, Richardson TQ (1961): Effect of hematocrit on venous return. *Circ Res* 9: 157–163.
31. Messmer K, Goernandt L, Jesch F, Sinagowitz E, Sunder-Plassman L, Kessler M (1973): Oxygen transport and tissue oxygenation during hemodilution with Dextran. *Adv Exp Med Biol* 37B: 669–677.
32. Parmley WW, Talbot L (1979): Heart as a pump, in: Berne RM (ed), *Handbook of Physiology,* Section 1. The Cardiovascular System, Vol 1: *The Heart,* pp 429–460. Bethesda: American Physiological Society.
33. Noresson E, Ricksten SE, Hallback-Nordlander M, Thoren P (1979): Performance of the hypertrophied left ventricule in spontaneously hypertensive rats. *Acta Physiol Scand* 107: 1–8.
34. Gilmore JP, Weisfeld ML (1965): Contribution of intravascular receptors to the renal responses following intravascular volume expansion. *Circ Res* 17: 144–154.
35. Weaver LC (1977): Cardiopulmonary sympathetic afferent influences on renal nerve activity. *Am J Physiol* 233: H 592–599.
36. Vatner SF, Boettcher DH (1978): Regulation of cardiac output by stroke volume and heart rate in conscious dogs. *Circ Res* 42: 557–561.
37. Bishop VS, Lombardi F, Malliani A, Pagani M, Recordati G (1976): Reflex sympathetic tachycardia during intravenous infusion in chronic spinal cats. *Am J Physiol* 230: 25–29.
38. Thames MD, Abboud FM (1979): Interaction of somatic and cardiopulmonary receptors in control of renal circulation. *Am J Physiol* 237: H 560–565.
39. Gribbin B, Pickering TG, Sleight P, Peto R (1971): Effect of age and high blood pressure on baroreflex sensitivity in man. *Circ Res* 29: 424–431.
40. Mancia G, Ludbrock J, Ferrari A, Gregorini L, Zanchetti A (1978): Baroreceptor reflexes in human hypertension. *Circ Res* 43: 170–177.
41. Grassi G, Gavazzi C, Ramirez A, Sabadini E, Turolo L, Mancia R (1984): Role of cardiopulmonary receptors in reflex control of renin release in man. *J of Hypertension* 2 (suppl 3): 263–265.
42. Folkow B, Hallback M, Lundgreen Y, Siertsson R, Weiss L (1973): Importance of adaptive changes in vascular design for establishment of primary hypertension, studied in man and in spontaneously hypertensive rats. *Circ Res* 32 (suppl 1): 2–15.

18. Systolic function and inotropism of the heart in borderline and sustained essential hypertension

JAMES CONWAY

Left ventricular hypertrophy and cardiac performance

Increased aortic impedance provides a powerful stimulus to cardiac hypertrophy [71, 99] and the association of left ventricular hypertrophy with hypertension in both human and experimental hypertension has long been recognised [8, 20, 37, 46, 51, 61, 64, 87, 95, 103]. This hypertrophy compensates for the additional stress imposed on the heart by the arterial pressure and as the increased wall thickness develops it matches the increased work load so that the wall stress in relation to wall thickness is restored to normal or slightly reduced levels [1, 12, 36, 73, 77, 79, 87, 92, 97, 98]. End-diastolic volume remains normal or perhaps slightly diminished [17, 39, 62, 68]. The force of cardiac contraction then is increased by myocardial hypertrophy but the adaptive processes ensure that cardiac output remains normal [3, 7, 10, 24, 33, 52, 65, 66, 69, 86, 106] although the external indices of contraction such as systolic time intervals (pre-ejection period, ejection time) may be increased in duration [19, 32, 44, 56, 81, 108].

While overall function at rest is well maintained in hypertension, under the increased stress of exercise or raised arterial pressure, stroke volume and cardiac output may become inadequate [3, 4, 9, 32, 72, 98, 99] indicating a reduced cardiac reserve. This can also be demonstrated experimentally where it can be shown that the Starling curve is shifted to the right [28, 38, 77].

The suggestion has been made that the compensatory hypertrophy may not be 'turned off' properly when the wall stress has matched the augmented strain. Excessive hypertrophy would then lead to a substantially lower wall stress and this would be manifested by an increased inotropic state [9, 17, 98]. This suggestion has not been supported by experimental studies [87, 105].

It was thought that a phase of increased myocardial contractility (Dp/dt 40) occurred in conscious dogs as hypertension developed [41]. However, in these

M.E. Safar & F. Fouad-Tarazi (eds.), The heart in hypertension.
© *1989 Kluwer Academic Publishers, Dordrecht –*

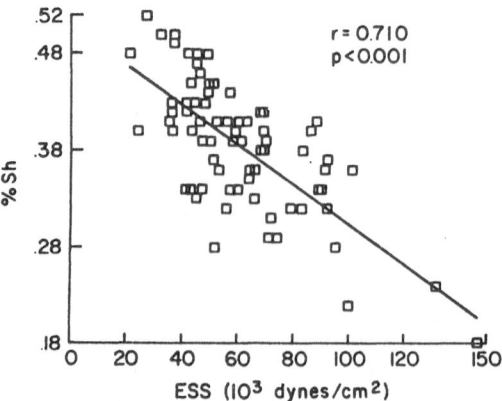

Figure 1. The relationship established by echocardiography between end-systolic left ventricular wall stress (ESS) and percent shortening (% sh) in 74 hypertensive subjects. From Abi et al. [1] with permission. This demonstrates that ventricular performance is strongly dependant upon afterload in hypertension.

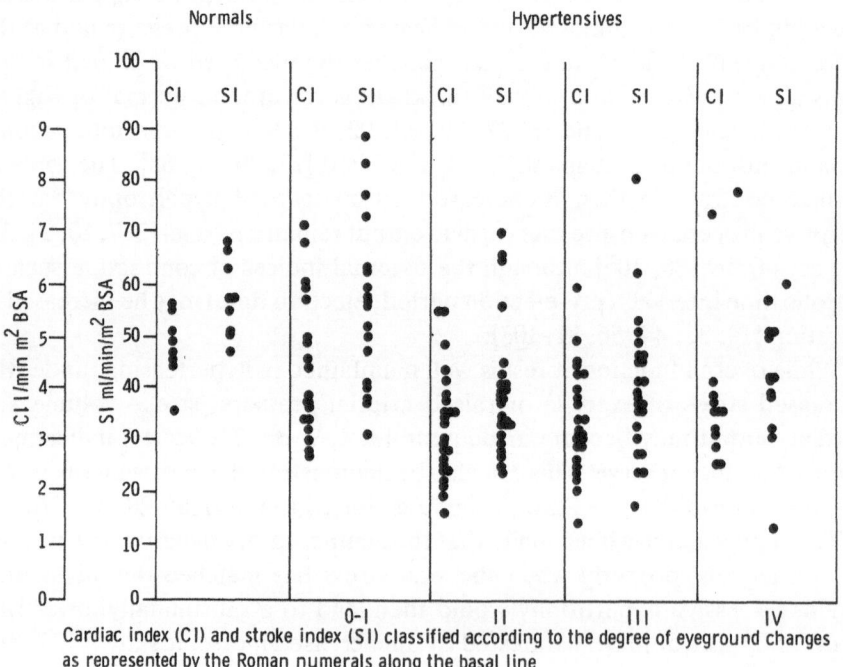

Figure 2. A cross-sectional study of cardiac output in different levels of severity as depicted by fundal change. This early study shows that subjects with established hypertension have a normal cardiac output but when the condition is more severe performance declines. It was further shown that in subjects with the mildest hypertension (without fundal change) cardiac output varies considerably but the mean in higher than it is in established hypertension. From Varnanskas [106].

experiments pre-load and after-load conditions could not be controlled. In anaesthetised preparations, where this can be done, maximum Dp/dt is higher in hypertensive animals but when contractility is related to wall thickness the contractility is normal [12, 53]. It seems therefore that in experimental hypertension a phase of increased myocardial contractility cannot be demonstrated.

Cardiac performance is critically affected by afterload [1, 38] (Figure 1) and in experimental hypertension over a period of time a decline in left ventricular function becomes evident [23, 28, 38, 64]. When hypertrophy is extreme, the transport of oxygen to myocardial cells may become compromised. Abnormalities in diastolic function also occur. These will be discussed elsewhere in this volume (editor note). Diminished contractility is also probably associated with collagen deposition around the myocardial fibers [91]. The same thing appears to occur in human hypertension. With time or increased severity of hypertension and contractility falls and with it stroke volume declines and cardiac dilatation emerges [50, 66, 67, 96, 99, 106, 107, 112]. (Figure 2) Sustained hypertrophy appears therefore to trigger processes that lead to the eventual deterioration in cardiac function. Therefore prevention of hypertrophy is an important goal of therapy in hypertension.

While the physiology of the compensated state is well understood, closer examination of the heart in hypertension reveals a rather more complicated situation. It had been pointed out by Tarazi's group that asymmetrical hypertrophy is common in hypertension suggesting a picture more akin to the cardiomyopathies. Hypertrophy may be inappropriate to the level of pressure and the stimulus to it may be something other than the pressure load. The relationship between blood pressure level and left ventricular hypertrophy is not as close as one would expect if hypertension were the chief stimulus for its development. The incidence of left ventricular hypertrophy, whether detected by electrocardiography or by echocardiography, is surprisingly low [13, 14, 15, 39, 94] and the correlation between blood pressure level and left ventricular hypertrophy only a loose one (r = 0.4 approx) [1, 16, 17, 30, 82, 44, 87]. The correlation can be improved when ambulatory blood pressure monitoring is used to estimate the blood pressure level but the correlation is still low (r = 0.6) [17, 18, 78]. A substantial proportion of subjects with mild labile hypertension have echocardiographic evidence for left ventricular hypertrophy [16, 81] and it can be found in adolescents with minimal elevation of blood pressure [89, 90]. This situation resembles the findings in spontaneously hypertensive rats in which left ventricular hypertrophy can be shown to be present at birth when blood pressure is minimally elevated above that in normotensive controls [38, 75, 92, 110].

Hyperdynamic circulation

There has long been evidence for the presence of a hyperdynamic circulation in a substantial proportion of hypertensive subjects. These are usually young mild and labile hypertensives [5, 6, 21, 24, 26, 29, 47, 65, 67, 69, 70, 83, 84, 104, 106, 109]. (Figure 2) In these subjects systolic time intervals are shortened [43, 81] and heart rate increased [29, 32, 52, 54] giving a haemodynamic pattern very much like that seen with mental stimulation [10, 11]. In younger subjects this may present clinically as isolated systolic hypertension [2]. There is also an increase in oxygen consumption in some labile hypertensives which correlates with increased cardiac output [47, 86]. By using the appropriate blocking agents increased sympathetic activity and reduced vagal tone [48, 49] has been demonstrated and it has been suggested that some patients with this condition represents a hyperbeta-adrenergic state since the haemodynamic pattern is very similar to that seen after the infusion of isoprenaline [31]. It has not been

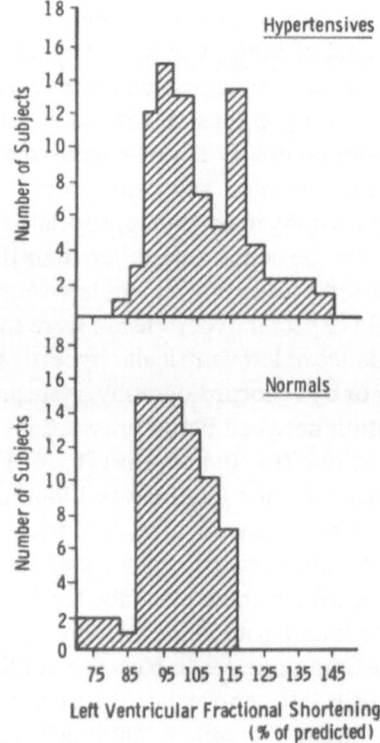

Figure 3. Frequence of increased left ventricular fractional shortens in a group of hypertensive as compared to normal subjects. Note the double hum in the distribution of LV fractional shortening with approximately 23% of patients having increased contractility. Redrawn from Lutas et al. [68] with permission.

easy however to demonstrate an increase in catecholamines in the blood in hypertensives. Though it can be seen in a group of younger male hypertensives [22, 34, 35, 70]. The excretion of noradrenaline tends to be higher in patients with established hypertension and this increase has been correlated with left ventricular muscle mass [40, 45]. The integrated activity of the sympathetic system in young hypertensives appears to be directed preferentially to the heart and the kidneys since there is evidence for increased noradrenaline spillover to these organs [22].

Echocardiographic studies have also confirmed the increase in contractility in some young hypertensive subjects [88, 111]. In a large study of 87 individuals it was shown that 23% of hypertensive subjects showed an increase in left ventricular fractional shortening which was greater than that seen in normal subjects (Figure 3). Cardiac index, estimated from echocardiography, was also elevated. In this study, as in many others, the increase in cardiac output in these mild hypertensives is associated with the low peripheral resistance [68].

There is ample evidence then for increased cardiac contractility in mild hypertension. This is associated with evidence for increased sympathetic activity not only to the heart but to the capacitance system; there is a reduced compliance of the veins and a redistribution of blood from the periphery to the central circulation which increases cardiopulmonary blood volume [63, 69, 80, 82, 84, 102] and therefore preload.

Cardiogenic hypertension?

The increased myocardial contractility and cardiac output in mild hypertension cannot be accounted for an increase in plasma volume but the pre-load is elevated slightly by diversion of blood from the peripheral veins to the thorax leading to a small increase in end-diastolic volume [68, 80, 81]. In addition to increased pre-load as a stimulus to increased output, sympathetic activity shifts Starling's curve to the left [80, 101, 102] leading to a higher output at all end-diastolic pressure.

The question therefore arises as to whether the heart itself could be *causally* involved in hypertension [101]. Cardiac function ordinarily reacts to changes in pre-load and after-load produced by the central stimulation mental and physical activity. For a variety of reasons isolated cardiac stimulation would not in itself be expected to increase blood pressure or peripheral resistance. However experimental evidence shows this is not the case. Prolonged stimulation of cardiac sympathetic nerves in conscious dogs leads to hypertension [60]. Furthermore prolonged infusion of dobutamine into the left coronary artery leads to hypertension in which there is a transient increase in cardiac output to be followed by an increase in peripheral resistance [58] (Figure 4). This

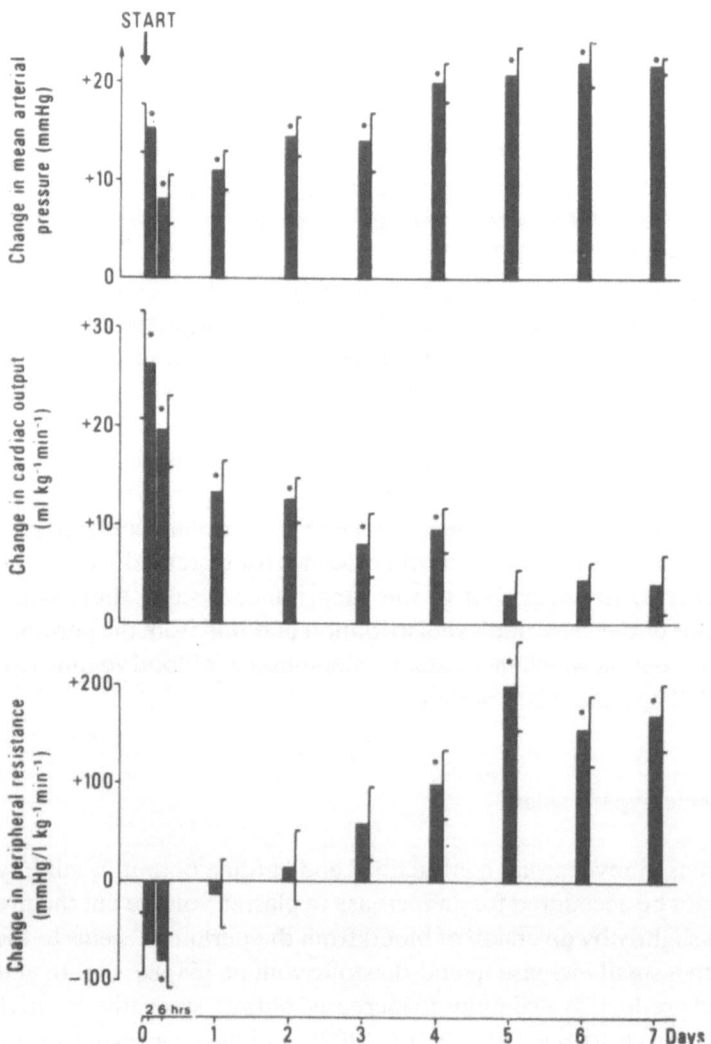

Figure 4. The haemodynamic changes which result from a sustained intra-coronary perfusion of dobutamine. Note that arterial pressure rises immediately. Cardiac output is elevated initially but it falls towards the control level on the 5th day. Peripheral resistance falls initially but after 4 days is above control. From Liard et al. [58] with permission.

hypertension can be prevented by beta-blockade [59]. Sympathetic stimulation then, particularly if it is directed to the heart, can increase cardiac performance and lead to hypertension with increased resistance with both cardiac and vascular hypertrophy [52].

In addition to its direct effect noradrenaline has an independent action as a trophic hormone, and the infusion of sub pressor doses of noradrenaline leads to ventricular hypertrophy [55]. The sympathetic system is also essential for the hypertrophy of physical training to occur [76]. Noradrenaline may therefore be responsible for inappropriate hypertrophy seen in a proportion of hypertensives, particularly those with inappropriate hypertrophy in relation to their blood pressure. Hypertrophy therefore results partly as a reaction to the stimulus of raised pressure and partly from trophic influences of noradrenaline. It should also be mentioned that angiotensin can be an independent stimulus to hypertrophy [93]. In the face of multiple stimuli it is not surprising that cardiac hypertrophy should correlate poorly with blood pressure in hypertension and it can be present when pressure is minimally elevated. Control of blood pressure with specific agents can prevent or reverse the hypertrophy, an effect which is not closely related to the achieved pressure [27].

Conclusion

The force of cardiac contraction increases with the development of hypertension. This is brought about by cardiac hypertrophy which matches the increased load with the result that ventricular wall stress remains normal as is cardiac output. With the passage of time or the increase in severity of hypertension cardiac contractility decreases, cardiac dilatation occurs and stroke volume falls.

In a proportion of young mild hypertensives there is evidence for enhanced sympathetic stimulation which leads to increased contractility and cardiac output. Trophic effects of noradrenaline and perhaps angiotensin, can then independently induce cardiac hypertrophy. It can be shown experimentally that isolated cardiac stimulation can lead to hypertension in which there is transient increase in cardiac output with a later rise in peripheral resistance.

The heart itself may therefore be aetiologically involved in development in hypertension in some individuals.

References

1. Abi-Samra F, Fouad FM, Tarazi RC (1983): Determinants of left ventricular hypertrophy and function in hypertensive patients: An echocardiographic study. *Am J Med* 75: 26–33.
2. Adamopoulus PN, Chrysanthakopoulis SG, Frohlich ED (1975): Systolic hypertension: Nonhomogeneous diseases. *Am J Cardiol* 36: 697–701.
3. Amery AS, Julius S, Whitlock LS, Conway J (1967): Influence of hypertension response to exercise. *Circulation* 36: 231–237.
4. Averill DB, Ferario CM, Tarazi RC, et al. (1976): Cardiac performance in rats with renal hypertension. *Circ Res* 38: 280–288.

5. Bello CT, Sevy RW, Harakal C (1965): Varying hemodynamic patterns in essential hypertension. *Am J Med Sci* 250: 24–35.
6. Bello CT, Sevy RW, Harakal C, Hillyer PN (1967): Relationship between clinical severity of disease and hemodynamic patterns in essential hypertension. *Am J Med Sci* 253: 194–208.
7. Blumgart HL, Weiss S (1927): Studies on the velocity of blood flow, IV: The velocity of blood flow and its relation to other aspects of the circulations in patients with arteriosclerosis and in patients with arterial hypertension. *J Clin Invest* 4: 173–197.
8. Bolomey AA, Michie AJ, Michie C, Breed ES, Schreiner GE, Lauson HD (1949): Simultaneous measurement of effective renal blood flow and cardiac output in resting normal subjects and patients with essential hypertension. *J Clin Invest* 28: 10–12.
9. Borer JS, Jason M, Devereux RB, Pickering T, Erle S, Laragh JH (1983): Left ventricular performance in the hypertensive patient: Exercise-mediated non-invasive separation of loading influences from intrinsic muscle dysfunction. *Chest* 83: 314–316.
10. Brod J, Fencl V, Hejl Z, Jirka J (1959): Circulatory changes underlying blood pressure elevation during acute emotional stress (mental arithmetic) in normotensive and hypertensive subjects. *Clin Sci* 18: 269–279.
11. Brod J, Fencl V, Hejl Z, Jirka J, Ulrych M (1962): General and regional hemodynamic pattern underlying essential hypertension. *Clin Sci* 23: 339–349.
12. Broughton A, Korner PI (1983): Basal and maximal inotropic state in renal hypertensive dogs with cardiac hypertrophy. *Am J Physiol* 245 (*Heart Circ Physiol* 14): H 33–41.
13. Carr AA, Prisant LM, Watkins LO (1985): Detection of hypertensive left ventricular hypertrophy. *Hypertension* 7: 948–954.
14. Cohen A, Hagan AD, Watkins J, Mitas J, Schvartzman M, Mazzoleni A, Cohen IM, Warren SE, Vioeweg WVR (1981): Clinical correlates in hypertensive patients with left ventricular hypertrophy diagnosed with echocardiography. *Am J Cardiol* 47: 335–341.
15. Corea L, Bentivoglio M, Verdecchia P (1983): Echocardiographic left ventricular hypertrophy as related to arterial pressure and plasma norepinephrine concentration in arterial hypertension: Reversal by atenolol treatment. *Hypertension* 5: 837–843.
16. Devereux RB, Pickering TG, Alderman MH, Chien S, Borer JS, Laragh JH (1987): Left ventricular hypertrophy in hypertension. Prevalence and relationship to pathophysiologic variables. *Hypertension* 9 (suppl II): II 53–60.
17. Devereux RB, Savage DD, Sachs I, Laragh JH (1983): Relation of hemodynamic load to left ventricular hypertrophy and performance in hypertension. *Am J Cardiol* 51: 171–176.
18. Drayer JIM, Gardin JM, Brewer DD, Weber MA (1987): Disparate relationships between blood pressure and left ventricular mass in patients with and without left ventricular hypertrophy. *Hypertension* 9 (suppl II): II 61–64.
19. Dodek A, Burg JR, Kloster FR (1975): Systolic time intervals in chronic hypertension: Alterations and response to treatment. *Chest* 68: 51–55.
20. Dunn FG, Chandraratna P, De Cavalho JGR, Basta LL, Frohlich ED (1977): Pathophysiologic assessment of hypertensive heart disease with echocardiography. *Am J Cardiol* 39: 789–795.
21. Eich RH, Cuddy RP, Smulyan H, Lyons RH (1966): Hemodynamics in labile hypertension: A follow up study. *Circulation* 34: 299–307.
22. Esler M, Jennings G, Biriano B, Lambert G, Hasking (1986): Mechanism of elevated plasma noradrenaline in the course of essential hypertension. *J Cardiovasc Pharmacol* 8 (suppl): 539–544.
23. Ferrario CM, Spech MM, Tarazi RC, Doi Y (1979): Cardiac pumping ability in rats with experimental renal and genetic hypertension. *Am J Cardiol* 44: 979–985.
24. Finkielman S, Worcel M, Agrest A (1965): Hemodynamic patterns in essential hypertension. *Circulation* 31: 356–368.

25. Folkow B (1982): Physiological aspects of primary hypertension. *Physiol Rev* 62: 347–504.
26. Fouad FM, Tarazi RC, Dustan HP, Bravo EL (1978): Hemodynamics of essential hypertension in young subjects. *Am Heart J* 96: 646–654.
27. Fouad FM, Nakashima Y, Tarazi RC, Salcedo EE (1982): Reversal of left ventricular hypertrophy in hypertension treated with methyldopa. *Am J Cardiol* 49: 795–801.
28. Friberg P (1985): Structural and functional adaptation in the rat myocardium and coronary vascular bed caused by changes in pressure and volume load. *Acta Physiol Scand* 124 (suppl 540).
29. Frohlich ED, Kozul VJ, Tarazi RC, Dustan HP (1970): Physiological comparison of labile and essential hypertension. *Circ Res* 26: 1–55.
30. Frohlich ED, Tarazi RC (1979): Is arterial pressure the sole factor responsible for hypertensive cardiac hypertrophy? *Am J Cardiol* 44: 959–963.
31. Frohlich ED, Tarazi RC, Dustan HP (1969): Hyperdynamic beta-adrenergic circulatory state: Increased beta-receptor responsiveness. *Arch Intern Med* 123: 1–7.
32. Frohlich ED, Tarazi RC, Dustan HP (1971): Clinical physiological correlations in the development of hypertensive heart disease. *Circulation* 44: 446–455.
33. Glazer GA, Lediashova GA (1975): Changes in general hemodynamics and renal function during exercise in patients with arterial hypertension. *Cor Vasa* 17: 1–13.
34. Goldstein DS (1981): Plasma norepinephrine in essential hypertension: A study of the studies. *Hypertension* 3: 48–52.
35. Goldstein DS (1983): Plasma catecholamines and essential hypertension: An analytical review. *Hypertension* 5: 86–89.
36. Grossman W, Jones D, McLaurin LP (1975): Wall stress and patterns of hypertrophy in the human left ventricle. *J Clin Invest* 56: 56–64.
37. Hallback-Nordlander M (1980): Left/right ventricular weight ratio: An estimate of 'cardiac adaptation to hypertension'. *Clin Sci* 59: 415s–417s.
38. Hallback-Nordlander M, Noresson E, Thoien P (1979): Hemodynamic consequences of left ventricular hypertrophy in spontaneously hypertensive rats. *Am J Cardiol* 44: 986–1001.
39. Hammond IW, Devereux RB, Alderman MH, Lutas EM, Spitzer MC, Crowley JS, Laragh JH (1986): The prevalence and correlates of echocardiographic left ventricular hypertrophy among employed patients with uncomplicated hypertension. *J Am Coll Cardiol* 7: 639–650.
40. Hartford M, Wikstrand J, Wallentin I, Ljungman S, Wilhelmsen L, Berland G (1983): Left ventricular mass in middle-aged men. *Clin & Exper Hyper – Theory and Practice* A5 (9): 1429–1451.
41. Hawthorne EW, Hinds JE, Crawford WJ, Tearney RJ (1974): Left ventricular myocardial contractility during the first week of renal hypertension in conscious instrumented dogs. *Circ Res* 34/35 (suppl I): 223–234.
42. Hofman A, Ellison RC, Newburger J, Miettinen O (1982): Blood pressure and haemodynamics in teenagers. *Br Heart J* 48: 377–380.
43. Ibrahim MM, Tarazi RC, Dustan HP, Bravo EL (1974): Cardiogenic factor in hypertension. *Am Heart J* 88: 724–732.
44. Inoue K, Smulyan H, Young GM, Grierson AL, Eich RH (1973): Left ventricular function in essential hypertension. *Am J Cardiol* 32: 264–270.
45. Izzo Jr JL, Smith RJ, Larrabee PS, Kallay MC (1987): Plasma norepinephrine and age as determinants of systemic hemodynamics in men with established essential hypertension. *Hypertension* 9: 415–419.
46. Jones RS (1953): The weight of the heart and its chambers in hypertensive cardiovascular disease with and without failure. *Circulation* 7: 357–369.
47. Julius S, Conway J (1968): Hemodynamic studies in patients with borderline blood pressure elevation. *Circulation* 38: 282–288.

48. Julius S, Esler M (1975): Autonomic nervous cardiovascular regulation in borderline hypertension. *Am J Cardiol* 36: 685–696.
49. Julius S, Pascual AV, London R (1971): Role of parasympathetic inhibition in the hyperkinetic form of borderline hypertension. *Circulation* 44: 413–418.
50. Kannel WB, Castelli WP, McNamara PM, McKee PA, Feinleib M (1972): Role of blood pressure in the development of congestive heart failure. *N Engl J Med* 287: 781–787.
51. Karliner JS, Williams D, Gorwit J, Crawford MH, O'Rourke RA (1977): Left ventricular performance in patients with left ventricular hypertrophy caused by systemic arterial hypertension. *Br Heart J* 39: 1239–1245.
52. Korner PI (1982): Causal and homestatic factors in hypertension. *Clinical* 63: 5s–26s.
53. Korner PI (1983): The role of the heart in hypertension, in: Robertson JIS (ed), *Handbook of Hypertension, Vol 1: Clinical Aspects of Essential Hypertension,* pp 97–131.
54. Korner PI, Shaw J, Uther JB, West MJ, McRitchie RJ, Richards JG (1973): Autonomic and non-autonomic circulatory components in essential hypertension in man. *Circulation* 48: 107–117.
55. Laks MM, Morady F, Swan HJC (1973): Myocardial hypertrophy produced by chronic infusion of subhypertensive doses of norepinephrine in the dog. *Chest* 64: 75.
56. Lehner JP, Safar MR, Dimitriu UM, Simon A Ch, Carrez JP, Plainfosse MT (1979): Systolic time intervals and echocardiographic findings in borderline hypertension. *Eur J Cardiol* 9: 319–331.
57. Lequime J (1940): Le debit cardiaque. Etudes experimentales et cliniques. *Acta Med Scand* Suppl 7: 151–223.
58. Liard JF (1978): Hypertension induced by prolonged intracoronary administration of dobutamine in conscious dogs. *Clinical Science* 54: 153–160.
59. Liard JF, (1980): Cardiogenic hypertension: experimental evidence from a comparison between intravenous and intracoronary administration of dobutamine in conscious dogs. *Clincial Science* 58: 271–277.
60. Liard JF, Tarazi RC, Ferrario CM, Manger WM (1975): Hemodynamic and humoral characteristics of hypertension induced by prolonged stellate ganglion stimulation in conscious dogs. *Circ Res* 36: 455.
61. Linzbach AJ (1960): Heart failure from the point of view of quantitative anatomy. *Am J Cardiol* 5: 370–382.
62. Logan AG, Gilbert BW, Haynes RB, Milne BJ, Flanagan PT (1981): Early effect of mild hypertension on the heart: A longitudinal study. *Hypertension* 3 (suppl II): II 187–190.
63. London GM, Safar ME, Simon AC, Alexandre JM, Levenson JA, Weiss YA (1978): Total effective compliance, cardiac output and fluid volumes in essential hypertension. *Circulation* 57: 995–1000.
64. Lundgren J, Hallback M, Weiss L, Folkow B (1974): Rate and extent of adaptive cardiovascular changes in rats during experimental renal hypertension. *Acta Physiol Scand* 91: 103–115.
65. Lund-Johansen P (1968): Hemodynamics in early essential hypertension. *Acta Med Scand* Suppl 482: 1–105.
66. Lund-Johansen P (1977): Hemodynamic alternations in hypertension – spontaneous changes and effects of drug therapy: A review. *Acta Med Scand* Suppl 603: 1–14.
67. Lund-Johansen P (1980): State of the art review: Hemodynamics in essential hypertension. *Clin Sci* 59 (suppl): 343s–354s.
68. Lutas EM, Devereux RB, Reis G, Alderman MH, Pickering TG, Borer JS, Laragh JH (1985): Increased cardiac performance in mild essential hypertension: Left ventricular mechanics. *Hypertension* 7: 979–988.
69. Messerli FH, De Carvalho JGR, Christie B, Frohlich ED (1978): Systemic and regional

hemodynamics in low, normal and high cardiac output borderline hypertension. *Circulation* 58: 441–448.

70. Messerli FH, Frohlich ED, Suarez DH, Reisin E, Dreslinski GR, Dunn FG, Cole FE (1981): Borderline hypertension: Relationship between age, hemodynamics and circulating cate-cholamines. *Circulation* 64: 760–764.

71. Meerson FZ (1969): The myocardium in hyperfunction, hypertrophy and heart failure. *Circ Res* 25: II 1–163.

72. Miller DD, Ruddy TD, Zusman RM, Okada RD, Strauss HW, Kanarek DJ, Christensen D, Federman EB, Boucher CA (1987): Left ventricular ejection fraction response during exercise in asymptomatic systemic hypertension. *Am J Cardiol* 59: 409–413.

73. Nichols AB, Sciacca RR, Weiss MB, Blood DK, Brennan DL, Cannon PJ (1980): Effect of left ventricular hypertrophy on myocardial blood flow and ventricular performance in systemic hypertension. *Circulation* 62: 329–340.

74. Olivari MT, Florenti C, Polese A, Guazzi MD (1978): Pulmonary hemodynamics and right ventricular function in hypertension. *Circulation* 57: 1185–1190.

75. Oparil S, Bishop SP, Clubb Jr FJ (1984): Myocardial cell hypertrophy or hyperplasia. *Hypertension* 6 (suppl III): III 38–43.

76. Ostman-Smith I (1981): Cardiac sympathetic nerves as the final common pathway in the induction of adaptive cardiac hypertrophy. *Clin Sci* 61: 265.

77. Pfeffer J, Pfeffer M, Fletcher P, Braunwald E (1979): Alterations of cardiac performance in rats with established spontaneous hypertension. *Am J Cardiol* 44: 994.

78. Rowlands DB, Ireland MA, Glover DV, McLeay AB, Stallard TJ, Littler WA (1981): The relationship between ambulatory blood pressure and echocardiographically assessed left ventricular hypertrophy. *Clin Sci* 61 (suppl): 101s–103s.

79. Safar ME, Chau NP, Weiss YA, London GM, Milliez PL (1976): Control of cardiac output in essential hypertension. *Am J Cardiol* 38: 332–336.

80. Safar ME, Chau NP, Weiss YA, London GM, Simon AC, Milliez PL (1976): The pressure-volume relationship in normotensive and permanent essential hypertensive patients. *Clin Sci Mol Med* 50: 207–212.

81. Safar ME, Lehner JP, Vincent MI, Planfosse MT, Simon AC (1979): Echocardiographic dimensions in borderline and sustained hypertension. *Am J Cardiol* 44: 930–935.

82. Safar ME, London GM, Levenson JA, Simon AC, Chau NP (1979): Rapid dextran infusion in essential hypertension. *Hypertension* 1: 615–623.

83. Safar ME, Weiss YA, Levenson JA, London GM, Milliez PL (1973): Hemodynamic study of 85 patients with borderline hypertension. *Am J Cardiol* 31: 315.

84. Safar ME, Weiss YA, London GM, Frackowiak RF, Milliez PL (1974): Cardiopulmonary blood volume in borderline hypertension. *Clin Sci Mol Med* 47: 153–164.

85. Sannerstedt R (1966): Hemodynamic response to exercise in patients with arterial hyperten-sion. *Acta Med Scand* Suppl 458: 1–83.

86. Sannerstedt R, Wasir H, Henning R, Werko L (1973): Systemic hemodynamics in mild arterial hypertension before and after physical training. *Clin Sci* 45 (suppl): 145s–149s.

87. Sasayama S, Ross Jr J, Franklin D, Bloor CM, Bishop S, Dilley RB (1976): Adaptations of the left ventricle to chronic pressure overload. *Circ Res* 38: 172–178.

88. Savage DD, Drayer JIM, Henry WL, Mathews ED, Ware JH, Gardin JM, Cohen ER, Epstein SE, Laragh LH (1979): Echocardiographic assessment of cardiac anatomy and function in hypertensive subjects. *Circulation* 59: 623–632.

89. Schieken RM (1987): Measurement of left ventricular wall mass in pediatric populations. *Hypertension* 9 (suppl II): II 47–52.

90. Schieken RM, Clarke WR, Lauer RM (1981): Left ventricular hypertrophy in children with blood pressures in the upper quintile of the distribution. *Hypertension* 3: 669–675.

91. Sen S, Bumpus FM (1979): Collagen synthesis in the development and reversal of cardiac hypertrophy in spontaneously hypertensive rats. *Am J Cardiol* 44: 954–958.

92. Sen S, Tarazi RC, Khairallah PA, Bumpus FM (1974): Cardiac hypertrophy in spontaneously hypertensive rats. *Circ Res* 35: 775–781.

93. Sen S, Tarazi RC, Bumpus FM (1977): Cardiac hypertrophy and antihypertensive therapy. *Cardiovasc Res* 11: 427–431.

94. Sokolow M, Werdegar D, Kain HK, Hinman AT (1966): Relationship between level of blood pressure measured casually and by portable recorders and severity of complications in essential hypertension. *Circulation* 34: 279–298.

95. Spotnitz HM, Sonnenblick EH (1973): Structural conditions in the hypertrophied and failing heart. *Am J Cardiol* 32: 398–406.

96. Strauer BE (1977): Ventrikelfunktion und Kornare Hamodynamic bei der essentiellen Hypertonie. *Verh Dtsch Ges Kreislaufforsch* 43: 41–55.

97. Strauer BE (1979): Myocardial oxygen consumption in chronic heart disease: Role of wall stress, hypertrophy and coronary reserve. *Am J Cardiol* 44: 730–740.

98. Strauer BE (1979): Ventricular function and coronary hemodynamics in hypertensive heart disease. *Am J Cardiol* 44: 999–1006.

99. Strauer BE (1980): *Hypertensive Heart Disease.* Berlin-Heidelberg: Springer Verlag.

100. Sugishita Y, Susumu K, Matsuda M, Yamaguchi T, Ito I (1983): Myocardial mechanics of athletic hearts in comparison with diseased hearts. *Am Heart J* 105: 273–280.

101. Tarazi RC (1982): Role of the heart in hypertension. *Clin Sci* 63, Suppl: 347s–358s.

102. Tarazi RC, Ibrahim MM, Dustan HP, Ferrario CM (1974): Cardiac factors in hypertension. *Circ Res* 34: I 213–221.

103. Tarazi RC, Nuler A, Frohlich ED, Dustan HP (1966): Electrocardiographic changes reflecting left atrial abnormality in hypertension. *Circulation* 34: 818–822.

104. Tsuchiya M (1972): Hemodynamic studies on hypertension: Hemodynamic characteristics in the resting supine position. *Jpn Circ J* 36: 267–274.

105. Tubau JF, Wikman-Coffelt J, Massie B, Sievers R, Parmley WW (1987): Improved myocardial efficiency in the working perfused heart of the spontaneously hypertensive rat. *Hypertension* 10: 396–403.

106. Varnauskas E (1955): Studies in hypertensive cardiovascular disease, with special reference to cardiac function. *Scand J Clin Lab Invest* Suppl 7: 1–117.

107. Weiss YA, Safar ME, London GM, Simon AC, Levenson JA, Milliez PL (1978): Repeat hemodynamic determination in borderline hypertension. *Am J Med* 64: 382–387.

108. Weissler AM, Peeler RG, Roehll WH (1961): Relationships between left ventricular ejection time, stroke volume and heart rate in normal individuals and patients with cardiovascular disease. *Am Heart J* 62: 367–378.

109. Widimsky J, Jandova R, Ressl J (1981): Hemodynamic studies in juvenile hypertensives at rest and during supine exercise. *Eur Heart J* 2: 307–315.

101. Yamori Y, Mori C, Nishio T, et al. (1979): Cardiac hypertrophy in early hypertension. *Am J Cardiol* 44: 964.

111. Wikstrand J (1984): Left ventricular function in early primary hypertension. Functional consequences of cardiovascular structural changes. *Hypertension* 6 (suppl III): III 108–116.

112. Yurchak PM, Hood WB, Rolett ET, et al. (1964): Effect of systemic hypertension on mean left ventricular ejection rate. *Am J Med Sci* 247: 76.

19. Left ventricular diastolic function in hypertension

FETNAT M. FOUAD-TARAZI

Introduction

Interest in left ventricular relaxation in hypertensive patients has increased in the past decade as a result of the availability of non-invasive techniques to examine indices of cardiac function in man [1–8]. Moreover, in contrast to alterations in left ventricular passive stiffness, changes in early diastol were shown to be dependent on modifiable factors such as heart rate [8, 9, 12], adrenergic tone [2, 13], end diastolic volume [14] and intracellular calcium kinetics [15–17]. Since left ventricular relaxation and filling influence left ventricular ejection and systolic performance [18], alterations of these determinants of relaxation may change the functional capacity of the heart as well as systemic hemodynamics.

Relationship between contraction and relaxation

The phenomenon of 'rhythmodiastolic dependence' demonstrates the importance of the contraction-relaxation relationship [19]. In a sense, it represents an indispensible link in cardiac adaptation to the organism's changing requirements [20, 21]. It is made possible by the interplay of several natural factors and mechanisms that influence both the process of contraction and the process of relaxation such as the frequency of cardiac stimulation and catecholamine levels. Indeed, these two stimuli not only increase calcium entry and increase the number of calcium-troponin complexes (which will accentuate the inotropic state) but also increase cyclic AMP release from the sarcolemma leading to activation of protein kinases and calcium reuptake by the sarcoplasmic reticulum [22]. Also, in relation to the Starling curve, relaxation velocity was found to decrease even before the plateau is reached in the concentration

M.E. Safar & F. Fouad-Tarazi (eds.), The heart in hypertension.
© *1989 Kluwer Academic Publishers, Dordrecht –*

curve [22]. Since these modulating factors may be altered by a number of physiologic situations, it is conceivable that the relationship between contraction and relaxation is not static. Indeed, a disproportionate increase in the velocity of relaxation vs velocity and amplitude of contraction takes place when the heart is exposed to increasing frequency of stimulation or to increased catecholamines.

The complexity of the interrelationship between contraction and relaxation of the heart under natural physiologic conditions is compounded by pathological situations. Thus, immediate adapatation of the heart to an acute increase in hemodynamic load or to disturbances in oxygen supply, may be different from chronic adaptive mechanisms that occur under similar but sustained hemodynamic or metabolic alterations. For example, contrary to findings described above, both cytosolic calcium overload and impaired calcium transport by the sarcoplasmic reticulum were described during long-term adaptation by the overloaded heart [17].

Left ventricular diastolic function in hypertension

Whereas alteration in left ventricular diastolic function has not been studied in relation to acute left ventricular overload, several studies have been published describing the alterations in left ventricular relaxation and early filling in chronic hypertension. As early as 1980, we have reported that left ventricular peak filling rate is reduced in hypertensive patients at a time when ejection fraction, cardiac output and peak left ventricular ejection rate were still normal [2]. Our findings were soon confirmed by many others [3, 4] but the basic mechanisms underlying this abnormality are not yet fully understood. Neither blood pressure per se, nor the increase in left ventricular mass could explain the abnormality in left ventricular filling. Indeed, left ventricular filling rate was reported to be maintained within normal in the physiologic left ventricular hypertrophy of the athlete heart. In this respect, one may assume that the biological adaptation of the membrane systems that transport calcium, increases their ability to handle this ion and make the heart more capable of relaxing during exercise thereby enhancing its oxidative efficiency; it is possible that the increase in the frequency of contraction and of adrenergic nervous system activity during exercise play a role in this adaptive mechanism. Indeed, Katz [16] has pointed out the link between adrenergic stimulation, phosphorylated phospholamdan and the increase in calcium uptake by the sarcoplasmic reticulum accounting for the more rapid contraction and relaxation of cardiac muscle exposed to catecholamines. On the other hand, under pathological conditions such as hypertensive left ventricular hypertrophy, a decrease in the power of the cellular membrane systems to transport calcium may play a role in the observed impairment of the relaxation process and may on the long run reduce the efficiency of the heart. In relation to adrenergic activity, we have found that even in hypertensive patients, those exhibiting evidence of hyperkinetic circulation have normal left ventricular filling rate (Figure 1) compared with patients who have established 'high-resistance' hypertension [2].

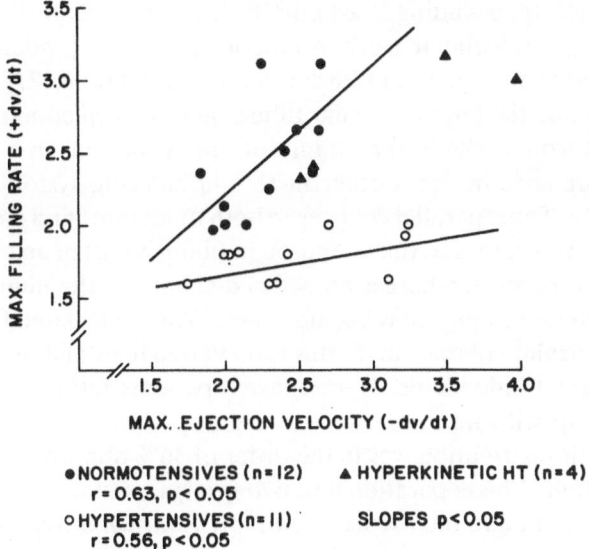

Figure 1. Correlation between LV maximum filling rate (+dv/dt) and LV maximum ejection rate (−dv/dt) obtained from radionuclide (99^mTc-HSA) gated blood pool scanning technique. Note that hypertensives with evidence of hyperkinetic circulation (▲) were closer to the normals (●) than to 'high-resistance' hypertensives (○). Permission from Fouad et al. [2].

Although calcium ion per se was found to play an important role in the relaxation of the left ventricle, it was paradoxically demonstrated that calcium entry blockade also improves left ventricular filling rate in the hypertensive heart [23]. It is of interest to note in this regard that Walsh and O'Rourke [24] have recently contrasted the impairment of LV relaxation induced by intracoronary administration of calcium entry blockers in normal dogs to the improvement of relaxation secondary to systemic administration of calcium entry blockers that induced reflex sympathetic stimulation.

No direct studies have been performed regarding the effects of alterations in myocardial perfusion on left ventricular diastole in hypertensive patients, but studies in patients with documented coronary artery disease and no myocardial infarction have shown a reduced peak rate of left ventricular filling [7, 25]. This diminished diastolic filling rate was corrected by successful coronary bypass surgery [7, 25] or coronary angioplasty [6]. Although suggestive, these findings did not prove, however, a direct relationship between impaired myocardial perfusion and abnormalities in LV diastolic function [6, 7, 25, 26].

Indices of left ventricular filling

In view of the complex interaction between different factors influencing both diastole and systole, including heart rate [8, 9, 12], adrenergic nervous system activity [2, 13], intracellular calcium kinetics [15–17, 27], adenylate cyclase system [16] and to a lesser extent cardiac loading conditions [27], we [12] have suggested relating the left ventricular filling rate to its ejection rate; the ratio thus obtained would take into account not only variations in left ventricular systolic performance but also other factors influencing systole and diastole simultaneously. Thus, parallel changes in both numerator and denominator in this ratio would suggest that the alteration in filling is part of an overall change in cardiac performance, whereas an isolated change in the numerator would point out a primary change in relaxation rate. When calculated from radionuclide left ventricular volume curve, this ratio varied in our laboratory from 0.9 to 1.37 in normal individuals. Hypertensive patients fell generally into two groups: a group with normal ratio and a group with reduced ratio. In our experience, this distribution was in the order of 36% abnormal: 64% normal. Factors underlying this separation into two groups are not clear; theoretically they could be related to the occurrence of left ventricular hypertrophy, duration of hypertension, coronary perfusion or intracellular changes.

Clinical importance of left ventricular diastolic dysfunction in hypertension

Although clinical implications of abnormalities of left ventricular compliance has been well recognized [28], little is known about the consequences of alterations in left ventricular relaxation and filling indices in hypertension. Since cardiopulmonary reflexes were reported to be blunted in patients with severe and established hypertension [29, 30], we hypothesized that this abnormality of the cardiopulmonary reflexes could be related to the abnormal diastolic function accompanying hypertension. Since it is not known yet whether this abnormality in left ventricular diastolic function in hypertension is limited to delayed early left ventricular filling and relaxation or extends to reduced left ventricular compliance in the same heart, any or all of these abnormalities could influence cardiopulmonary receptor sensitivity and adaptation, as has been demonstrated previously in the failing heart [31]. Using the ratio of positive dV/dt to negative dV/dt as an index of diastolic function we classified 13 hypertensive patients into two groups; one group had a normal

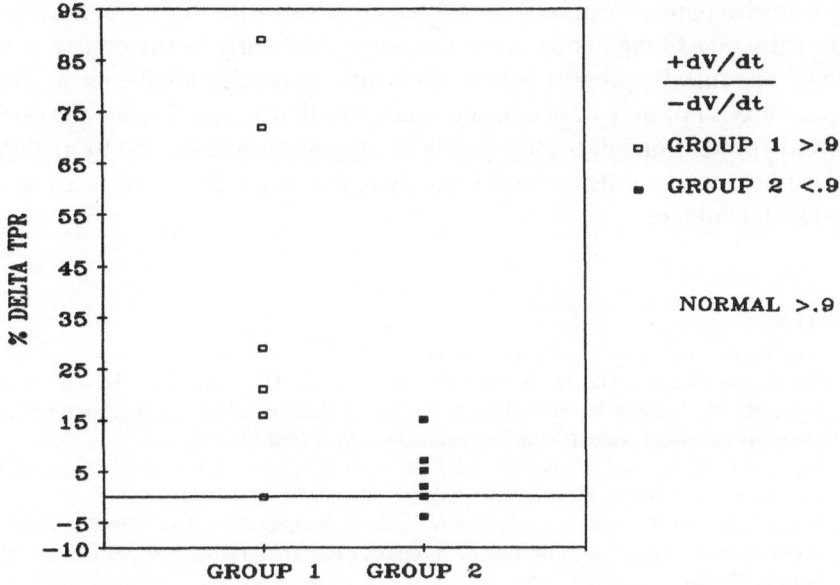

Figure 2. Effect of altered LV diastolic filling rate on reflex change in systemic resistance during head-up posture (45°–60°) in hypertensive patients. The ratio of maximum LV filling rate (+dv/dt) to maximum LV ejection rate (−dv/dt) was used to separate the hypertensive patients into 2 groups (above or below 0.9 which was found to be the lower limit in a contemporary series of normal volunteers). Permission from Fouad and Tarazi, [35].

ratio of +dV/dt to −dV/dt (>0.9), and the other group had an abnormal ratio of (<0.9). When these patients were subjected to head-up tilt the response of total peripheral resistance to the reduction in venous return and ventricular preload was reduced in the group with abnormal diastolic function compared with that in the other group (Figure 2). Thus, patients with abnormal left ventricular filling could not mobilize sufficient adrenergic vasoconstrictor activity in response to venous pooling. Since high pressure receptors have been reported to be reset early in hypertension [32], one may postulate that these observed differences in response between the two hypertensive groups are related to alterations in cardiopulmonary receptors. However, these studies should be repeated at low levels of lower body suction that are known to alter low pressure receptors without perturbation of high pressure receptors [33]. If this observation is confirmed, it would present an interesting and novel mechanism to explain resistant hypertension at least in some patients. The reversibility of the abnormality of the diastolic filling rate might be a valuable new aspect to be considered in the management of hypertension and hypertensive heart disease [34].

In conclusion, abnormalities in the diastolic function of the left ventricle in hypertensive patients can be assessed noninvasively with the use of indexes of left ventricular filling. They occur frequently and early in the course of the disease and may be present before other signs of cardiac involvement. Their importance is not only of diagnostic value, but they may influence the evolution of hypertension by altering systolic cardiac performance, and by modulating cardiovascular reflexes and hemodynamic responses to changes in intervascular volume.

References

1. Quereshi S, Wagner HN Jr, Alerson PO, Housholder DF, Douglass KH, Lotter MG, Nickoloff EL, Tanabe M, Knowles LG (1978): Evaluation of left ventricular function in normal persons and patients with heart disease. *J Nucl Med* 19: 135.
2. Fouad FM, Tarazi RC, Gallagher JH, MacIntyre WJ, Cook SA (1980): Abnormal left ventricular relaxation in hypertensive patients. *Clin Sci* 59: 411s.
3. Inouye I, Massie B, Loge D, Topic N, Silverstein D, Simpson P, Tubau J (1985): Abnormal left ventricular filling: an early finding in mild to moderate systemic hypertension. *Am J Cardiol* 53: 120.
4. Smith VE, Katz AM (1984): Relaxation abnormalities, Part II: Clinical aspects. *Hosp Prac* 19: 149.
5. Hartford M, Wikstrand J, Wallentin I, Ljungman S, Wilhelmsen L, Berglund G (1984): Diastolic function of the heart in untreated primary hypertension. *Hypertension* 6: 329.
6. Bonow RD, Vitale DF, Bacharach SL, Frederick TM, Kent KM, Green MV (1985): Asynchronous left ventricular regional function and impaired global diastolic filling in patients with coronary artery disease: reversal after coronary angioplasty. *Circulation* 71: 197.
7. Abi-Mansour P, Fouad FM, Rincon G, Kramer JR, Tarazi RC, Loop FD (1984): Improvement of left ventricular diastolic filling following coronary bypass surgery (CBPS). *Tenth European Congress of Cardiology*. Dusseldorf 1984.
8. Fifer MA, Borow KM, Colan S, Lorell BH (1983): Left ventricular diastolic filling rate: contributions of heart rate, age, and extent of systolic shortening. *Circulation* 68 (suppl III): III 101.
9. Williams LE, Loken MK, Forstrom LA, Ponto RA, Frick MP (1979): Radionuclide left-ventricular dV/dt and its dependence on cardiac rate. *J Nucl Med* 20: 997.
10. Upton MT, Gibson DG, Brown DJ (1976): Echocardiographic assessment of abnormal left ventricular relaxation in man. *Br Heart J* 38: 1001–1009.
11. Paulsen W, Magid N, Sagar RK, Mastillo A, Wolfgang TC, Lower RR, Hess H (1985): Left ventricular function of heart allografts during acute rejection. An echocardiographic assessment. *Heart Transpl* 19: 525–528.
12. Fouad FM (1987): Left ventricular diastolic function in hypertensive patients. *Circulation* 75 (suppl I): I 48–55.
13. Sonnenblick EH, Siegel JH, Sarnoff SJ (1963): Ventricular distensibility and pressure-volume curve during sympathetic stimulation. *Am J Physiol* 204: 1.
14. Hammermeister KE, Warbassee JR (1974): The rate of change of left ventricular volume in man, II: Diastolic events in health and disease. *Circulation* 49: 739.
15. Katz AM (1977): *Physiology of the Heart,* 434 pp. New York: Raven Press Books.
16. Katz AM (1979): Role of the contractile proteins and sarcoplasmic reticulum in the response of the heart to catecholamines: An historical review. *Adv Cyclic Nucleotide Res* 11: 303.

17. Limas CJ, Spier SS (1980): Effect of antihypertensive therapy on calcium transport by cardiac sarcoplasmic reticulum of SHRs. *Cardiovasc Res* 14: 692.
18. Bahler RC, Martin P (1985): Effects of loading conditions and inotropic state on rapid filling phase of left ventricle. *Am J Physiol* 248: 523.
19. Udelnov MG (1968): Autoregulatory mechanism of the heart (in Russian). *Nauchn Kokl Bysshei Shkoly Biol Nauki* 5: 37–55.
20. Meerson FZ, Kapelko VI (1974): Role of the interconnection between the intensity of the contractile function and the velocity of relaxation of the cardiac muscle in the adaptation of the heart to a great load (in Russian). *Kardiologiia* 7: 43–53.
21. Meerson FZ, Kapelko VI (1975): The significance of the interrelationship between the intensity of the contractile state and the velocity of relaxation in adapting cardiac muscle to function at high work loads. *J Mol Cell Cardiol* 7: 793–806.
22. Meerson FZ (1983): The failing heart: Adaptation and deadaptation, in: Katz AM (ed). New York: Raven Press.
23. Fouad FM, Slominski MJ, Bravo EL, Tarazi RC (1985): Effect of calcium entry blockade on left ventricular filling in hypertension. *Twelfth Interamerican Congress of Cardiology*, 1985.
24. Walsh RA, O'Rourke RA (1985): Direct and indirect effects of calcium entry blocking agents on isovolumic left ventricular relaxation in conscious dogs. *J Clin Invest* 75: 1426.
25. Carroll JD, Hess OM, Hirzel HO, Turina M, Krayenbuehl HP (1985): Left ventricular systolic and diastolic function in coronary artery disease: Effects of revascularization on exercise-induced ischemia. *Circulation* 72: 119.
26. Templeton GH, Wildenthal K, Mitchel JH (1972): Influence of coronary blood flow on left ventricular contractility and stiffness. *Am J Physiol* 223: 1216.
27. Brutseart DL, Rademakers FE, Sys SU (1984): Triple control of relaxation: implications in cardiac disease (Editorial). *Circulation* 69: 190–196.
28. Gaasch WH, Levine HJ, Quinones MA, et al. (1976): Left ventricular compliance: Mechanisms and clinical implications. *Am J Cardiol* 38: 645–653.
29. Frohlich ED, Tarazi RC, Ulrych M, Dustan HP, Page I (1967): Tilt test for investigating a neural component in hypertension. *Circulation* 36: 387–393.
30. Mark AL, Kerber RE (1982): Augmentation of cardiopulmonary baroreflex control of forearm vascular resistance in borderline hypertension. *Hypertension* 4: 39.
31. Zucker IH, Gilmore JP (1981): Atrial receptor modulation of renal function in heart failure, in: Abboud FM, Fozzard HA, Gilmore JP, Reis DJ (eds), *Disturbances in Neurogenic Control of the Circulation*. Bethesda: American Physiological Society.
32. Abboud FM (1982): The sympathetic system in hypertension. State-of-the-Art Review. *Hypertension* 4 (suppl II): II 208–225.
33. Zoller RP, Mark AL, Abboud FM, Schmid PG, Heistad DD (1972): The role of low pressure baroreceptors in reflex vasoconstrictor responses in man. *J Clin Invest* 51: 2967–2972.
34. Fouad-Tarazi FM (1987): Factors contributing to resistant hypertension. Cardiac considerations. *Hypertension* 11 (suppl II): II 84–87.
35. Fouad FM, Tarazi RC (1986): The sympathetic drive to the heart and hypertension, in: Lown B, Malliani A, Prosdocimi M (eds), *Neural Mechanisms and Cardiovascular Disease*, pp 225–232. Padova (Italy): Liviana Press; Berlin-Heidelberg-New York-Tokyo: Springer Verlag (Fidia Research Series, Vol 5).

20. The right ventricle and the lesser circulation in essential hypertension

MAURIZIO D. GUAZZI

The dynamics of the right side of the heart and of the lesser circulation in systemic hypertension have been poorly investigated in the past and the results were somewhat discordant. Normal values of pulmonary pressure in hypertensive subjects have been reported in some studies [1, 2]. Elevated values were detected in patients with hypertension and left ventricular dysfunction and were interpreted as a backward effect of the latter [3]. On the contrary, it has been reported that in a considerable number of cases of arterial hypertension without clinical signs of heart failure, pressure in the pulmonary artery is somewhat higher than the highest recorded in cases with normal circulation [4].

If one calculates the right ventricular function characteristics in hypertension the performance of the right ventricle seems to be impaired, because the filling pressure is augmented and the right ventricular stroke output is diminished or changed little from normal [5]. If the concept is accepted that in hypertensive subjects hemodynamic variations in the pulmonary artery and the right side of the heart occur secondarily to left ventricular failure, the mechanism of right ventricular dysfunction is not clear. The classical theory that prolonged pulmonary pressure rise secondary to left ventricular failure causes failure of the right ventricle [6] is unsatisfactory because it does not seem entirely reasonable that the right ventricle would fail after relatively short-term exposure to only modest elevation of pulmonary arterial pressure.

Pulmonary hemodynamics and right ventricular function

In a pilot study [7] we investigate 33 primary hypertensive men with repeated readings of blood pressure above 180/100 mmHg, and 14 healthy volunteers or patients without circulatory disorders (control group). At an ultrasound eval-

M.E. Safar & F. Fouad-Tarazi (eds.), The heart in hypertension.
© 1989 Kluwer Academic Publishers, Dordrecht –

uation of the left ventricle the end-diastolic minor axis in 17 hypertensive subjects (Group 1) was similar to that in normotensive controls (4.85 ± 0.2 cm) and significantly exceeded this value in the remaining 16 cases (5.42 ± 0.22 cm) (Group 2). In Group 1 (1.22 ± 0.17 cm) and in Group 2 (1.25 ± 0.14 cm) the left ventricular posterior wall was thicker (p< 0.01) than in control subjects (1 ± 0.12 cm) suggesting that both groups had some degree of left ventricular hypertrophy associated or not with enlargement of the ventricular cavity.

Figure 1 summarizes the results of the hemodynamic evaluation performed at rest in these subjects. Pulmonary systolic, diastolic and mean wedge pressures were equivalent between the hypertensives and significantly higher than in normotensives. Cardiac output was normal in Group 1 and reduced in Group 2; since the driving pressure across the lungs was augmented in either group, pressure elevation in the pulmonary artery depended on an increased pulmonary arteriolar resistance.

Respiratory gases, pH of the blood and pulmonary blood volume did not seem to be responsible for an altered pulmonary vasomotility, because all of these variables were comparable between hypertensive and control subjects. Probably blood flow was also unrelated to changes in pulmonary arteriolar resistance since it was normal in Group 1 and reduced in Group 2, while pulmonary resistance was elevated in either group. Pleural pressure, as estimated by an esophageal balloon during quiet regular respiration, was equivalent in the three groups; alveolar pressure was not determined, but no reason was seen for an increase in hypertensive patients. Extramural pressures, therefore, could be excluded as important determinants of the differences in intramural pressure and arteriolar resistance between controls and hypertensives. Elevation of left ventricular diastolic pressure might well account for a rise in pulmonary arteriolar resistance; however, only a sustained elevation of back pressure from the left heart is documented to assume increasing importance in determining pulmonary vascular resistance in hypertension [8]. A high degree of correlation has been proven between pulmonary vascular resistance and wedge pressures exceeding 20 mmHg, the correlation is lost at lower wedge pressures, although many of these subjects may still present an increased pulmonary vascular resistance [8]. In our patients the left ventricular filling pressure was moderately elevated (lower than 20 mmHg in each subject) and, in keeping with the findings of above, was not related to the level of pulmonary vascular resistance. Pulmonary resistance, in fact, was significantly higher in Group 2, while the wedge pressure was equal in the two hypertensive groups, suggesting that the former variable was not fully dependent upon the latter.

From all these considerations and on the basis of the relationship observed between elevation in systemic and in pulmonary vascular resistance (both of

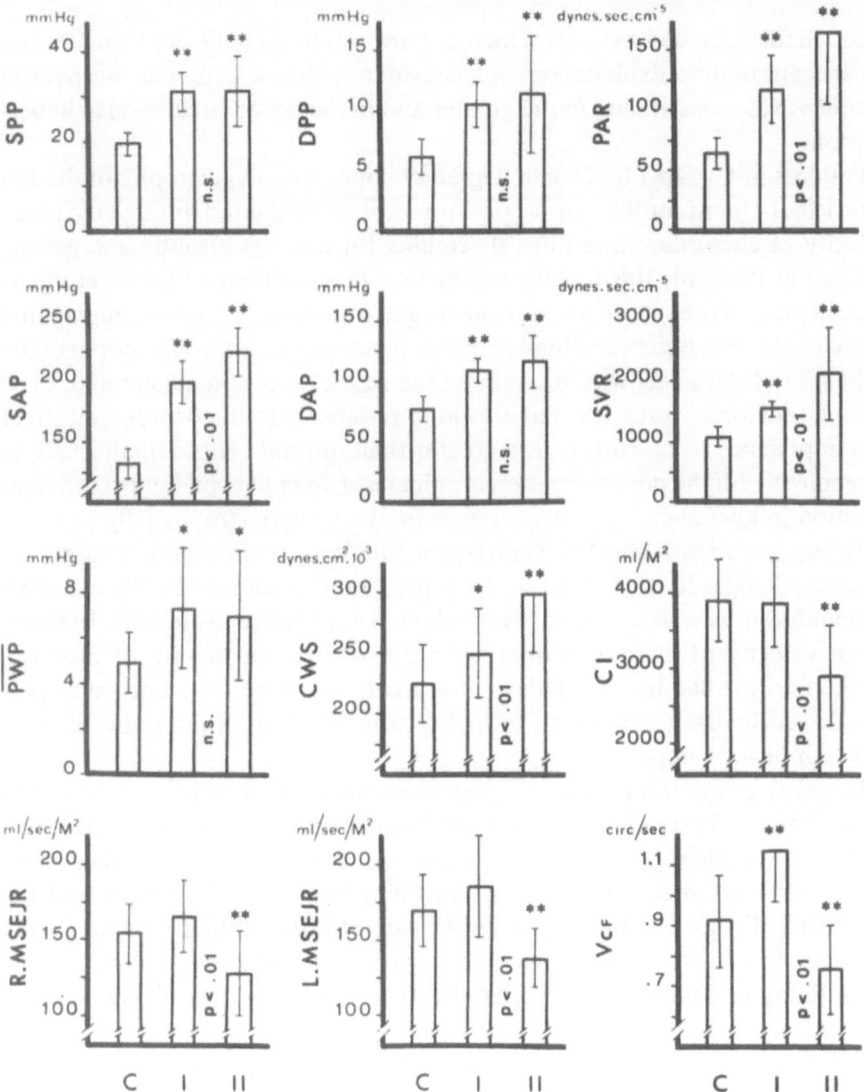

Figure 1. Hemodynamic functions in normotensive control subjects (c) and in two groups of essential hypertensive patients: Group I, patients with left ventricle hypertrophy; Group II, patients with increased left ventricular wall thickness and with enlargement of the ventricular cavity. Bars represent the mean for the group (SD). * and ** indicate p values of < 0.05 and < 0.01, respectively, for differences between the hypertensive groups and the control subjects. p values for differences between the hypertensive groups are indicated in the figure.

SPP = systolic pulmonary pressure; DDP = diastolic pulmonary pressure; PAR = pulmonary arteriolar resistance; SAP = systolic arterial pressure; DAP = diastolic arterial pressure; SVR = systemic vascular resistance; $\overline{PWP}$ = mean pulmonary wedge pressure; CWS = left ventricular circumferential wall stress; CI = cardiac index; R.MSEJR and L.MSEJR = right and left mean systolic ejection rate; V_{CF} = left ventricular mean velocity of circumferential fiber shortening. From Olivari et al. [7] by permission.

them, in fact, showed a stepwise increase from controls to Group 1 and Group 2), the alternative explanation was considered that a common mechanism produces vasoconstriction in the greater and in the lesser circulation in hypertension.

Patients in Group 1 had some degree of concentric hypertrophy of the left ventricle. In them cardiac muscle performance, as evaluated through the mean velocity of circumferential fiber shortening [9] was significantly and greatly enhanced. Probably this was the mechanism that maintained in this group or even increased the rate of ejection and the stroke index, in spite of augmented systolic wall stress, pressure load and impedance to ejection. The output of the right side of the heart was normal and the rate of ejection augmented, even though pulmonary pressure and arteriolar resistance (and possibly wall stress and impedance to ejection) were greater than normal. These findings are in agreement with the documentation in animals of an enhanced right ventricular function following systemic hypertension-induced hypertrophy [10].

Group 2 patients had left ventricular enlargement in addition to hypertrophy. Compared to Group 1, they presented a larger rise in afterload (circumferential wall stress) and, probably, in impedance to ejection. In them, mean velocity of circumferential fiber shortening, mean rate of ejection, stroke and cardiac indexes indicated a greatly reduced left ventricular performance. Similarly, the mean rate of systolic ejection of the right ventricle was significantly depressed.

In either group, the functional pattern of the right ventricle, as evaluated through the variations in the mean systolic ejection rate, was similar to the one of the left ventricle. The same conclusion was suggested by the analysis of the relationship between stroke index and filling pressure of the right and left ventricles (Figure 2). In fact, in either side elevated filling pressures were associated with a somewhat augmented stroke index in Group 1, while comparable filling pressures were associated with a greatly reduced stroke index in Group 2.

All these findings indicate that left ventricular hypertrophy alone, and hypertrophy associated with enlargement of the cavity have a well defined pathophysiological significance. They reflect different hemodynamic changes in the right and left ventricles, as well as in the systemic and pulmonary circulations. It may be postulated that in the presence of left ventricular pressure overload a stimulus is generated in response to the increased functional requirements of the myocardium. As suggested by Meerson [11], this stimulus, which is maintained as long as the left ventricle is under stress, initially improves the function of the ventricle, but is subsequently overwhelmed by the adverse effects of direct exposure to an increasing stress. The pressure overload interpretation does not fit findings in the right side of the heart for two reasons: the right ventricle is exposed to only modest elevation of

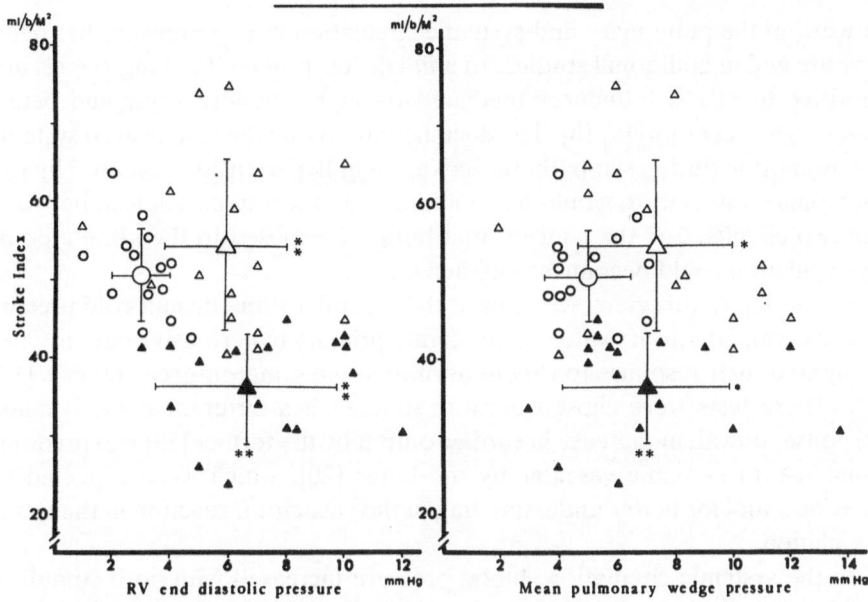

Figure 2. Relationship between filling pressure and stroke index of the right and left ventricle in normal (○) and hypertensive (△ Group I; ▲ Group II) subjects.
Averages (± SD) are indicated by the large symbols. * and ** indicate differences from the normal group significant at p < 0.05 and p < 0.01, respectively.
From Olivari et al. [7] by permission.

pulmonary arterial pressure; at equivalent levels of pressure loading its performance may be either enhanced (Group 1) or reduced (Group 2) in parallel with the performance of the left ventricle.

A functional interdependence of the two sides of the heart was documented in animals by Taylor and collaborators [12]. It has been proven that these experimental principles can well influence the hemodynamic conditions in disease states such as acute myocardial infarction [13]. The present study suggests that a chronic increase of left ventricular afterload may have important effects on the whole heart, and again proposes the concept that the right and the left sides represent a single functional unit. Their relationship in the same anatomical framework [14] can be regarded as a reasonable mechanism of interpretation.

Reactivity of the pulmonary vessels to adrenergic activation and exogenous catecholamines

The possibility that a common factor responsible for vasoconstriction may be at work in the pulmonary and systemic circulation in hypertension has been investigated in additional studies. In animals it is proven that lung vessels are sensitive to neural influences mediated through alfa-adrenergic and beta$_2$-adrenergic receptors [15, 16]. The documentation that the emphasized systemic vasomotion during sympathetic activation in hypertension is shared by the pulmonary vasculature would be an additional aspect of parallelism between the two circuits, and the concept that both are exposed to the same type of dysregulation could become strengthened.

According to this view, we utilized the mental arithmetic and cold pressor tests as sympathetic activators in moderate primary hypertensive patients and compared their response to that in normotensive symptom-free subjects [17, 18]. These tests were chosen because they elicit a different hemodynamic response, prevalent increase in cardiac output by the former [19] and predominant rise of systemic vascular by the latter [20], which were expected to provide a tool for better understanding of the vasomotor reaction in the lesser circulation.

In the systemic circulation, blood pressure increased with both stimuli in both groups, but to a greater extent in the hypertensive one; in either group the systemic pressure increase during mental arithmetic was mediated through a similar increase in cardiac index, associated with a tendency of the vascular resistance to decrease, while a raised systemic vascular resistance (which was greater in hypertensives) with hardly noticeable changes in cardiac index characterized the systemic hemodynamic response to cold. In the pulmonary circuit, neither stimulus affected pressure and arteriolar resistance in the normotensive subjects, while both stimuli augmented pulmonary pressure, systolic and diastolic, to similar levels in hypertensive patients; the increase was mediated through increments in both flow and resistance during mental arithmetic and exclusively through the latter during the cold pressor test (Figure 3). Plasma concentrations of epinephrine and norepinephrine were higher in the hypertensive group in the steady state and were augmented to a larger extent during both stimuli. The increase in epinephrine was more pronounced during the mental test, and that of norepinephrine during the physical cold stimulus.

In many respects the hemodynamic responses to exogenous epinephrine and norepinephrine [18, 21] were similar to the responses recorded during the mental arithmetic and the cold pressor test, respectively. As specifically referred to the pulmonary circulation, the finding was duplicated that either compound was ineffective in normotensive subjects and unequivocally increased pulmonary pressure and resistance in hypertensive subjects. Dose-response curves (Figure 4) showing the increase of systemic and pulmonary arteriolar resistance with increasing doses of norepinephrine had similar shaped configurations in normotensives and hypertensives, but the curves for

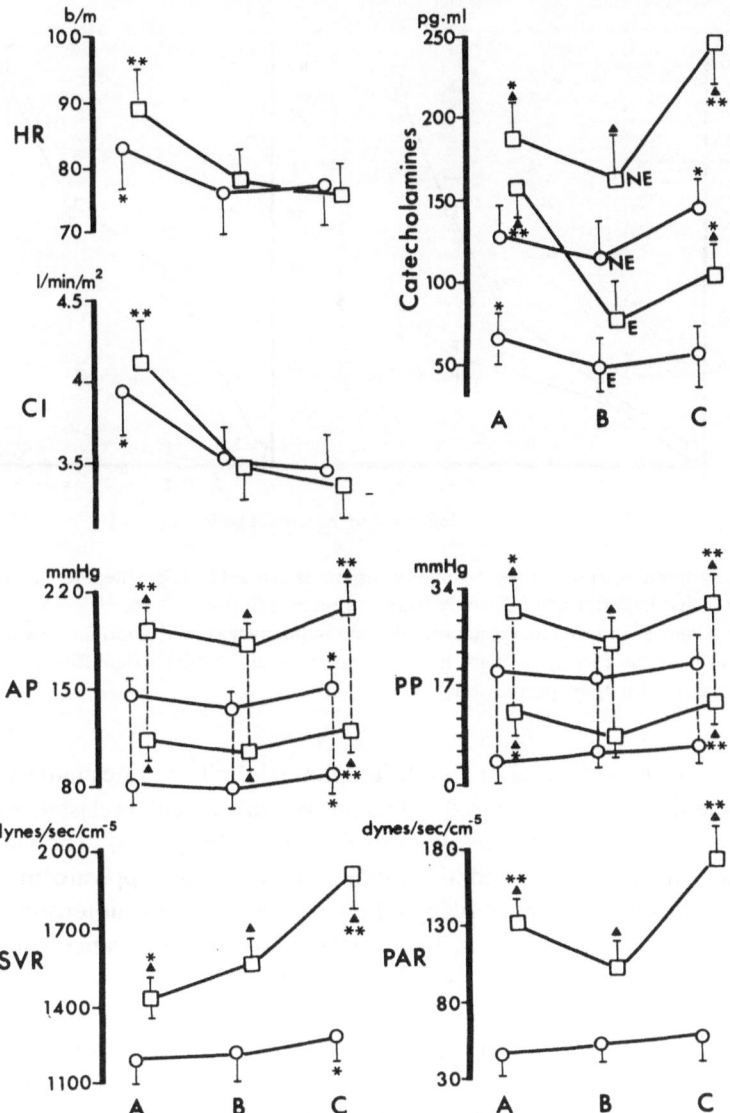

Figure 3. Hemodynamic values and plasma catecholamine concentrations at baseline (B) and during arithmethic (A) and cold pressor (C) tests in the normotensive (O) and hypertensive (□) study patients (mean ± SD).

AP = aortic pressure (systolic and diastolic); CI = cardiac index; HR = heart rate; PAR = pulmonary arteriolar resistance; PP = pulmonary pressure (systolic and diastolic); SVR = systemic vascular resistance; ▲ = differences from the corresponding value in the normotensive group significant at p < 0.01; * and ** indicate differences from baseline significant at p < 0.05 and p < 0.01, respectively. E = Epinephrine; NE = Norepinephrine.

From Guazzi et al. [18] by permission.

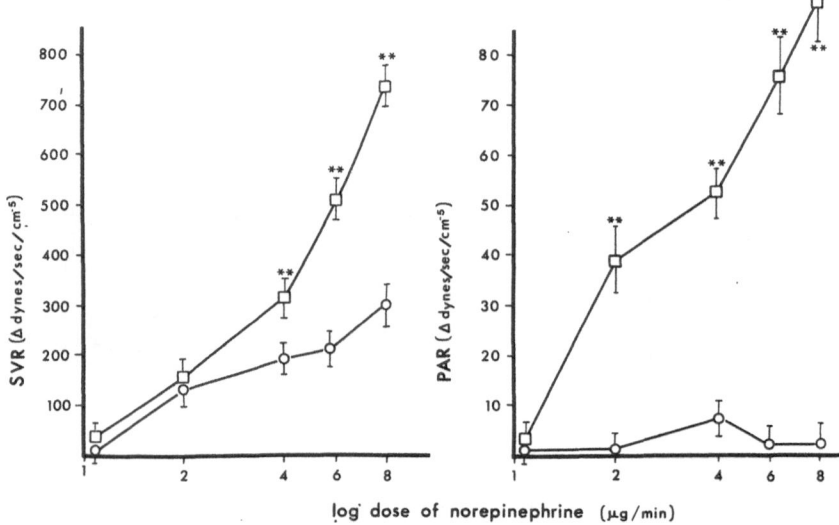

Figure 4. Systemic and pulmonary vasomotor responses evoked by norepinephrine in the normotensive (O) and hypertensive (□) study patients (mean ± SD).
Ordinate: Changes in systemic vascular (SVR) and pulmonary (PAR) arteriolar resistance; ** = differences from the corresponding value in the normotensive subjects significant at p < 0.01. From Guazzi et al. [18] by permission.

the latter group were steeper and shifted to the left. The same analysis showed that epinephrine had a depressor effect on systemic vascular resistance and this was more pronounced in the hypertensive group (Figure 5). The vasomotor influence of epinephrine on the pulmonary bed was opposite in the two groups, arteriolar resistance being mildly depressed in normotensive subjects and substantially enhanced in hypertension, so that differences in changes were significant at any step beyond the threshold.

Among the factors controlling the flow of blood through the pulmonary circuit, those of mechanical origin are predominant, and knowledge of the passive relation between pressure and flow is essential in the interpretation of pharmacologic and physiologic interventions that also involves the heart and the systemic circuit. If this relation is not linear, changes in resistance when flow is also changing may not necessarily reflect an active vasomotion. In the study reported above, the increase in pulmonary blood flow promoted by the endogenously released (mental arithmetic) and exogenously administered epinephrine slightly reduced the baseline difference between the pulmonary artery and wedge pressures in the normotensives, while a similar increase in flow by the same stimuli in hypertensives was associated with a substantial increase in the driving pressure across the lungs. It follows that changes in pulmonary arteriolar resistance under the influence of epinephrine, endoge-

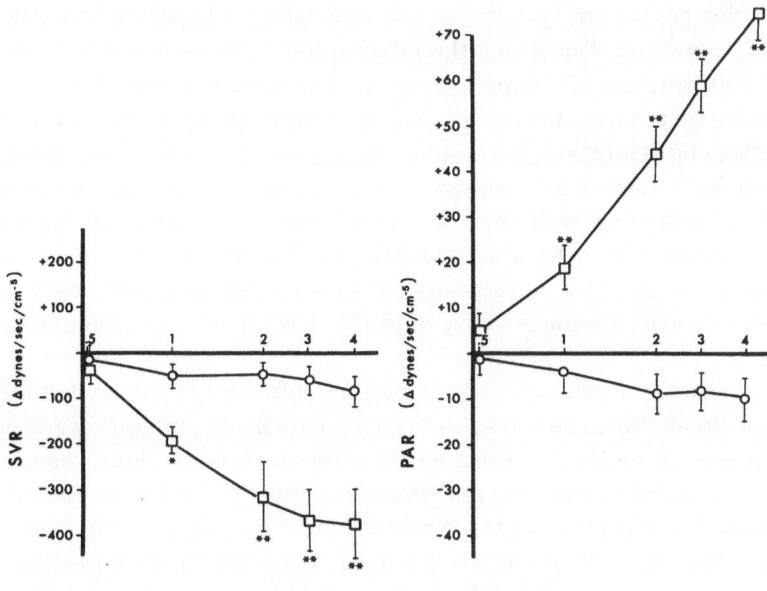

log dose of epinephrine (μg/min)

Figure 5. Systemic and pulmonary vasomotor responses evoked by epinephrine in the normotensive (O) and hypertensive (□) study patients (mean ± SD).
* and ** = differences from the corresponding value in the normotensive subjects significant at p < 0.05 and p < 0.01, respectively; abbreviations and format as in Figure 4.
From Guazzi et al. [18] by permission.

nous or exogenous, actually reflected active vasoconstriction in this group. The response to norepinephrine, either infused or released during the cold test, is of particular significance. In both circumstances, blood flow tended to become reduced to a similar extent in the two patient groups; however, in hypertensives, the driving pressure through the lungs became as great as under the influence of epinephrine, suggesting that an even greater vasomotion had occurred.

There are good reasons to be cautious about the application of catecholamine concentrations in body fluids for assessing neurogenic contributions [22], so that no inference can be drawn as to whether the underlying mechanism of the obvious pulmonary vasoconstriction and pressor responses to adrenergic activation during arithmetic and cold tests take origin from an excessive neural vascular activation in hypertension. The dose-response plot showing the increase in resistance with increasing doses of norepinephrine documented the existence of vascular overreactivity. Although some evidence has been reported of a tendency to increase the pulmonary artery medial thickness in spontaneous hypertensive rats [23], there is no information in human subjects concerning the possibility of duplication in the lesser circulation of the structural vascular changes occurring in the greater circulation in hypertension [24]. The question, therefore, concerning the relationship between constrictor overre-activity and structure of the pulmonary vessels remains open. However, the observation that, during the release of endogenous epinephrine and especially during exogenous infusion, normotensive subjects responded with vasodilata-tion while hypertensive patients developed substantial vasoconstriction is not in favor of increased wall thickness and lumen encroachment, because a greater decrease rather than an increase in resistance would be anticipated. This opposite vasomotor pattern suggests that a constrictor pulmonary vascu-lar supersensitivity becomes active with the development of systemic hyper-tension.

A review of the studies concerned with the influence of catecholamines on the lesser circulation in humans shows an increase in the pulmonary artery and wedge pressures under the influence of norepinephrine without remarkable changes in arteriolar resistance and blood flow through the lungs. The balance of evidence is against the existence of substantial pulmonary vasoconstriction in normal humans. This pattern is interpreted as resulting from passive vaso-dilatation as a consequence of displacement of blood from the periphery and some vasoconstriction caused by stimulation of alpha-adrenergic receptors [25]. On this basis one should deduce that in hypertension, in addition to an impedance to the pulmonary passive dilatation, there is an enhancement of active pulmonary vasoconstriction. These changes may derive from abnormal-ities in the number or quality [26] of adrenergic receptors or other regulatory components [27], or in the biochemistry of the excitation-contraction cou-pling.

Enhanced hypoxic pulmonary vasoconstriction

Alveolar hypoxia is a physiological stimulus that causes local vasoconstriction of the pulmonary arteries, probably by affecting excitation, contraction, or the coupling of the two [28]. A role of increased slow channel calcium entry into vascular smooth muscle in mediating hypoxic pulmonary vasoconstriction is suggested by the observation that verapamil inhibits such vasoconstriction [29] and that nifedipine reduces pulmonary vascular resistance in patients with respiratory failure [30, 31]. The influences of alveolar hypoxia on the pulmo-nary vessels investigated in the absence and in the presence of calcium channel blockade (nifedipine), was seen as a means to shed light upon the background of the disordered vasomotility and catecholamine hypersensitivity of the lesser circulation in high blood pressure.

The pulmonary arteriolar resistance has been evaluated in 43 hypertensive and 17 normotensive men during air respiration and after 15 min of breathing

17, 15 and 12% oxygen in nitrogen. Curves relating changes in pulmonary arteriolar resistance to oxygen breathing contents had similar shaped configuration in the two populations, but those in hypertension were steeper and significantly shifted to the left, reflecting a lower threshold and an enhanced vasoconstrictor reactivity.

The pattern was not related to differences in severity of the hypoxic stimulus, degree of hypocapnia and respiratory alcalosis induced by hypoxia, plasma levels of catecholamines, and was not mediated through alpha-adrenergic receptor activation (the pulmonary vasomotor reactions, in fact, persisted identical with those before alpha-adrenergic receptor blockade with phonoxybenzamine). Calcium channel blockade was able to abolish both the normotensive and the hypertensive pulmonary vasoconstriction reaction to each of the low oxygen breathing steps.

If, as it has been prospected, the final step in hypoxic vasomotion of the lungs consists of an increased flux of calcium through the vascular smooth muscle cell membrane, then these findings suggest that the influx of calcium ions into the contractile elements of the lung vessels is facilitated with the development of systemic high blood pressure.

References

1. Richards DW Jr (1946): Recording of right heart pressure in normal subjects and in patients with chronic pulmonary disease and various types of cardiocirculatory diseases. *J Clin Invest* 25: 639.
2. Gregory R (1953): Effect of epinephrine, norepinephrine, angiotonin and tetraethylammonium bromide on pulmonary and systemic arterial pressures in normotensive and hypertensive subjects. *Proc Soc Exp Biol Med* 83: 847–850.
3. Nelson RA, May LG, Bennett A, Kobayashi M, Gregory R (1955): Comparison of the effects of pressor and depressor agents and influences on pulmonary and systemic pressures of normotensive and hypertensive subjects. *Am Heart J* 50: 172–187.
4. Werkö L, Lagerlöf H (1949): Studies on the circulation in man, IV: Cardiac output and blood pressure in the right auricle, right ventricle and pulmonary artery in patients with hypertensive cardiovascular disease. *Acta Med Scand* 133: 427–436.
5. Cohn JN, Limas CJ, Guiha NH (1974): Hypertension and the heart. *Arch Intern Med* 133: 969–979.
6. Friedberg CK (1956): *Diseases of the Heart*, p 277. Philadelphia: WB Saunders.
7. Olivari MT, Fiorentini C, Polese A, Guazzi MD (1978): Pulmonary hemodynamics and right ventricular function in hypertension. *Circulation* 57: 1185–1190.
8. Atkins JM, Mitchell HC, Pettinger WA (1977): Increased pulmonary vascular resistance with systemic hypertension: Effect of Minoxidil and other antihypertensive agents. *Am J Cardiol* 39: 802–807.
9. Fortuin NJ, Hood WP Jr, Craige E (1972): Evaluation of left ventricular function by echocardiography. *Circulation* 46: 26–35.
10. Pool PE, Piggott WJ, Seagren SC, Skelton CL (1976): Augmented right ventricular function in systemic hypertension-induced hypertrophy. *Cardiovasc Res* 10: 124–128.

11. Meerson FZ (1969): The myocardium in hyperfunction, hypertrophy, and heart failure. *Circ Res* 24 (suppl 2): 1.
12. Taylor RR, Covell JW, Sonnenblick EH, Ross J Jr (1967): Dependence of ventricular distensibility on filling of the opposite ventricle. *Am J Physiol* 213: 711–718.
13. Cohn JN, Tristani FE, Khatri IM (1969): Studies in clinical shock and hypertension, VI: Relationship between left and right ventricular function. *J Clin Invest* 48: 2008–2018.
14. Brecher GA, Galletti PM (1963): Functional anatomy of cardiac pumping, in: Dow P (ed), *Handbook of Physiology,* 48: Section 2: Circulation, Vol 2, p. 759. Washington: American Physiological Society.
15. Ingram RH, Szidon JP, Skalak R, Fishman P (1968): Effects of sympathetic nerve stimulation on the pulmonary arterial tree of the isolated lobe perfused in situ. *Circ Res* 22: 801–815.
16. Hyman AL, Nandiwada P, Knight DS, Kadowitz PJ (1981): Pulmonary vasodilator responses to catecholamines and sympathetic nerve stimulation in the cat. *Circ Res* 407–415.
17. Fiorentini C, Barbier P, Galli C, Loaldi A, Tamborini G, Tosi E, Guazzi MD (1985): Pulmonary vascular overreactivity in systemic hypertension: A pathophysiological link between the greater and the lesser circulation. *Hypertension* 7: 995–1002.
18. Guazzi MD, De Cesare N, Fiorentini C, Galli C, Montorsi P, Pepi M, Tamborini G (1986): Pulmonary vascular supersensitivity to catecholamines in systemic high blood pressure. *J Am Coll Cardiol* 8: 1137–1144.
19. Guazzi M, Fiorentini C, Polese A, Magrini F, Olivari MT (1975): Stress-induced and sympathetically-mediated electrocardiographic and circulatory variations in the primary hyperkinetic heart syndrome. *Cardiovasc Res* 9: 342–354.
20. Cuddy RP, Smulyan H, Keghley JF, Markanson CR, Eich RH (1966): Hemodynamic and catecholamine changes during standard cold pressor test. *Am Heart J* 71: 446–454.
21. Guazzi MD, Alimento M, Fiorentini C, Pepi M, Polese A (1986): Hypersensitivity of lung vessels to catecholamines in systemic hypertension. *Br Med J* 293: 291–294.
22. Floras J, Jones JV, Hassan MO, Osikowska BA, Sever PS, Sleight P (1986): Failure of plasma norepinephrine to consistently reflect sympathetic activity in humans. *Hypertension* 8: 641–649.
23. McMurtry IF, Petrun MD, Tucker A, Reeves JT (1979): Pulmonary vascular reactivity in the spontaneously hypertensive rats. *Blood Vessels* 16: 61–70.
24. Schwartz SM (1984): Smooth muscle proliferation in hypertension. State-of-the-art lecture. *Hypertension* 6 (suppl I): I 56–61.
25. Harris P, Heath D (1977): *The Human Pulmonary Circulation,* pp 129–130, 182–188. New York: Churchill Livingstone.
26. Ohsuru F, Strauss HW, Homcy CJ (1984): The lung beta-receptor in the spontaneous hypertensive rat. *Jpn Circ J* 48: 1203–1209.
27. Ellsworth ML, Gregory TJ, Newell JC (1983): Pulmonary prostacyclin production with increased flow and sympathetic stimulation. *J Appl Physiol Respirat Environ Exercise Physiol* 55: 1225–1231.
28. Harris P, Heath D (1986): *The Human Pulmonary Circulation,* pp 145, 474–476. Edinburgh: Churchill Livingstone (Rev ed of [25]).
29. McMurtry IF, Davidson AB, Reeves JT, Grover RF (1976): Inhibition of hypoxic pulmonary vasoconstriction by calcium antagonist in isolated rat lungs. *Circ Res* 38: 99–104.
30. Simonneau G, Escourron P, Duroux P, Lockhart A (1981): Inhibition of hypoxic pulmonary vasoconstriction by nifedipine. *New Engl J Med* 304: 1582–1585.
31. Kennedy TP, Michael JR, Huang CK, Kallman CH, Zahkak, Schlott W, Summer W (1984): Nifedipine inhibits hypoxic pulmonary vasoconstriction during rest and excercise in patients with chronic obstructive pulmonary disease. *Am Rev Respir Dis* 129: 544–551.

21. Management of hypertensive patients with cardiac problems

RAY W. GIFFORD, Jr.

Many of the therapeutic principles described in this chapter resulted from investigations carried out by Dr. Robert Tarazi and his associates. Our understanding of the complex inter-relationships of the heart and hypertension has been enriched by his many contributions.

Introduction

The presence of cardiac complications in hypertensive patients should not only influence the selection of antihypertensive agents and the urgency with which they are administered but may also require consideration of ancillary therapeutic and dietary measures.

This chapter will consider appropriate treatment of hypertension complicated by atherosclerotic heart disease and/or left ventricular hypertrophy with or without left ventricular failure (Table 1).

Evidence of target organ disease, whether cardiac, renal or cerebral compromises the prognosis for the hypertensive patient, even with appropriate antihypertensive therapy [1]; nevertheless, the outlook is better with treatment than without but is not as good as it would have been had treatment been initiated before there was evidence of complications [1]. Postponing antihypertensive therapy until there is evidence of target organ disease cannot be condoned. However, the presence of target organ disease when the patient first presents is an urgent indication for antihypertensive therapy, even in patients with mild hypertension (diastolic 90 to 104 mmHg) [2].

M.E. Safar & F. Fouad-Tarazi (eds.), The heart in hypertension.
© *1989 Kluwer Academic Publishers, Dordrecht –*

Evaluation of the hypertensive patient for evidence of cardiac disease

One of the most important objectives of pretreatment evaluation of the hypertensive patient is to evaluate the status of the target organs because this has a profound effect on prognosis, the decision to treat and the selection of drugs.

With respect to the heart, it is important to elicit a history of angina pectoris and/or prior myocardial infarction, dependent edema and unusual dyspnea or orthopnea suggesting congestive heart failure or compromised myocardial reserve.

During physical examination the physician should listen for a fourth heart sound indicative of early left ventricular hypertrophy, evaluate the neck veins and look for hepatomegaly, peripheral edema, basilar rales and a third heart sound.

The laboratory investigation should include, as a minimum, a standard electrocardiogram. For patients with angina pectoris or a history of myocardial infarction, an exercise stress test is indicated and under some circumstances a coronary angiogram may be desirable. Routine stress tests, chest X-rays, echocardiograms and Holter monitoring without some indication other than hypertension are not advocated at this time, except for hypertensive children for whom the Task Force Report on Pediatric Hypertension recommended that a baseline echocardiogram be performed whenever drug therapy is seriously being considered [3].

Atherosclerotic heart disease

Stable angina pectoris

Antihypertensive regimens for patients who have stable angina pectoris without evidence of myocardial infarction should include either a beta blocking or a calcium channel blocking agent to take advantage of the dual beneficial effects of these drugs on hypertension and angina (Table 1). Usually one of these drugs is used as monotherapy to initiate treatment. In some cases with particularly resistant hypertension or angina pectoris, a drug from each class may be prescribed. While there are relative contraindications to combining a beta blocking agent and a calcium channel blocking drug in the same regimen, this applies mainly to verapamil which has a negative inotropic effect and depresses conduction similar to the beta blockers. For patients with normal conduction and good myocardial reserve adverse effects are unlikely from this combination [4]. If there is doubt, nifedipine can be preecribed with a beta blocker because it has very little effect on cardiac conduction and contractility but is an excellent coronary vasodilator.

The combination of a beta blocker and a calcium channel blocker is particularly effective in reducing the frequency of episodes of ST segment depression during ambulatory blood pressure monitoring in patients with silent myocardial ischemia [4].

A diuretic, a centrally or peripherally acting adrenergic blocking agent or an ACE inhibitor may be added to the regimen if necessary to control hypertension.

Isosorbide is indicated in addition to antihypertensive agents for most patients with angina pectoris, although it may be less important if a calcium channel blocking agent is incorporated in the regimen because both are coronary vasodilators. Isosorbide in large doses will reduce afterload thus decreasing the oxygen requirements of the heart, although the latter effect is not as dramatic as it is with calcium channel blockers. Sublingual nitroglyc-

Table 1. Selection of drugs for hypertensive patients with cardiac disease.

Heart disease	Preferred drug	Relatively contraindicated
Atherosclerotic heart disease with angina pectoris	Beta blockers Ca channel blockers	Direct vasodilators without an adrenergic blocker
Remote myocardial infarction	Non-ISA beta blocker	
Acute myocardial infarction with severe hypertension	Nitroglycerine IV Sodium nitroprusside IV Labetalol IV	Diazoxide Hydralazine Nifedipine
Left ventricular hypertrophy without congestive heart failure	Ca channel blockers Beta blockers ACE inhibitors Diuretics Methyldopa	Direct vasodilators without an adrenergic blocker
Congestive heart failure – Chronic	Diuretics ACE inhibitors Isosorbide Hydralazine	Beta blockers* Verapamil Diltiazem
– Acute	Furosemide IV Sodium nitroprusside IV Nitroglycerine IV	Diazoxide Labetalol

* It has been suggested that beta blocking drugs may be beneficial in some patients with congestive cardiomyopathy [81].

erine should be used on a PRN basis. Transdermal nitroglycerine can be prescribed in addition to or instead of isosorbide. It is well to remember that sustained-release isosorbide dinitrate can decrease systolic blood pressure [5] which might lead to a cumulative effect when combined with antihypertensive agents, especially the calcium channel blocking agents or the alpha-1 adreno-receptor blocking drugs.

Cruickshank and colleagues [6] have reported a paradoxical increase in the incidence of fatal myocardial infarction when diastolic blood pressure was reduced to < 85 mmHg in hypertensive patients with evidence of pre-existing ischemic heart disease or intermittent claudication. The optimal range for diastolic blood pressures seemed to be 85–90 mmHg. This J-shaped curve was not evident for systolic blood pressure, however.

Samuelsson et al. [7] also found a slight increase in the incidence of coronary events when blood pressure was reduced below 150/85 mmHg in men, whether or not they had clinical evidence of coronary atherosclerosis. In the HAPPHY trial there was an inverse relationship between mean in-study blood pressure and coronary events, whereas there was a direct relationship between mean in-study blood pressure and the incidence of stroke and total mortality [8]. However, none of the large randomized controlled trials have demonstrated the J-shaped curve for coronary morbidity and mortality during antihypertensive therapy. In the IPPPSH study, ischemic changes in the electrocardiogram were least likely to develop for participants whose diastolic blood pressure was reduced to less than 85 mmHg [9].

Because most patients who have atherosclerotic heart disease also have abnormal serum lipids, it is important to measure serum cholesterol and its fractions to determine whether dietary restriction of saturated fats and/or anticholesterolemic drugs are indicated in addition to antihypertensive therapy.

In this regard there is some concern about the use of thiazide and related diuretics and some beta blockers in patients with atherosclerotic heart disease because of their potential adverse effects on blood lipids. The diuretics have been studied more extensively than the beta blockers in this respect, but both can elevate serum cholesterol, LDL cholesterol and triglycerides, and the beta blocking drugs may depress HDL cholesterol in some cases [10].

The hyperlipidemic effect of the diuretics seems to be dose-related and was observed in susceptible patients only [11], was apparent within six weeks of initiating therapy [11], was blunted or reversed by a low-fat diet [12], was not observed in elderly patients [13, 14], was more likely to affect patients with low or normal serum cholesterol than patients with high serum cholesterol [15, 16] and it seems to be temporary, lasting less than a year in most long-term studies [15, 17, 18]. The potassium-sparing diuretics (spironolactone, triamterene and amiloride) do not affect blood lipids but they aren't very potent antihypertensive agents. Indapamide is said to have a lesser effect on serum lipids than conventional thiazides [19].

The adverse effect of beta blockers on serum lipids may persist longer than that of the diuretics [17]. Beta blockers with intrinsic sympathomimetic activity (ISA) and the combined beta and alpha blocking drug (labetalol) do not seem to alter blood lipids as much as conventional beta blockers do [10].

Unstable angina pectoris and acute myocardial infarction

A syndrome of paroxysmal hypertension associated with unstable angina pectoris or acute myocardial infarction has been described [20]. James and colleagues, using a dog model, attributed the sudden rise in blood pressure to a chemo-reflex arising from an area of ischemic myocardium surrounding the main left coronary artery, possibly mediated by serotonin released from aggregated platelets in this area [21].

Hypertension, whether chronic and stable, or acutely precipitated by the ischemic event, is an unnecessary and costly burden, adding to the oxygen demands on an already ischemic left ventricle. When blood pressure is ≥ 180/110 mmHg, prompt but judicious reduction of blood pressure is indicated. This constitutes a hypertensive emergency and the drug of choice is usually nitroglycerine by intravenous infusion (Table 1). Nitroglycerine is preferred to sodium nitroprusside for this emergency because it dilates coronary arteries [22]; however it is not as potent as sodium nitroprusside in reducing afterload, so if the blood pressure does not come down with an infusion of nitroglycerine, sodium nitroprusside should be substituted. Hypotension and/or rapid reduction of blood pressure should be avoided as this might jeopardize coronary perfusion. Consequently drugs that are given by bolus injection such as diazoxide and labetalol are relatively contraindicated as is the sublingual administration of nifedipine [23]. Direct vasodilators, including diazoxide and hydralazine may induce tachycardia reflexly and thereby increase myocardial oxygen consumption.

As a result of the First International Study of Infarct Survival (ISIS-1) [24], many cardiologists are now using a beta blocker such as metoprolol intravenously during the acute phase of myocardial infarction to limit infarct size unless there is a contraindication. Except for labetalol, beta blockers administered intravenously have minimal or unpredictable effects on blood pressure and cannot be relied on to bring blood pressure down if it is greater than 180/110 mmHg. Below this level it is reasonable to observe the effect of the beta blocker given intravenously and if it doesn't bring blood pressure down to desired levels, an infusion of nitroglycerine or sodium nitroprusside should be added cautiously, because there may be a synergistic effect on blood pressure when both types of agents are administered simultaneously.

Adjunctive therapy with nitrates, either orally or transdermally, is not necessary if nitroglycerine is administered intravenously. If sodium nitroprusside or a beta blocker is given intravenously, oral or transdermal nitrates can be used to dilate the coronary vascular bed but the bloodpressure should be monitored closely to avoid hypotension from the combination of agents.

Post myocardial infarction

Only beta blockers have been shown to have a cardioprotective effect when administered after a myocardial infarction. In the Norwegian Study the cumulative mortality rate was significantly lower in men receiving a beta blocker (timolol) than in a control group receiving placebo for up to six years afterthe infarct [25].

Unless there is a contraindication, a beta blocker should be prescribed and continued indefinitely for most patients who have had a myocardial infarction. If the patient also has hypertension, it is reasonable to use the beta blocker as step one in the antihypertensive regimen. Additional agents, usually a diuretic, can be added subsequently if needed to keep the blood pressure at normotensive levels.

The evidence to date would suggest that only the non-ISA beta blockers without alpha blocking properties have this cardioprotective effect.

Post coronary bypass hypertension

Hypertension occurring immediately after coronary bypass operations was recognized early in the experience with this type of open heartprocedure. It can occur in previously normotensive as well as hypertensive patients [26]. Whileit is usually mild to moderate (eg < 160/110 mmHg) it can be detrimental to the recently revascularized myocardium. It is characterized by an increase in plasma catecholamines, total peripheral vascular resistance and heart rate suggesting hyperactivity of the adrenergic nervous system, which may be due to an afferent sympathetic reflex ornating in the heart, great vessels or coronary arteries [27]. An infusion of nitroglycerine or sodium nitroprusside is usually thetreatment of choice[22, 28].

Left ventricular hypertrophy

Electrocardiographic evidence of left ventricular hypertrophy (ECG-LVH) is associated with an increased incidence of ventricular arrhythmias including runs of ventricular tachycardia [29–31], and sudden death [32], especially where there are repolarization (ST-T) changes as well as voltage criteria [29, 32].

The echocardiogram is a more sensitive and specific modality for the diagnosis of LVH than is the ECG. Many patients with echocardiographic evidence of LVH do not have ECG evidence of it. Is prognosis compromised for this group as it is for patients with ECG-LVH? Casale et al. [33] have reported that seven of 29 men with hypertension and echocardiographic evidence of LVH had a morbid event within a mean follow-up period of 4.8 years compared to seven of 111 hypertensive men who had no evidence of LVH on echocardiogram. The seven events in men with LVH included two deaths (one from myocardial infarction), two nonfatal myocardial infarctions and three coronary bypass operations. The seven events in men without LVH included one death due to myocardial infarction, two nonfatal myocardial infarctions, one of whom also had a stroke, two strokes and two coronary bypasses. Only five of the 29 men with echocardiographic evidence of LVH had ECG evidence of LVH by the Romhilt-Estes score ≥ 5. Three patients without echocardiographic evidence of LVH had ECG-LVH by this criteria.

Echocardiographic evidence of LVH was present in 16% of men and 19% of women in the Framingham study [34]. Prevalence increased dramatically with age, systolic blood pressure and obesity. Other risk factors included valve disease and myocardial infarction. The relationship between systolic blood pressure and echocardiographic evidence of LVH begins below 140 mmHg. There is a closer relationship between systolic blood pressure and LVH than there is between diastolic blood pressure and LVH [35]. Echocardiographic evidence of LVH has been noted in adolescents with borderline blood pressure [36] and is a criterion to be considered before prescribing drug therapy in children [3].

Evidence of LVH, whether by ECG or echocardiogram, is an urgent indication for drug therapy, even when hypertension is mild. While nonpharmacologic therapy should be prescribed as an adjunct to drug therapy for such patients, it is a mistake to lose several months in an unsuccessful attempt to control hypertension with hygienic measures alone.

Our friend and colleague, Dr. Robert Tarazi, in whose memory this book is being published was the first to show that all antihypertensive drugs did not reverse echocardiographic evidence of LVH even though blood pressure was reduced to similar levels [37, 38] (Table 2). In general, adrenergic inhibiting agents [37, 39], calcium channel blockers [40, 41] and ACE inhibitors [42, 43] tend to reverse LVH while diuretics [39] and direct vasodilators (hydralazine [37], minoxidil [40, 44]) do not, even though blood pressureis well controlled, suggesting that hypertrophy cannot be explained solely on a hemodynamic basis [45]. There are exceptions, however. Beta blockers do not prevent or reverse hypertension or LVH in spontaneously hypertensive rats (SHR)[46] or renal hypertensive rats [47] but the non-ISA beta blockers do reverse LVH in hypertensive patients [48–50]. Methyldopa has consistently reversed LVH in rats and man [37, 39], yet clonidine, a drug with similar action on the adrenergic nervous system does not [51, 52] unless doses large enough to exert a peripheral adrenergic agonist effect were used [51]. Furthermore, diuretics have not been shown to reverse LVH [39], yet they reduce vascular reactivity to norepinephrine infusions [53].

In an editorial in 1983, Tarazi and I [54] questionedwhether reversal of LVH should be a goal of antihypertensive therapy. Subsequently, in a paper published posthumously, Tarazi and his coauthor Frohlich [55] suggested that reversal of LVH which is an adaptive mechanism to an increased afterload might not be desirable if it leaves the left ventricle less capable of sustaining a resurgence of hypertension should it occur.

Until that controversy is settled, any of the drugs proposed by the Fourth Joint National Committee [2] for initial monotherapy would be appropriate to

Table 2. Effect of antihypertensive drugs on preventing or reversing echocardiographic evidence of LVH.

Drug	Rats	Man
Methyldopa	+ [37, 51, 52]	+ [39]
Methyldopa and diuretic		+ [39]
Methyldopa and minoxidil	+ [44]	
Diuretic	0 [42]	0 [39]
Metoprolol		+ [48]
Propranolol	± [44] 0 [46]	
Atenolol	0 [47]	+ [49]
Timolol	0 [46]	+ [50]
Hydralazine	0 [37]	
Minoxidil	0 [40, 44]	
Propranolol + minoxidil	0 [44]	
Calcium channel blockers	+ [40]	+ [41]
ACE inhibitors	+ [42]	+ [43]
Clonidine	0 [51, 52]	
Clonidine (high dose)	+ [51]	
ACE inhibitors + diuretic	+ [42]	

+ = reversal of LVH demonstrated.
0 = reversal of LVH not demonstrated.
± = partial reversal of LVH demonstrated.

treat hypertension associated with echocardiographic evidence of LVH (Table 1). These include diuretics, beta blockers, calcium channel blockers and ACE inhibitors. Of these, only diuretics have not been shown to reverse LVH. There is no temptation to use hydralazine or minoxidil as initial monotherapy because they lead to reflex tachycardia and fluid retention unless a sympathetic inhibitor and diuretic are in the regimen, but they are appropriate Step 3 drugs. Any of the drugs proposed for Step 1 can also be used for Step 2, as can central alpha agonists, alpha₁ blockers and drugs which inhibit norepinephrine release from adrenergic neurons. With two exceptions noted subsequently, usual antihypertensive regimens are appropriate for patients with echocardiographic evidence of LVH.

Numerous studies have shown that reduction of blood pressure, irrespective of which drugs were prescribed, can improve or reverse ECG/LVH [56–59] (Figure 1), even when hypertension is suboptimally controlled [9]. Whether this improves prognosis is not known, but based on results from the HDFP trial it is unlikely to reduce risk to the level of uncomplicated but treated hypertension [1].

A word of caution is warranted for two unusual situations which require special regimens.

Hypertensive hypertrophic cardiomyopathy of the elderly is characterized by severe concentric cardiac hypertrophy and a small left ventricular cavity by echocardiogram and supernormal indexes of systolic function [60]. Patients present with dyspnea and atypical chest pain but no evidence of coronary disease. Even when there is clinical evidence of congestive heart failure, these patients respond better to beta blockers or calcium channel blockers than they do to hydralazine, nitrates, prazosin or ACE inhibitors, all of which have caused hypotension in some cases [60]. In one case, administration of nitroglycerine intravenously resulted in death.

Similar therapeutic precautions are applicable to hypertensive patients with *asymmetric septal hypertrophy and obstruction of the left ventricular outflow tract* (idiopathic hypertrophic subaortic stenosis). Beta blockers are the drugs of choice. Verapamil, because of its negative inotropic effect, has also been helpful but the predominantly vasodilating effect of nifedipine can lead to hypotension and cardiogenic shock. Nitrates, hydralazine, minoxidil, ACE inhibitors and to some extent diuretics are contraindicated. Obviously there is an inverse relationship between systemic blood pressure and severity of outflow obstruction, so that patients with significant hypertension are not likely to have much outflow obstruction. Nevertheless the outflow obstruction is a dynamic process and an ill-conceived antihypertensive regimen can suddenly exacerbate the pressure gradient in the outflow tract.

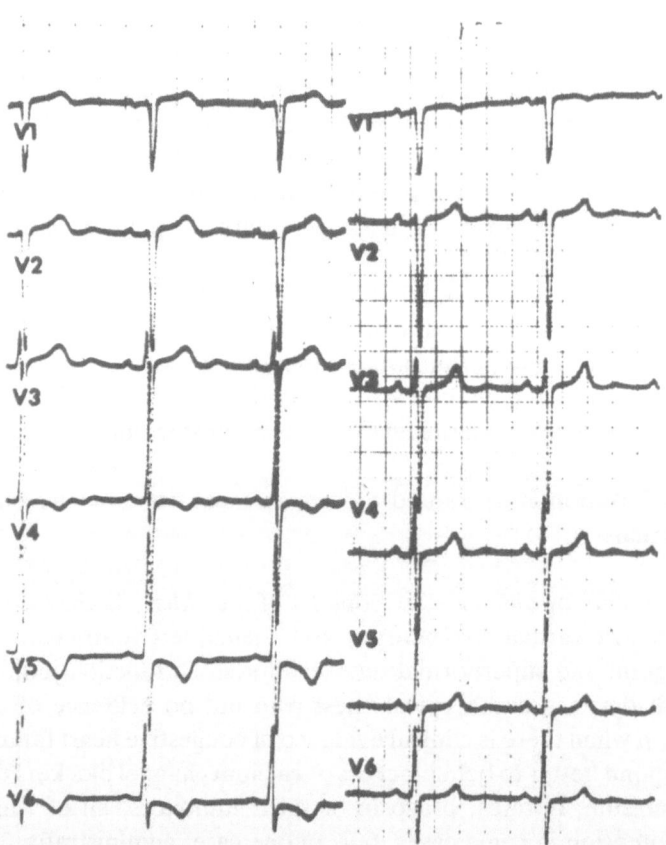

Figure 1. Precordial leads of the electrocardiogram of a 63-year-old man with Group 2 hypertension before (10/12/72) and during (1/14/74) effective antihypertensive treatment, showing reversion of ST-T abnormalities to normal. Note decrease in voltage of QRS.
Adapted from Gifford [82] with permission.

Congestive heart failure

Whether congestive heart failure is due to hypertensive heart disease or unrelated causes, reduction of total peripheral resistance (afterload) is beneficial [61] (Table 1) and is often as important, if not more important, than administering digitalis preparations. Even for patients who have normal blood pressure, vasodilating agents have been helpful in controlling the symptoms and correcting the hemodynamic perturbations of left ventricular failure, especially when it has been refractory to conventional therapy [61–65].

In 1974 Guiha et al. [62] first reported the successful treatment of patients with refractory left ventricular failure using intravenous infusions of sodium nitroprusside which is a potent arteriolar and venous vasodilator, thus reducing preload as well as afterload.

Other agents or combination of agents which dilate the venous as well as the arterial side of the circulation (Figure 2), and can be administered orally have been investigated for the chronic management of congestive heart failure.

Prazosin, an alpha$_1$ blocking agent has been effective in managing congestive heart failure for short periods but tachyphylaxis has been a problem in its long-term use [66].

In a double-blind randomized trial, the Veterans Administration Cooperative Study Group demonstrated that the addition of hydralazine and isosorbide dinitrate to a regimen of digoxin and diuretics produced a 28% reduction in mortality in patients with chronic congestive heart failure for periods ranging from 6 months to 5.7 years compared to a control group receiving a placebo plus digoxin and diuretics [67]. A third group, receiving prazosin in addition to diuretic and digoxin had a mortality rate similar to the placebo control group [67].

The ACE inhibitor, enalapril, has also been shown to decrease mortality (−27%, p = 0.003) for patients with severe congestive heart failure when added to conventional treatment in a double-blind placebo-controlled trial with a follow-up of one day to 20 months [65]. The control group received a placebo in addition to conventional therapy. Doses of enalapril ranged from 5 to 20 mg twice daily.

A multicenter, placebo-controlled trial has shown that captopril was more effective than digoxin when added to maintenance diuretic therapy in improving exercise time and decreasing ventricular premature beats, but digoxin increased ejection fraction slightly more than captopril did [68].

When renal blood flow is reduced by renal artery disease, hypovolemia or a decrease in cardiac output secondary to congestive heart failure, or a combination of these, glomerular filtration rate (GFR) is maintained by angiotensin II-mediated constriction of the efferent arterioles. Under these circumstances administration of an ACE inhibitor can decrease GFR with a resultant rise in serum creatinine and BUN which may be gradual and mild but on occasion can be abrupt and severe with acute renal failure. The latter is more likely to occur with severe bilateral renal artery stenosis or stenosis in the artery supplying a solitary kidney than in congestive heart failure.

Packer et al. [69] reported their observations in treating 104 patients with severe chronic heart failure with either enalapril or captopril. Seventy patients had no change or even an improvement in renal function while 34 developed functional insufficiency. Patients who developed renal insufficiency had a lower central venous pressure and were receiving a larger dose of furosemide

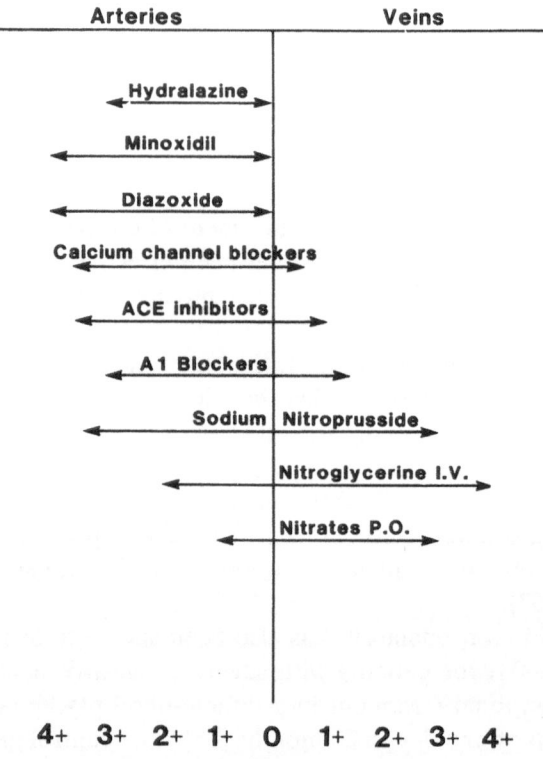

Figure 2. Semi-quantitative estimate of the spectrum of relative effects of vasodilators on arteries and veins. In the management of congestive heart failure which is characterized by an increase in afterload (total peripheral resistance) and preload (cardiac filling pressure), it is important to select drugs or combinations of drugs which have an effect on both the arteriolar and venous sides of the circulation. Sodium nitroprusside is the prototype. ACE inhibitors have also been effective in treatment of chronic congestive heart failure (see text). A combination of hydralazine (a pure arteriolar vasodilator) and isosorbide dinitrate which has its predominant effect on the venous side of the circulation has been shown to reduce mortality in patients with chronic congestive heart failure. It is entirely possible that the relative effects of these drugs on arteries and veins may be different in patients with congestive heart failure than in patients who have adequate cardiac compensation [61]. Oral nitrates must be given in relatively large doses (at least 40 mg of isosorbide QID) to dilate peripheral arterioles.

on the average than those who did not. Eighty-two percent of patients who had renal insufficiency with ACE inhibition had excessive reductions in left ventricular filling pressure (<15 mmHg) and/or mean arterial pressure (<60 mmHg) compared to only 31% of those who had no deterioration in renal function. Renal function was restored to pretreatment levels by reducing the dose of diuretic without altering the dose of the ACE inhibitor. ACE inhibitors with a long duration of action, such as enalapril seem to be more likely to induce deterioration of renal function and to increase serum potassium than shorter acting ACE inhibitors such as captopril [70].

In summary, diuretics and either ACE inhibitors or a combination of hydralazine and isosorbide dinitrate are particularly indicated in managing hypertension associated with chronic congestive heart failure. Beta blockers and verapamil are relatively contraindicated because of their negative inotropic effects. However, a history of congestive heart failure in a patient who no longer has manifestations of it is not a contraindication to therapy with beta blockers or verapamil. Calcium channel blockers with little or no cardiac effects (eg, nitrendipine, nifedipine) may ultimately prove to be beneficial in managing congestive heart failure because of their potent vasodilating effect which reduces afterload, but a venodilator such as isosorbide might be necessary to reduce preload by relaxing the large veins.

Serum creatinine and potassium should be monitored closely when an ACE inhibitor is included in the regimen for patients with chronic heart failure. Hypovolemia and excessive reduction of blood pressure may lead to a decrease in GFR. If this occurs, reducing the dose of diuretic may be even more important than reducing the dose of the ACE inhibitor.

An intravenous infusion of sodium nitroprusside or nitroglycerine, along with intravenous furosemide is the regimen of choice for emergency treatment of patients with acute left ventricular failure and pulmonary edema. In the absence of coronary insufficiency, sodium nitroprusside is preferable to nitroglycerine because it is a more potent arteriolar dilator (Figure 2) and hence is more effective in reducing afterload. On the other hand, if there is evidence of coronary insufficiency, nitroglycerine might be preferred because of its ability to dilate coronary arteries.

Diuretics and hypokalemia in patients with heart disease

Many patients with hypertension and heart disease, irrespective of etiology, will benefit from diuretic therapy but physicians are often reluctant to prescribe diuretics, especially since the Multiple Risk Intervention Trial (MRFIT) study showed an excess of sudden unexpected deaths in the Special Intervention (SI) group of hypertensive men with resting electrocardiographic abnormalities who received oral diuretics, compared to the Usual Care (UC) group who had resting electrocardiographic abnormalities and hypertension, many of whom also received diuretics [71]. Although the implication is that these sudden deaths may have resulted from acute arrhythmias induced by hypokalemia, this has not been documented [72] and may never be.

Some authors have demonstrated a relationship between diuretic-induced hypokalemia and ventricular ectopy [73–76], but others have not [29, 77–80], even in the presence of LVH [29, 79]. The Medical Research Council (MRC) study has shown a correlation between thiazide therapy and ventricular ectopic activity, but this could not be attributed to serum potassium concentration [80].

Until this controversy is resolved, it is reasonable to prescribe a combination thiazide-potassium sparing diuretic to prevent hypokalemia for most patients who have cardiac disease of any type or an abnormal ECG without definite evidence of heart disease. Certain precautions must be observed, however, because hyperkalemia is more lethal than hypokalemia. Potassium-sparing diuretics should be used with caution, if at all, in patients with chronic renal failure or who are also taking potassium supplements or ACE inhibitors. In this regard it is important to remember that most salt substitutes contain a variety of potassium salts. Potassium-retaining diuretics can cause hyperkalemia in patients with hyporeninemic hypoaldosteronism which sometimes occurs in elderly patients, often with non-insulin dependent diabetes mellitus. Their serum potassium concentration is usually in the high normal range before any treatment is given.

Keeping the diuretic dose at the minimal effective level and prescribing a potassium-sparing diuretic with the thiazide are the most effective methods of preventing hypokalemia. Increasing dietary potassium, reducing dietary sodium and prescribing supplements of potassium chloride are much less reliable.

Cardiac arrhythmias and conduction disturbances

Certain antihypertensive drugs may be especially indicated or relatively contraindicated when hypertension is complicated by cardiac arrhythmias or conduction disturbances.

Non-ISA beta blockers may be helpful in controlling paroxysmal supraventricular tachycardia and premature ventricular contractions due to adrenergic hyperactivity. On the other hand, by slowing the heart rate, they can actually increase premature ventricular contractions arising from an irritable focus.

Verapamil is even more effective than beta blockers in treating and preventing recurrences of paroxysmal supraventricular tachycardia. Intravenous verapamil is recommended for terminating an acute episode of paroxysmal supraventricular tachycardia.

Beta blockers and verapamil slow AV conduction and therefore are often effective in controlling the ventricular rate in patients with atrial fibrillation or flutter. For the same reason, however, they are contraindicated in the presence of greater than first degree AV block, but may be used in patients with intraventricular block and bundle branch block. Both are contraindicated for patients with sick sinus syndrome unless a functioning ventricular pacemaker is in place. Special precautions must be observed in using either verapamil or beta blockers in patients with an accessory bypass tract (Wolff-Parkinson-White or Lown-Ganong-Levine syndromes). Verapamil can convert atrial flutter or atrial fibrillation to ventricular tachyarrhythmias including ventricular fibrillation when administered to patients with accessory bypass tracts. Rare instances of severe bradycardia requiring a demand pacemaker have been reported when beta blockers have been given to patients with paroxysmal atrial tachycardia in the presence of Wolff-Parkinson-White syndrome.

Valvular heart disease

Arteriolar vasodilating agents such as calcium channel blockers and ACE inhibitors are helpful in minimizing the regurgitant flow in patients with either mitral or aortic insufficiency [61].

References

1. Hypertension Detection and Follow-up Program Cooperative Group (1982): Results of the Hypertension Detection and Follow-up Program: The effect of treatment on mortality in 'mild' hypertension. *New Engl J Med* 307: 976–980.
2. The 1988 report of the Joint National Committee on Detection, Evaluation and Treatment of High Blood Pressure (1988). *Arch Intern Med* 148: 1023–1038.
3. Task Force on Blood Pressure Control in Children (1987): Report of the Second Task Force on Blood Pressure Control in Children – 1987. *Pediatrics* 79: 1–25.
4. Dargie HJ (1986): Combination therapy with beta-adrenoceptor blockers and calcium antagonists. *Br J Clin Pharmacol* 21: 155S–160S.
5. Duchier J, Iannascoli F, Safar M (1987): Antihypertensive effect of sustained-release isosorbide dinitrate for isolated systolic systemic hypertension in the elderly. *Am J Cardiol* 60: 99–102.
6. Cruickshank JM, Thorp JM, Zacharias FJ (1987): Benefits and potential harm of lowering high blood pressure. *Lancet* 1987/1: 581–584.
7. Samuelsson O, Wilhelmsen L, Andersson OK, Pennert K, Berglund G (1987): Cardiovascular morbidity in relation to change in blood pressure and serum cholesterol levels in treated hypertension. *JAMA* 258: 1768–1776.
8. Wilhelmsen L, Berglund G, Elmfeldt D, Fitzsimons T, Holzgreve H, Hosie J, Hornkvist PE, Pennert K, Tuomilehto J, Wedel H (1987): Beta-blockers versus diuretics in hypertensive men: Main results from the HAPPHY trial. *J Hypertension* 5: 561–574.
9. Bolli P, Burkart F, Vesanen K, Baker JL, Pinto M, Buhler FR (1987): Electrocardiographic changes during antihypertensive therapy in the International Prospective Primary Prevention Study in Hypertension. *Hypertension* 9 (suppl III): 69–74.
10. Weidmann P, Gerber A, Mordasini R (1983): Effects of antihypertensive therapy on serum lipoproteins. *Hypertension* 5 (suppl III): 120–131.
11. Ames RP, Hill P (1976): Elevation of serum lipid levels during diuretic therapy of hypertension. *Am J Med* 61: 748–757.

12. Grimm RH, Leon AS, Hunninghake DB, Lenz K, Hannan P, Blackburn H (1981): Effects of thiazide diuretics on plasma lipids and lipoproteins in mildly hypertensive patients. A double-blind controlled trial. *Ann Intern Med* 94: 7–11.

13. Amery A, Birkenhager W, Bulpitt C, Clement D, Deruyttere M, De Schaepdryver A, Dollery C, Fagard R, Forette F, Forte J, Hamdy R, Leonetti G, O'Mally K, Tuomilehto J (1982): Influence of antihypertensive therapy on serum cholesterol in elderly hypertensive patients: Results of trial by the European Working Party on High Blood Pressure in the Elderly (EWPHE). *Acta Cardiologica* 37: 235–244.

14. Hulley SB, Furberg CD, Gurland B, McDonald R, Perry HM, Schnaper HW, Schoenberger JA, Smith WM, Vogt TM (1985): The Systolic Hypertension in the Elderly Program (SHEP): Antihypertensive efficacy of chlorthalidone. *Am J Cardiol* 56: 913–920.

15. Williams WR, Schneider KA, Borhani NO, Schnaper HW, Slotkoff LM, Ellefson RD (1986): The relationship between diuretics and serum cholesterol in Hypertension Detection and Follow-up Program participants. *Am J Prev Med* 2: 248–255.

16. Goldman AI, Steele BW, Schnaper HW, Fritz AE, Frohlich ED, Perry HM (1980): Serum lipoprotein levels during chlorthalidone therapy. A Veterans Administration-National Heart, Lung, and Blood Institute cooperative study on antihypertensive therapy. *JAMA* 244: 1691–1695.

17. Veterans Administration Cooperative Study Group on Antihypertensive Agents (1982): Comparison of propranolol and hydrochlorothiazide for the initial treatment of hypertension, II: Results of long-term therapy. *JAMA* 248: 2004–2011.

18. Berglund G, Andersson O (1981): Beta-blockers or diuretics in hypertension? A six-year follow-up of blood pressure and metabolic side effects. *Lancet* 1981/1: 744–747.

19. Meyer-Sabellek W, Gotzen R, Heitz J, Arntz HR, Schulte KL (1985): Serum lipoprotein levels during long-term treatment of hypertension with indapamide. *Hypertension* 7 (suppl II): 170–174.

20. Horwitz D, Sjoerdsma A (1965): Some inter-relationships between elevation of blood pressure and angina pectoris. Proc Counc High Blood Pressure Res, *Am Heart Assoc* 13: 39–48.

21. James TN, Isobe JH, Urthaler F (1975): Analysis of components in a cardiogenic hypertensive chemoreflex. *Circulation* 52: 179–192.

22. Flaherty JT, Magee PA, Gardner TL, Potter A, MacAllister NP (1982): Comparison of intravenous nitroglycerin and sodium nitroprusside for treatment of acute hypertension developing after coronary artery bypass surgery. *Circulation* 65: 1072–1077.

23. O'Mailia JJ, Sander GE, Giles TD (1987): Nifedipine-associated myocardial ischemia or infarction in the treatment of hypertensive urgencies. *Ann Intern Med* 107: 185–186.

24. First International Study of Infarct Survival Collaborative Group (1986): Randomised trial of intravenous atenolol among 16,027 cases of suspected acute myocardial infarction: ISIS-1. *Lancet* 1986/2: 57–66.

25. Pedersen TR, For the Norwegian Multicenter Study Group (1985): Six-year follow-up of the Norwegian Multicenter Study on Timolol After Acute Myocardial Infarction. *New Engl J Med* 313: 1055–1058.

26. Estafanous FG, Tarazi RC, Viljoen JF, El Tawil MY (1973): Systemic hypertension following myocardial revascularization. *Am Heart J* 6: 732–738.

27. Fouad FM, Estafanous FG, Bravo EL, Iyer KA, Maydak JH, Tarazi RC (1979): Possible role of cardioaortic reflexes in postcoronary bypass hypertension. *Am J Cardiol* 44: 866–872.

28. Stinson EB, Holloway EL, Derby G, Oyer PE, Hollingsworth H, Griepp RB, Harrison DC (1975): Comparative hemodynamic responses to chlorpromazine, nitroprusside, nitroglycerin, and trimethaphan immediately after open-heart operations. *Circulation* 51 (suppl I): 26–33.

29. McLenachan JM, Henderson E, Morris KI, Dargie HJ (1987): Ventricular arrhythmias in patients with hypertensive left ventricular hypertrophy. *New Engl J Med* 317: 787–792.
30. Frohlich ED (1986): Left ventricular hypertrophy as a risk factor. *Cardiology Clinics* 4: 137–144.
31. Messerli FH, Ventura HO, Elizardi DJ, Dunn FG, Frohlich ED (1984): Hypertension and sudden death. Increased ventricular ectopic activity in left ventricular hypertrophy. *Am J Med* 77: 18–22.
32. Kannel WB (1983): Prevalence and natural history of electrocardiographic left ventricular hypertrophy. *Am J Med* 75 (suppl 3A): 4–11.
33. Casale PN, Devereux RB, Milner M, Zullo G, Harshfield GA, Pickering TG, Laragh JH (1986): Value of echocardiographic measurement of left ventricular mass in predicting cardio-vascular morbid events in hypertensive men. *Ann Intern Med* 105: 173–178.
34. Levy D, Anderson KM, Savage D, Kannel WB, Christiansen JC, Castelli WP (1988): Echocardiographically detected left ventricular hypertrophy: Prevalence and risk factors. *Ann Intern Med* 108: 7–13.
35. Drayer JIM, Weber MA, DeYoung JL (1983): BP as a determinant of cardiac left ventricular muscle mass. *Arch Intern Med* 143: 90–92.
36. Laird WP, Fixler DE (1981): Left ventricular hypertrophy in adolescents with elevated blood pressure: Assessment by chest roentgenography, electrocardiography, and echocardio-graphy. *Pediatrics* 67: 255–259.
37. Sen S, Tarazi RC, Khairallah PA, Bumpus FM (1974): Cardiac hypertrophy in spontaneously hypertensive rats. *Circ Res* 35: 775–781.
38. Tarazi RC, Fouad FM (1984): Reversal of cardiac hypertrophy in humans. *Hypertension* 6 (suppl III): 140–146.
39. Wollam GL, Hall WD, Porter VD, Douglas MB, Unger DJ, Blumenstein BA, Cotsonis GA, Knudtson ML, Felner JM, Schlant RC (1983): Time course of regression of left ventricular hypertrophy in treated hypertensive patients. *Am J Med* 75 (suppl 3A): 100–110.
40. Kazda S, Garthoff B, Thomas G (1982): Antihypertensive effect of calcium antagonists in rat differs from that of vasodilators. *Clin Sci* 63: 363s–365s.
41. Smith VE, White WB, Meeran MK, Karimeddini MK (1986): Improved left ventricular filling accompanies reduced left ventricular mass during therapy of essential hypertension. *J Am Coll Cardiol* 8: 1449–1454.
42. Sen S, Tarazi RC, Bumpus FM (1980): Effect of converting enzyme inhibitor (SQ12,225) on myocardial hypertrophy in spontaneously hypertensive rats. *Hypertension* 2: 169–176.
43. Nakashima Y, Fouad FM, Tarazi RC (1984): Regression of left ventricular hypertrophy from systemic hypertension by enalapril. *Am J Cardiol* 53: 1044–1049.
44. Sen S, Tarazi RC, Bumpus FM (1977): Cardiac hypertrophy and antihypertensive therapy. *Cardiovasc Res* 11: 427–433.
45. Frohlich ED, Tarazi RC (1979): Is arterial pressure the sole factor responsible for hyperten-sive cardiac hypertrophy? *Am J Cardiol* 44: 959–963.
46. Pfeffer MA, Pfeffer JM, Weiss AK, Frohlich ED (1977): Development of SHR hypertension and cardiac hypertrophy during prolonged beta blockade. *Am J Physiol* 232: H639–H643.
47. Lindpainter K, Sen S (1987): Role of Beta$_1$ adrenoceptors in hypertensive cardiac hyper-trophy. *J Hypertension* 5: 663–669.
48. Franz IW, Behr DW, Ketelhut R (1986): Regression of myocardial hypertrophy in hyperten-sives on long-term treatment with beta-blockers. *Dtsch Med Wschr* 111: 530–534.
49. Dunn FG, Venntura HO, Messerli FH, Kobrin I, Frohlich D (1987): Time course of regres-sion of left ventricular hypertrophy in hypertensive patients treated with atenolol. *Circulation* 2: 254–258.
50. Rowlands DB, Glover DR, Stallard TJ, Littler WA (1982): Control of blood pressure and

reduction of echocardiographically assessed left ventricular mass with once-daily timolol. *Br J Clin Pharmacol* 14: 89–95.

51. Ishise S, Pegram BL, Frohlich ED (1980): Disparate effects of methyldopa and clonidine on cardiac mass and haemodynamics in rats. *Clin Sci* 59 (suppl 6): 449–452.

52. Pegram BL, Ishise S, Frohlich ED (1982): Effect of methyldopa, clonidine, and hydralazine on cardiac mass and haemodynamics in Wistar Kyoto and spontaneously hypertensive rats. *Cardiovasc Res* 16: 40–46.

53. Feisal K, Eckstein JW, Horsley AW, et al. (1961): Effects of chlorothiazide on forearm vascular responses to norepinephrine. *J Applied Physiol* 16: 549–552.

54. Tarazi RC, Gifford RW Jr (1983): Left ventricular hypertrophy and hypertension (editorial). *JAMA* 250: 1319.

55. Tarazi RC, Frohlich ED (1987): Is reversal of cardiac hypertrophy a desirable goal of antihypertensive therapy? *Circulation* 75 (suppl I): 113–117.

56. Freis ED (1983): Electrocardiographic changes in the course of antihypertensive treatment. *Am J Med* 75 (suppl 3A): 111–115.

57. Hypertension Detection and Follow-Up Program Cooperative Group (1985): Five-year findings of the Hypertension Detection and Follow-up Program. Prevention and reversal of left ventricular hypertrophy with antihypertensive drug therapy. *Hypertension* 7: 105–112.

58. Dorph S, Leth A, Degnbol B, et al. (1970): Visceral changes in severe hypertension and their response to drug treatment. *Acta Med Scand* 187: 411–417.

59. Farmer RG, Gifford RW Jr, Hines EA Jr (1963): Effect of medical treatment on severe hypertension. *Arch Intern Med* 112: 118–128.

60. Topol EJ, Traill TA, Fortuin NJ (1985): Hypertensive hypertrophic cardiomyopathy of the elderly. *New Engl J Med* 312: 277–283.

61. Abrams J (1985): Vasodilator therapy for chronic congestive heart failure. *JAMA* 254: 3070–3074.

62. Guiha NH, Cohn JN, Mikulic E, Franciosa JA, Limas CJ (1974): Treatment of refractoory heart failure with infusion of nitroprusside. *New Engl J Med* 291: 587–592.

63. Romankiewicz JA, Brogden RN, Heel RC, Speight TM, Avery GS (1983): Captopril: An update review of its pharmacological properties and therapeutic efficacy in congestive heart failure. *Drugs* 25: 6–40.

64. Faxon DP, Creager MA, Halperin JL, Gavras H, Coffman JD, Ryan TJ (1980): Central and peripheral hemodynamic effects of angiotensin inhibition in patients with refractory congestive heart failure. *Circulation* 61: 925–930.

65. CONSENSUS Trial Study Group (1987): Effects of enalapril on mortality in severe congestive heart failure. *New Engl J Med* 316: 1429–1435.

66. Packer M, Meller J, Gorlin R, Herman MV (1979): Hemodynamic and clinical tachyphylaxis to prazosin-mediated afterload reduction in severe chronic congestive heart failure. *Circulation* 59: 531–539.

67. Cohn NJ, Archibald DG, Francis GS, Ziesche S, Franciosa JA, Harston WE, Tristani FE, Dunkman WB, Jacobs W, Flohr KH, Goldman S, Cobb FR, Shah PM, Saunders RS, Fletcher RD, Loeb HS, Hughes VC, Baker BB (1987): Veterans Administration cooperative study on vasodilator therapy of heart failure: Influence of prerandomization variables on the reduction of mortality by treatment with hydralazine and isosorbide dinitrate. *Circulation* 75 (suppl IV): 49–54.

68. Captopril-Digoxin Multicenter Research Group (1988): Comparative effects of therapy with captopril and digoxin in patients with mild to moderate heart failure. *JAMA* 259: 539–544.

69. Packer M, Lee WH, Medina N, Yusak M, Kessler PD (1987): Functional renal insufficiency during long-term therapy with captopril and enalapril in severe chronic heart failure. *Ann Intern Med* 106: 346–354.

70. Packer M, Lee WH, Yushak M, Medina N (1986): Comparison of captopril and enalapril in patients with severe chronic heart failure. *New Engl J Med* 315: 847–853.
71. Multiple Risk Factor Intervention Trial (1982): Risk factor changes and mortality results. *JAMA* 248: 1465–1477.
72. Multiple Risk Factor Intervention Trial Research Group (1985): Baseline resting electrocardiographic abnormalities, antihypertensive treatment, and mortality in the Multiple Risk Factor Intervention Trial. *Am J Cardiol* 55: 1–15.
73. Holland OB, Nixon JV, Kuhnert L (1981): Diuretic-induced ventricular ectopic activity. *Am J Med* 70: 762–768.
74. Hollifield JW, Slaton PE (1981): Thiazide diuretics, hypokalemia and cardiac arrhythmias. *Acta Med Scand* suppl 647: 67–73.
75. Stewart DE, Ikram H, Espiner EA, Nicholls MG (1985): Arrhythmogenic potential of diuretic induced hypokalaemia in patients with mild hypertension and ischemic heart disease. *Br Heart J* 54: 290–297.
76. Ragnarsson J, Hardarson T, Snorrason SP (1987): Ventricular dysrhythmias in middle-aged hypertensive men treated either with a diuretic agent or a beta blocker. *Acta Med Scand* 221: 143–148.
77. Madias JE, Madias NE, Gavras HP (1984): Nonarrhythmogenicity of diuretic-induced hypokalemia: Its evidence in patients with uncomplicated hypertension. *Arch Intern Med* 144: 2171–2176.
78. Lief PD, Belizon I, Matos J, Bank N (1984): Diuretic-induced hypokalemia does not cause ventricular ectopy in uncomplicated essential hypertension (abstract). *Kidney Int* 25: 203.
79. Papademetriou V, Price M, Notargiacomo A, Gottdiener J, Fletcher RD, Freis ED (1985): Effect of diuretic therapy on ventricular arrhythmias in hypertensive patients with or without left ventricular hypertrophy. *Am Heart J* 110: 595–599.
80. Greenberg G, Brennan PJ, Miall WE (1984): Effects of diuretic and beta blocker therapy in the Medical Research Council Trial. *Am J Med* 76 (suppl 2A): 45–51.
81. Shanes JG (1987): Beta blockade: rational or irrational therapy for congestive heart failure? *Circulation* 76: 971–973.
82. Gifford RW Jr (1975): Management and prognosis in complicated hypertension, in: Moser M (ed), *Hypertension: A Practical Approach*. Boston: Little, Brown and Company.

PART THREE

Coronary circulation, left ventricular hypertrophy, and hypertension

22. Coronary circulation, cardiac hypertrophy, and myocardial ischemia
Basic concepts

JULIEN I.E. HOFFMAN

Ventricular hypertrophy is a common consequence of most forms of heart disease. There is usually a period of compensated hypertrophy, often lasting many years in humans, but eventually there may be decompensation with congestive heart failure [1, 2]. During the compensated stage the increased wall thickness remains constant, and in concentric hypertrophy due to pressure overloads, the wall stress tends to be normal [2–4]. Because peak systolic wall tension is a good predictor of myocardial oxygen demand [5], the resting hypertrophied ventricle has an increased oxygen consumption in proportion to its increased mass. With exercise or sympathetic stimulation, its oxygen consumption will rise in proportion to the increased heart rate, contractility, and systolic pressure that result. If, however, the ventricle dilates, either because of excessive stresses placed on it or because of myocardial depression from drugs or surgical procedures, then the decreased mass:volume ratio will be associated with an increased peak wall stress [2]. Consequently, the myocardial oxygen demand will rise out of proportion to pressures and heart rates.

The major determinant of myocardial blood flow is myocardial oxygen consumption [6] because the heart has limited ability to increase oxygen extraction. As long as all parts of the ventricles can receive an adequate blood flow, there will be no ischemia and ventricular function will remain adequate. However, if flow is inadequate so that oxygen supply falls below demand, there will be impaired function [7, 8] that is manifest first in the subendocardium [9]. If the supply-demand imbalance is maintained for more than an hour, then subendocardial muscle cells will die because the myocardium cannot obtain enough energy from anaerobic glycolysis to survive; subendocardial necrosis and replacement fibrosis occur, as exemplified by the striking subendocardial fibrosis seen in patients with severe aortic stenosis [10, 11]. Although there is evidence that subendocardial muscle cells use about 15–20% more oxygen per gram of muscle than do more superficial muscle cells, it is

M.E. Safar & F. Fouad-Tarazi (eds.), The heart in hypertension.
© 1989 Kluwer Academic Publishers, Dordrecht –

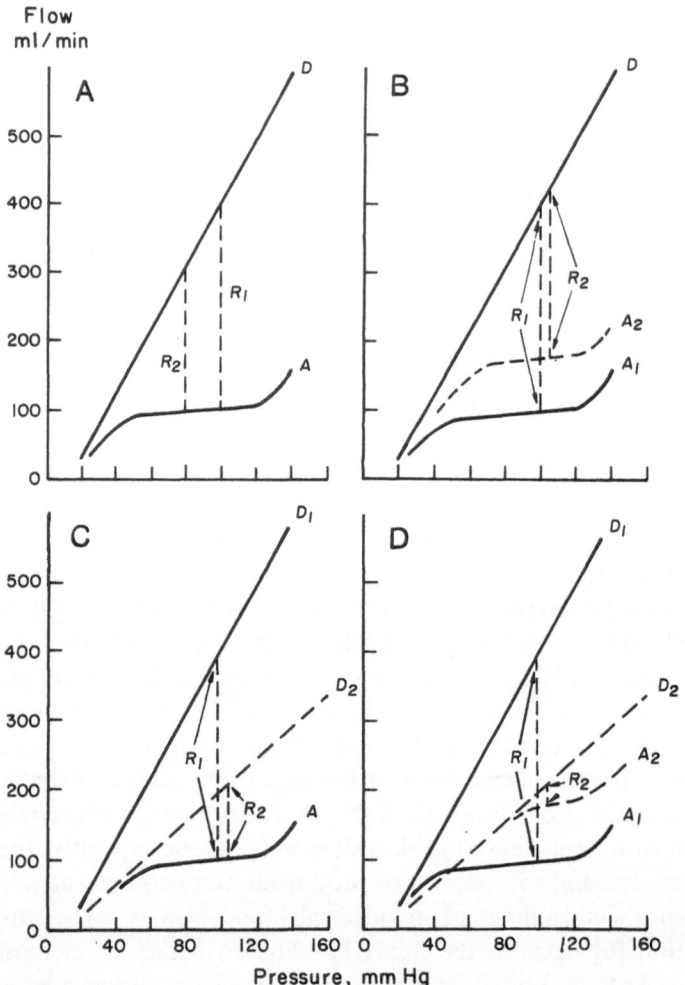

Figure 1. A (*upper left*): Diagram of left coronary pressure flow relations during autoregulation (labelled A) and with maximal vasodilatation (labelled D). The dashed vertical lines indicate the coronary flow reserve at two different coronary perfusing pressures. Note that a small change of perfusing pressure makes a big change in the flow reserve. Note, too, that at low perfusing pressures the autoregulated flow is not maximal.

B (*upper right*): Superimposed on the normal pressure-flow diagram, in which the normal autoregulated resting flow is labelled A_1, is a higher level of autoregulated flow indicated by the dashed line A_2. This increase in flow could be due to exercise, sympathetic stimulation, anemia, hypoxemia, thyrotoxicosis, or tachycardia. Because of the elevated resting flow, the normal coronary flow reserve (vertical dashed line R_1) is reduced to R_2. Note that because the resting flow is elevated, autoregulation begins to fail at a higher coronary perfusing pressure than when flow is normal.

C (*lower left*): On the normal pressure-flow diagram (solid lines labelled A and D_1) is superimposed a line of maximal pressure-flow relations with a decreased slope (dashed line D_2). Such a decrease in slope could be due to polycythemia, increased blood viscosity due to macroglobulinemia or hyperfibrogenemia, to increased stiffness of red cell membranes, or to tachycardia or a marked increased in aortic pressure. Because of the decrease in slope, the normal coronary flow reserve (dashed line R_1) is reduced to R_2.

clear that subendocardial ischemia is always due to an absolute or relative decrease in subendocardial flow [12, 13]. To understand the mechanisms responsible for subendocardial vulnerability to ischemia, a vulnerability common to most forms of heart disease [13, 14], it is necessary to review briefly the factors that control regional myocardial blood flow.

If the canine left coronary artery is cannulated so that coronary perfusion pressure can be varied while the left ventricle works at a constant heart rate and pressure, thereby keeping its myocardial oxygen demand constant, coronary flow remains relatively constant over a pressure range from about 60 to 120 mmHg. When perfusion pressure is raised, coronary vascular resistance increases, and when perfusion pressure is lowered, the coronary vascular resistance decreases. This phenomenon is termed *autoregulation,* and it is likely to be due to metabolic mechanisms associated with oxygen excess or deficit [6, 15, 16]. On the other hand, if myocardial metabolism is increased or decreased, then myocardial blood flow increases or decreases in proportion [6, 17, 18]; this is termed *metabolic regulation.*

When coronary vessels are maximally dilated, for example, by infusing adenosine, then all tonic vascular control is lost and flows are determined primarily by perfusing pressures. The relationship of flow to pressure has a steep slope, whereas during autoregulation the pressure-flow relation is almost horizontal (Figure 1A). In this diagram, first introduced in 1962 by Shaw et al. [19], the lines represent coronary vascular conductance, the reciprocal of resistance. At any given perfusion pressure, the difference between autoregulated and maximal flow is the coronary flow reserve. As shown in Figure 1A, when autoregulated flows decrease at low perfusing pressures, the flows remain below those obtained at the same pressures during maximal vasodilatation; in other words, even though there is severe ischemia at these low flows, the myocardial vessels are not maximally dilated [20–22], and there is still some flow reserve.

If autoregulation is examined regionally across the left ventricular wall as perfusion pressure is decreased, flows remain constant in all layers down to a pressure of about 60–70 mmHg, and then flows (per gram) decrease first in the subendocardial muscle, next in the midwall, and are preserved in the subepicardial muscle until perfusion pressure falls below 40 mmHg [23]. Therefore,

---

D (*lower right*): In this diagram, the normal autoregulated and maximally dilated pressure-flow lines (solid lines A_1 and D_1) have superimposed on them both a raised autoregulated flow line (dashed line A_2) and a maximal pressure-flow relation with a decreased slope (dashed line D_2). As a result, the normal coronary flow reserve (dashed line R_1) is greatly reduced to R_2. Note that in this presumed resting heart, there is almost no flow reserve to meet added stresses, and that autoregulation fails at what would be regarded as normal perfusing pressures. This adverse combination of events could occur with hypertrophy and combinations of one or more of the following: tachycardia, anemia, polycythemia, hypoxemia.

This figure is adapted from one published in the Proceedings of the Fifth Ettore Majorana Conference on Diastolic Myocardial Function.

coronary flow reserve decreases first in the subendocardial muscle and last in the subepicardium. As a corollary to this, if perfusion pressure is kept constant but myocardial work is increased by raising left ventricular systolic pressure or pacing the heart, flows increase in all layers up some critical pressure or heart rate, after which flows do not increase further in the subendocardium but continue to rise in the subepicardium [13, 24, 25]. Thus both decreased perfusion pressure or time, or increased myocardial work at constant perfusion pressure, eventually produce relative or absolute subendocardial hypoperfusion and ischemia.

The explanation for the earlier decrease of subendocardial flows was once ascribed to the effect that systolic intramyocardial pressures had on the perfusion time of different muscle layers [24, 26]. Because systolic intramyocardial pressures are highest under the endocardium and are almost atmospheric beneath the epicardium [27, 28], it was thought that the outer half of the ventricular wall was perfused continuously in systole and diastole, whereas the inner half was perfused only in systole. Therefore, any compromise of diastolic perfusion pressure or time would have its greatest effect on subendocardial flow. However, more recent studies have indicated that there is little systolic flow in the myocardium, so that other mechanisms have to be sought. At present, the likely explanation is that during systole the higher intramyocardial pressures in the subendocardium squeeze more blood out of the deep vessels than the lower subepicardial pressures squeeze out of the superficial vessels. Consequently, the deeper vessels are narrower than the superficial vessels at the end of systole, so that the time constant for reflow into the myocardium in diastole is longer in the deep than the superficial muscle; any compromise of diastolic pressure or duration will therefore decrease flow most in the deepest vessels [29–31]. An added impediment to subendocardial blood flow occurs if there is an elevated ventricular diastolic pressure or delayed ventricular relaxation [13].

In ventricular hypertrophy, the control of regional autoregulation is similar to that in normal hearts, but coronary flow reserve is reduced, sometimes drastically. Almost all experimental studies of ventricular hypertrophy have found that at rest the flow per gram is normal [32–37], so that the total ventricular flow is increased in proportion to the increased muscle mass. However, although the ventricular muscle mass increases, the maximal cross-sectional area of the myocardial vascular bed does not increase; that is, the minimal coronary vascular resistance per ventricle is unchanged by hypertrophy [32–38] because there is no new growth of conducting arteries and arterioles. Consequently, the increased total flow to the ventricle is achieved by vasodilatation, and the coronary flow reserve is reduced (Figure 1B). Note that if flows are measured per unit mass, the resting flow per gram would be the same in normal and hypertrophied muscle, but the maximal flow per gram would be less in the hypertrophied ventricle because the same absolute maximal flow is supplying more muscle. A reduction in coronary flow reserve at rest reduces the increment of coronary flow that can be attained at times of stress, and may explain why some of these patients develop subendocardial fibrosis.

The reduced coronary flow reserve that occurs in ventricular hypertrophy is decreased still more if myocardial oxygen consumption is increased by exercise, tachycardia, ventricular dilatation, or thyrotoxicosis, or if the resting flows are increased by anemia or hypoxemia [39]. Not only does the increase in autoregulated flow diminish the flow reserve, but with tachycardia and ventricular dilatation there is probably also a decrease in maximal flow at any pressure that exaggerates the reduction of coronary flow reserve. Many of these factors may occur at or just after cardiac surgery, with serious consequences for subendocardial viability. It is important to recognize that whenever the resting (autoregulated) flow is increased, the pressure at which autoregulation fails and at which subendocardial ischemia begins is also higher than normal because of the slope of the line of maximal pressure-flow relations.

Some of the observations made in animals have been confirmed in humans. Marcus and his colleagues [40, 41] have described reduced coronary flow velocity reserve in patients with left ventricular hypertrophy due to aortic stenosis and right ventricular hypertrophy due to atrial septal defects. In another study in patients with essential hypertension, Strauer [2] noted that the relative coronary resistance reserve (defined as the ratio of coronary vascular resistance at rest to that during maximal vasodilatation) decreased as peak wall stress increased.

The equivalence of experimental and human hypertrophy, however, is still undetermined. Almost all animal experiments are of relatively short duration and have relatively modest hypertrophy when compared with what occurs in human disease. Some studies in humans or dogs with congenital aortic stenosis or coarctation of the aorta have described abnormalities of the intramural arteries and arterioles [42–44]; the effect of these vascular lesions would be to decrease the maximal flows possible with maximal vasodilatation and so to make the coronary flow reserve lower in humans than would be predicted from experimental hypertrophy. On the other hand, one recent study observed a decreased minimal coronary vascular resistance (implying growth of conducting vessels) in adult dogs in which left ventricular hypertrophy due to renal hypertension was allowed to develop over six months [45]; this growth would partly or completely compensate for the increased muscle mass and help to restore coronary flow reserve. Until adequate measurements of coronary flow reserve can be made in humans, the importance of vascular growth and of vascular lesions will remain unknown.

The second major mechanism that can reduce coronary flow reserve is a reduced maximal coronary flow (Figure 1C). This reduction can occur because of coronary arterial disease, either extramural or intramural. Thus, the combination of occlusive coronary atheroma with hypertrophy due to hypertension or aortic stenosis is particularly likely to cause subendocardial ischemia. Another factor that reduces maximal coronary flow is increased blood viscosity, due to altered rigidity of red cell membranes, abnormalities of plasma proteins like macroglobulinemia or hyperfibrinogenemia, or (most commonly) due to polycythemia. In general, an increase of hematocrit to 70% approximately doubles blood viscosity and halves maximal coronary flow at any given perfusing pressure [46]. Thus, patients who have ventricular hypertrophy and polycythemia due to cyanotic heart disease, either congenital heart disease or cor pulmonale, have a major predisposition to reduced coronary flow reserve and subendocardial ischemia. The hypoxemia tends to raise autoregulated flow, while the increased blood viscosity reduces maximal flow. Therefore, these patients have a coronary flow reserve that may be very low or even absent at what seem to be normal perfusing pressures, and their risk of subendocardial damage is great (Figure 1D). Finally, an elevated ventricular diastolic pressure or delayed ventricular relaxation will also reduce maximal flow, particularly in the subendocardium [13, 14, 24].

The problems of coronary flow in hypertrophy apply to the right ventricle as well as to the left ventricle. Thus, in dogs with congenital pulmonic stenosis, the higher the right ventricular systolic pressure, the less the coronary flow reserve as measured by reactive hyperemia [47], and in both dogs and ponies with experimental right ventricular hypertrophy [48, 49], coronary flow reserve has been reduced because no growth of right ventricular myocardial vessels has occurred. However, when right ventricular hypertrophy has been produced in fetal or newborn animals [50–53], there has been an increase in the vascular bed in the right ventricle that increases maximal coronary flows and so prevents the decrease in coronary flow reserve that hypertrophy would otherwise produce. Increased growth of myocardial vessels was not found in the left ventricles of puppies with aortic banding at six to seven weeks of age [54]; this finding is at odds with the studies of hypertensive dogs cited before [45].

Summary

Ventricular hypertrophy increases myocardial oxygen consumption and therefore the demand for myocardial blood flow primarily because of the increase in myocardial mass and secondarily if changes occur that increase peak systolic wall stress. Flow to different layers of the ventricle can be maintained at the expense of a decreased coronary flow reserve in the subendocardium; this decrease may be compensated for in part by increased growth of intramural coronary arteries and arterioles, or it may be accentuated by pathologic changes in those intra-myocardial vessels. Coronary flow reserve is further decreased by factors that raise autoregulated flows (hypoxemia, anemia, exercise, tachycardia, thyrotoxicosis, sympathetic stimulation) or that decrease the maximal flows at any given pressures (polycythemia, tachycardia, coronary arterial lesions, elevated ventricular diastolic pressures, delayed ventricular relaxation). Because of these factors, hypertrophied ventricles are particularly susceptible to episodes of subendocardial ischemia that may eventually lead to cell death and replacement fibrosis. These episodes may or may not be accompanied by manifestations of ischemia like angina pectoris or electrocardiographic changes.

Acknowledgement

Supported in part by Program Project Grant HL-25847 from the United States Public Health Service.

References

1. Meerson FZ (1969): The myocardium in hyperfunction, hypertrophy and heart failure. *Circ Res* 25 (suppl II): 1–163.
2. Strauer BE (1980): *Hypertensive Heart Disease*. Berlin: Springer Verlag.
3. Sasayama S, Ross J Jr, Franklin D, Bloor CM, Bishop S, Dilley RB (1976): Adaptations of the left ventricle to chronic pressure overload. *Circ Res* 38: 172–178.
4. Grossman W, Jones D, McLaurin LP (1975): Wall stress and patterns of hypertrophy in human left ventricle. *J Clin Invest* 56: 56–64.
5. McDonald RH, Taylor RR, Cingolani HE (1966): Measurement of myocardial developed tension and its relation to oxygen consumption. *Am J Physiol* 211: 667–673.
6. Vergroesen I, Noble MIM, Wieringa PA, Spaan JAE (1987): Quantification of O_2 consumption and arterial pressure as independent determinants of coronary flow. *Am J Physiol* 252 (*Heart Circ Physiol* 21): H545–553.
7. Downey JM (1976): Myocardial contractile force as a function of coronary blood flow. *Am J Physiol* 230: 1–6.
8. Vatner SF (1980): Correlation between acute reductions in myocardial blood flow and function in conscious dogs. *Circ Res* 47: 201–207.
9. Gallagher KP, Kumada T, Koziol JA, McKown MD, Kemper WS, Ross J Jr (1980): Significance of regional wall thickening abnormalities relative to transmural myocardial perfusion in anesthetized dogs. *Circulation* 62: 1266–1274.
10. Marquis RM, Logan A (1955): Congenital aortic stenosis and its surgical treatment. *Br Heart J* 17: 373–390.
11. Schwarz F, Flameng W, Schaper J, Langebartels F, Thormann J, Hehrlein F, Schlepper M (1978): Myocardial structure and function in patients with aortic valve disease and their relation to postoperative results. *Am J Cardiol* 41: 661–669.
12. Bache RJ, Arentzen CE, Simon AB, Vrobel TR (1984): Abnormalities in myocardial perfusion during tachycardia in dogs with left ventricular hypertrophy: Metabolic evidence for myocardial ischemia. *Circulation* 69: 409–417.
13. Hoffman JIE (1987): Transmural myocardial perfusion. *Prog Cardiovasc Dis* 29: 429–464.
14. Hoffman JIE, Buckberg GD (1976): Transmural variations in myocardial perfusion, in: Yu P, Goodwin JF (eds), *Progress in Cardiology*, 5: 37–89. Philadelphia: Lea and Febiger.

15. Dole WP (1987): Autoregulation of the coronary circulation. *Prog Cardiovasc Dis* 29: 293–323.
16. Olsson RA, Bünger R (1987): Metabolic control of coronary blood flow. *Prog Cardiovasc Dis* 29: 369–387.
17. Drake-Holland AJ, Laird JD, Noble MIM, Spaan JAE, Vergroesen I (1984): Oxygen and coronary vascular resistance during autoregulation and metabolic vasodilatation in the dog. *J Physiol* (London) 348: 285–299.
18. Hoffman JIE (1987): A critical view of coronary reserve. *Circulation* 75 (suppl I) 6–11.
19. Shaw RF, Mosher P, Ross J Jr, Joseph JI, Lee ASJ (1962): Physiologic principles of coronary perfusion. *J Thorac Cardiovasc Surg* 44: 608–616.
20. Aversano T, Becker LC (1985): Persistence of coronary vasodilator reserve despite functionally significant flow reduction. *Am J Physiol* 248 (*Heart Circ Physiol* 17): H403–411.
21. Canty JM Jr, Klocke FJ (1985): Reduced regional myocardial perfusion in the presence of pharmacologic vasodilator reserve. *Circulation* 71: 370–377.
22. Grattan MT, Hanley FL, Stevens MB, Hoffman JIE (1986): Transmural coronary flow reserve pattern in dogs. *Am J Physiol* 250 (*Heart Circ Physiol* 19): H276–283.
23. Guyton RA, McClenethan JH, Newman GE, Michaelis LL (1977): Significance of subendocardial S-T segment elevation caused by coronary stenosis in the dog. *Am J Cardiol* 40: 373–380.
24. Buckberg GD, Fixler DE, Archie JP, Hoffman JIE (1972): Experimental subendocardial ischemia in dogs with normal coronary arteries. *Circ Res* 30: 67–81.
25. Bache RJ, Vrobel TR, Arentzen CE, Ring WS (1981): Effect of maximal coronary vasodilation on transmural myocardial perfusion during tachycardia in dogs with left ventricular hypertrophy. *Circ Res* 49: 742–750.
26. Moir TW (1972): Brief reviews: Subendocardial distribution of coronary blood flow and the effect of antianginal drugs. *Circ Res* 30: 621–627.
27. Hamlin RL, Levesque MJ, Kittelson MD (1982): Intramyocardial pressure and distribution of coronary blood flow during systole and diastole in the horse. *Cardiovasc Res* 16: 256–262.
28. Heineman FW, Grayson J (1985): Transmural distribution of intramyocardial pressure measured by micropipette technique. *Am J Physiol* 249 (*Heart Circ Physiol* 18): H1216–1223.
29. Hoffman JIE, Baer RW, Hanley FL, Messina LM, Grattan MT (1985): Regulation of transmural myocardial blood flow. *J Biomech Eng* 107: 2–9.
30. Arts T, Reneman, RS (1985): Interaction between intramyocardial pressure (IMP) and myocardial circulation. *J Biomech Eng* 107: 51–56.
31. Levy BI, Tedgui A, Michel JB (1985): A mechanical model of the dynamics of the coronary circulation in the dog. *J Theor Biol* 116: 225–242.
32. Marchetti GV, Merlo L, Noseda V, Visioli O (1973): Myocardial blood flow in experimental hypertrophy in dogs. *Cardiovasc Res* 7: 519–527.
33. Mueller TM, Marcus ML, Kerber RE, Young YA, Barnes RW, Abboud FM (1978): Effect of renal hypertension and left ventricular hypertrophy on the coronary circulation in dogs. *Circ Res* 42: 543–549.
34. O'Keefe DD, Hoffman JIE, Cheitlin R, O'Neill MJ, Allard JR, Shapkin E (1978): Coronary blood flow in experimental canine left ventricular hypertrophy. *Circ Res* 43: 43–51.
35. Holtz J, von Restorff W, Bard P, Bassenge E (1977): Transmural distribution of myocardial blood flow and coronary reserve in canine left ventricular hypertrophy. *Basic Res Cardiol* 72: 286–292.
36. Borkon AM, Jones M, Bell JH, Pierce JE (1982): Regional myocardial blood flow in left ventricular hypertrophy: An experimental investigation in Newfoundland dogs with congenital aortic stenosis. *J Thorac Cardiovasc Surg* 84: 876–885.
37. Bache RJ, Vrobel TR, Ring WS, Emery RW, Anderson RW (1981): Regional myocardial

blood flow during exercise in dogs with chronic left ventricular hypertrophy. *Circ Res* 48: 76–87.

38. Wicker P, Tarazi RC (1982): Coronary blood flow in left ventricular hypertrophy: A review of experimental data. *Eur Heart J* 3 (suppl A): 111–118.
39. Hoffman JIE, Grattan MT, Hanley FL, Messina LM (1983): Total and transmural perfusion of the hypertrophied heart, in: ter Keurs HEDJ, Schipperheyn JJ (eds), *Cardiac Left Ventricular Hypertrophy*, pp 131–151. Dordrecht-Boston-Lancaster: Martinus Nijhoff Publishers (Series DICM, Volume 33).
40. Marcus ML, Doty DB, Hiratzka LF, Wright CB, Eastham CL (1982): Decreased coronary reserve. A mechanism for angina pectoris in patients with aortic stenosis and normal coronary arteries. *New Engl J Med* 307: 1362–1366.
41. Doty D, Wright C, Eastham C, Marcus ML (1980): Coronary reserve in atrial septal defect. *Circulation* 62 (suppl III): 115.
42. Naeye R, Liedtke AJ (1976): Consequences of intramyocardial arterial lesions in aortic valvular stenosis. *Am J Pathol* 85: 569–580.
43. Vlodaver Z, Neufeldt HN (1968): The coronary arteries in coarctation of the aorta. *Circulation* 37: 449–454.
44. Flickinger GL, Patterson DF (1967): Coronary lesions associated with congenital subaortic stenosis in the dog. *J Path Bact* 93: 133–140.
45. Tomanek RJ, Schalk KA, Nadle T, Harrison DG (1987): Coronary vascular growth in dogs with long-term hypertension. *Circulation* 76 (suppl IV): 328.
46. Baer RW, Vlahakes GJ, Uhlig PN, Hoffman JIE (1987): Maximal myocardial oxygen transport during anemia and polycythemia in dogs. *Am J Physiol* 252 (*Heart Circ Physiol* 21): H1086–1095.
47. Lowensohn HS, Khouri EM, Gregg DE, Pyle RL, Patterson RE (1976): Phasic right coronary artery flow in conscious dogs with normal and elevated right ventricular pressures. *Circ Res* 39: 760–766.
48. Murray PA, Vatner SF (1981): Reduction of maximal coronary vasodilator capacity in conscious dogs with severe right ventricular hypertrophy. *Circ Res* 48: 27–33.
49. Manohar M, Bisgard GE, Bullard V, Rankin JHG (1981): Blood flow in the hypertrophied right ventricular myocardium of unanesthetized ponies. *Am J Physiol* 240 (*Heart Circ Physiol* 19): H881–888.
50. Archie JP, Fixler DE, Ullyot DJ, Buckberg GD, Hoffman JIE (1974): Regional myocardial blood flow in lambs with concentric right ventricular hypertrophy. *Circ Res* 34: 143–154.
51. Manohar M, Thurmon JC, Tranquilli WJ, Devous MD Sr, Theodorakis MC, Shawley RV, Feller DL, Benson JG (1981): Regional myocardial blood flow and coronary vascular reserve in unanesthetized young calves with severe concentric right ventricular hypertrophy. *Circ Res* 48: 785–796.
52. Botham MJ, Lemmer JH, Gerren RA, Long RW, Behrendt DM, Gallagher KP (1984): Coronary vasodilator reserve in young dogs with moderate right ventricular hypertrophy. *Ann Thorac Surg* 38: 101–107.
53. Vlahakes GJ, Turley K, Verrier ED, Hoffman JIE (1980): Greater maximal coronary flow in conscious lambs with experimental congenital right ventricular hypertrophy. *Circulation* (suppl III): 111.
54. Bache RJ, Alonyo D, Sublett E, Dai X-Z (1986): Myocardial blood flow in left ventricular hypertrophy developing in young and adult dogs. *Am J Physiol* 251 (*Heart Circ Physiol* 20): H949–956.

23. Coronary circulation and coronary reserve in the hypertensive heart

PIERRE WICKER

Introduction

The occurrence of symptoms suggestive of myocardial ischemia such as angina pectoris or ST-T segment depression during exercise [1, 2] or the greater severity of myocardial infarction in patients or animals with hypertension [3, 4] has long prompted investigators to study the coronary circulation in hypertensive cardiac hypertrophy. Interest in this field and more generally in the cardiac consequences of increased blood pressure has heightened over the past decade because of a number of factors including (1) the demonstration that hypertension was the dominant etiology for left ventricular hypertrophy (LVH), (2) advances in noninvasive techniques, such as echocardiography, allowing a precise and reproducible assessment of cardiac mass, and (3) the possibility of reversing the cardiovascular structural changes of hypertension with treatment.

The concept of coronary reserve is currently used extensively to assess the ability of the coronary vasculature to dilate and to provide an adequate flow supply in response to changes in myocardial oxygen needs [5]. Coronary reserve is defined as the maximal coronary flow (coronary flow reserve) or the minimal coronary resistance (coronary vasodilator reserve) measured after maximal vasodilation. Some studies have expressed coronary reserve in relative terms, i.e. as the ratio or difference between peak and baseline flow or resistance. This approach yields determinations that are influenced by baseline values and may not reflect the actual coronary vasodilatory capacities. For these reasons, computations of coronary reserve based on absolute rather than relative measurements should be preferred. Unfortunately, this is not always possible in clinical studies because of the lack of reliable and noninvasive methods for measuring coronary blood flow in absolute terms in man, although substantial advances in this direction have been recently reported [6].

M.E. Safar & F. Fouad-Tarazi (eds.), The heart in hypertension.
© *1989 Kluwer Academic Publishers, Dordrecht –*

A large body of data, originating mostly from animal studies, is available on coronary reserve in hypertensive heart disease [7–9]. Coronary vasodilator reserve has consistently been found to be depressed in this situation and it is generally agreed that these abnormalities contribute to the development of ischemia and ultimately to the increased risk of cardiac complications and sudden death in hypertensive patients with LVH. However, a direct cause-effect relationship between these coronary alterations and the cardiac complications of hypertension has never been conclusively demonstrated. Furthermore, this view ignores the possible participation of coronary microcirculation abnormalities in the emergence of hypertension-related cardiac complications.

This chapter will summarize the evidence presently available regarding coronary reserve and the coronary microcirculation in hypertensive cardiac hypertrophy. In addition, the effects of antihypertensive treatment on these two aspects of the coronary circulation will be reviewed.

1. Coronary reserve during the development of hypertensive cardiac hypertrophy

1.1 *Left ventricular coronary vasodilator reserve*

Following the introduction of the microsphere technique in the early 1970s, coronary reserve has been extensively studied in animals with various types of experimental hypertension and different degrees of cardiac hypertrophy. In the majority of these studies, maximal coronary dilation has been obtained by pharmacological means. In contrast, very few clinical studies are available. All have utilized the inert gas technique to measure flow and a pharmacological agent (dipyridamole) was also used to induce maximal coronary dilation. Results of these investigations, which are summarized in Table 1, indicate that coronary vasodilator reserve is consistently depressed both in human and animal hypertension. Such a basic agreement is remarkable in view of the differences in species, in experimental models of hypertension, in the extent of cardiac hypertrophy and in the types of vasodilatory stimuli used.

1.2 *Right ventricular coronary vasodilator reserve*

Results of several clinical studies have suggested that pulmonary resistance is increased in systemic arterial hypertension [22–24]. One study reported a correlation between the increment in pulmonary and peripheral resistance [24]. Some studies have documented a small, but significant, increase in right ventricular mass in experimental [13, 25, 26] or human [27] hypertension. Changes in right ventricular function have also been described, but there is still controversy as to whether right ventricular performance is depressed [23, 28] or augmented [26, 28]. Because of these findings suggesting that the right side of the heart is not immune to the effects of systemic hypertension, various studies have investigated the right coronary circulation in this situation. Similarly to the left ventricle, the results show that right ventricular coronary vasodilator reserve is limited in experimentally induced or genetic models of hypertension (Table 2).

Table 1. Coronary total or transmural (endo/epi) flow reserve and coronary vasodilator reserve in experimental and human hypertensive left ventricular hypertrophy (LVH).

Author [Ref]	Animal/model or patient characteristics	LV mass	Coronary flow reserve		Coronary vasodilator reserve
			Total	endo/epi	
Clinical Studies					
Opherk [1]	AP, no CAD	↑ (+62%)	↓ (−79%)	–	↓ (−117%)
Strauer [10]	± CAD	↑ (+33 to +109%)	–	–	↓↓
Animal Studies					
Pharmacological dilatation					
Mueller [11]	Dog/1K–1C	↑ (+50%)	NS	NS	↓ (−14%)
Marcus [12]	Dog/2K–1C	↑ (+28%)	↓	NS	↓ (−50 to −56%)
Wangler [13]	Rat/SHR 7 mos	↑ (+28%)	NS	↑ (+38%)	↓ (−13 to −20%)
	3, 15 mos	↑ (+14 to +29%)	NS	↑ (+26 to +39%)	NS
Kobayashi [14, 15]	Rat/2K–1C, SHR-SP	↑ (+48 to +39%)	NS	–	–
Yamamoto [16]	Dog/DOCA	↑ (+32 to +42%)	NS	NS	↓ (−37 to −46%)
Tomanek [17]	Rat/SHR	↑ (+23%)	NS	NS	↓
Tomanek [18]	Dog/1K–1C	↑ (+27%)	NS	NS	↓ (−67%)
Wicker [19, 20]	Rat/2K–1C	↑ (+50 to +58%)	NS	NS or ↓ (−24%)	↓ (−36 to −64%)
Ischemia (Transient coronary occlusion)					
Peters [21]	Rat/SHR 3, 7 mos	↑ (+17 to +29%)	↓	–	–
	15 mos	↑ (+30%)	NS	–	–

1K–1C, 2K–1C, 2K–2C: one kidney – one clip, two kidney – one clip, two kidney – two clip Goldblatt hypertension; 1K–1W: one kidney – one wrapped Page Hypertension; DOCA = Doca salt hypertension; SHR: Spontaneously hypertensive rats; SP: Stroke prone; AP: Angina pectoris; CAD: Coronary artery disease.
NS: Not statistically different from controls.
↑ or ↓ : significantly greater or lower than controls.
–: not reported or not measured.

1.3 *Factors modulating the response of the coronary circulation to hypertension*

Although the vast majority of studies have shown that coronary vasodilator reserve is limited in hypertensive LVH, the extent of this reduction is by no means identical. Various factors, such as the animal species, the age, the severity and duration of hypertrophy may modulate the response of the coronary circulation to hypertension.

Clinical vs animal studies. One important finding from the studies summarized in Table 1 is that coronary vasodilator reserve is usually more depressed in humans than in animals. The inclusion in these clinical studies of subjects with chest pain may account for these discrepancies. Coronary reserve is impaired in patients with angina pectoris and normal coronary angiograms [29, 30] and the changes in coronary reserve reported in hypertensive patients may rather reflect intrinsic coronary abnormalities than a deleterious effect of hypertension per se. Moreover, the degree of LVH in these patients was larger than usually observed in unselected hypertensive subjects [31] or in animals (Table 1). Hence, these patients may not have been representative of the general hypertensive population and it remains unclear whether the results documented in this subset can be generalized.

Role of the severity of cardiac hypertrophy. A further analysis of the data in Table 1 reveals a significant ($r = 0.60$; $n = 13$; $p < 0.05$) correlation between the increase in cardiac mass and the limitation in coronary reserve, suggesting that the magnitude of hypertrophy is an important factor modulating the response of the coronary circulation to hypertension. However, this correlation is based on the average value(s) reported in each study rather than on the

Table 2. Coronary flow and vasodilator reserve in experimental hypertensive right ventricular hypertrophy (RVH).

Author [Ref]	Animal/Model	RV mass	Coronary flow reserve	Coronary vasodilator reserve
Wangler [13]	Rat/SHR 3 mos	NS	NS	NS
	7 mos	NS	NS	↓(−50%)
	15 mos	↑(+29%)	NS	↓(−50%)
Tomanek [17]	Rat/SHR 6–7 mos	NS	NS	↓
Yamamoto [16]	Rat/DOCA	NS	NS	↓(−82%)
Wicker [20, 25]	Rat/2K–1C	↑(+10 to +16%)	NS	NS or +50 to +75%

Abbreviations as in Table 1.

individual raw data and this conclusion remains to be demonstrated by more direct studies.

Role of the duration of cardiac hypertrophy. The effects of the duration of cardiac hypertrophy on coronary reserve are uncertain. On one hand, some studies have reported an improvement or a near normalization in coronary reserve when hypertension had been present for more than one year in spontaneously hypertensive rats (SHR) [13, 21]. This amelioration in coronary reserve was associated with anatomical evidence of capillary growth [13]. On the other hand, a study from the same group of investigators in dogs with renovascular hypertension reached an opposite conclusion as the decrement in coronary reserve was found to persist up to six months following the induction of hypertension [12]. Similarly, Friberg et al. measured coronary reserve in isolated rat hearts from 4- and 19-month-old WKY and SHR and found that coronary reserve was reduced by 15 to 25 percent both in young and senescent rats as compared to age-matched controls [32]. Finally, our own investigations could not document any improvement in coronary reserve in rats with long standing renovascular [19] or genetic [33] hypertensive cardiac hypertrophy. In addition to these functional studies, two anatomical studies could not find any evidence for a normalization of myocardial capillarity in aging SHR [34, 35]. Taken together, these data favor the view that the coronary circulation abnormalities observed in developing hypertensive hypertrophy persists for the entire course of the disease and that, if some vascular growth does occur, it is not of a sufficient magnitude to significantly improve the limitation in coronary reserve observed in this situation.

Effects of aging. In normal rats, aging is associated with a 30–40 percent reduction in the dilatory capacities of the coronary circulation [33]. Hypertension accentuates this age-related decline in coronary reserve and only 30 percent of the initially available reserve in young normal rats remains present in senescent (22 months old) SHR [33]. However, because blood pressure starts to rise at an early age, these studies in SHR could not dissociate the effects of aging from those of long standing hypertension. To the best of our knowledge, there are no published reports on the changes in coronary reserve when relatively short term hypertension develops or is induced in young or elderly patients and animals. Experimental studies performed in other forms of pressure overload hypertrophy indicate that coronary reserve remains normal when the stimulus is applied in utero or immediately following birth, suggesting that the adaptive capacities of the coronary circulation are appropriate early in life [36]. Whether this is also the case in hypertensive cardiac hypertrophy remains to be elucidated. Because of the increasing recognition of cardiac involvement in juvenile hypertension [37] and because of the prevalence of hypertension in the elderly population, these issues are not of pure academic interest.

1.4 *Mechanisms accounting for the limitation in coronary reserve*

Ten years ago, Mueller and his colleagues proposed to compute minimal coronary resistance for the whole left ventricle (usually referred to as total minimal coronary resistance) [11]. This approach has provided a very useful conceptual framework to analyze the effects of cardiac hypertrophy on the coronary circulation since it allows to separate changes in the total coronary cross-sectional area, i.e. the total area available for blood transport, from changes in cardiac mass. The vast majority of studies have found that total minimal coronary resistance is unchanged in hypertensive left ventricular hypertrophy [11, 13–20], suggesting that vascular growth is not commensurate with the development of hypertrophy. On theoretical and experimental grounds, this lack of expansion of the coronary resistance bed may result from alterations in the structural properties of the coronary arterioles, such as a decrease in arteriolar density (defined as the number of arterioles per unit cross sectional area) or an increase in vessel wall thickness encroaching upon the lumen and diminishing vessel diameter at maximal dilatation [38]. Until recently, the few studies that had attempted to address these issues were based uniquely on limited histological observations or had restricted the scope of their investigation to middle sized arteries, a questionable approach because coronary resistance appears to be distributed throughout the entire coronary bed [39]. In more recent investigations by our group [40] or others [18], the entire coronary bed was evaluated. Furthermore, in our studies, a large number of arterioles were analyzed. Large samples are required to detect small but physiologically significant alterations in wall thickness to lumen ratio. Using these methodological guidelines, we measured the lumen to wall thickness lumen ratio and arteriolar density in rats with eight weeks duration renovascular hypertension and LVH. Approximately 1,000 arterioles per heart were evaluated and all arterioles with a diameter equal to or larger than 10 microns were included. Results indicate that, with the exception of arterioles 20 μ or less in diameter, the lumen to wall thickness ratio was moderately but significantly decreased in coronary arterioles from hypertensive animals as compared to their sham-operated controls (Figure 1). In contrast, arteriolar density was similar in both groups. However, this lack of difference does not mitigate against the role of vascular rarefaction in the diminished coronary reserve of hypertensive LVH, since there was a significant ($r = 0.56$; $p < 0.05$) correlation between the product of arteriolar density by the average luminal area (an index of the anatomical coronary cross-sectional area per unit mass)

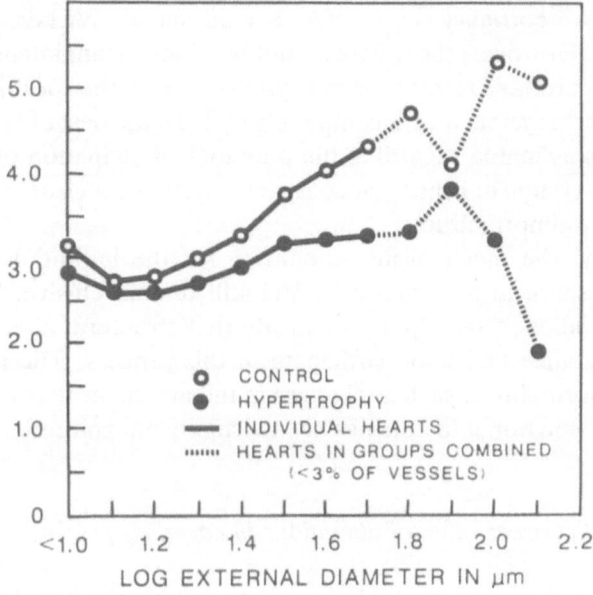

Figure 1. Coronary arteriole lumen to wall thickness ratio (y axis) plotted as a function of the external vessel size expressed in log units (x axis). In control rats, the lumen to wall thickness ratio increases with increasing vessel diameter, i.e. wall thickness tends to augment proportionately less than vessel size. In renovascular hypertensive rats with LVH, the arteriole wall is thicker in relation to vessel size, a difference which becomes significant in vessels larger than 16 μ in diameter. From Rakusan [40].

and coronary vasodilator reserve simultaneously measured in the same animal [40].

Two other investigations in an experimental canine model of renovascular hypertension reported no alterations in arteriolar density [41] or in the wall thickness to lumen ratio [18]. However, in the latter study, the wall thickness to lumen ratio was actually increased by approximately 10 percent in all, but two, luminal diameter classes.

Besides these anatomical alterations, functional factors may also be involved in the limitation of the coronary vasodilatory capacities seen in hypertensive hearts [11], more specifically the sympathetic nervous and angiotensin systems. These two systems have been involved in the development and maintenance of hypertension [42, 43] and stimulation of their activity can cause coronary vasoconstriction of limit pharmacologically induced coronary vasodilation [44, 45]. Data from our laboratory in rats suggest that the activation of the renin angiotensin system associated with 1-clip 2-kidney Goldblatt hypertension does not significantly participate in the coronary abnormalities seen in this model, since complete converting enzyme inhibition by captopril did not improve coronary reserve (A. Samad and P. Wicker, unpublished observations). However, these data do not preclude an angiotensin mediated restriction in coronary reserve since captopril blocks the local intravascular renin angiotensin system only incompletely [46]. To the best of knowledge, no information is available regarding the potential participation of the sympathetic nervous system or other vasoconstrictor systems, such as vasopressin, in these coronary abnormalities.

In summary, the mechanisms accounting for the limitation of coronary vasodilator reserve in hypertensive LVH still remain elusive. Some of the histological studies so far reported indicate that structural alterations of the coronary resistance bed may participate in this process. The role of other structural abnormalities, such as changes in the arteriolar network branching pattern, or of functional factors has been virtually unexplored.

1.5 *Functional consequences of alterations in coronary reserve*

The functional consequences of the coronary reserve abnormalities of hypertensive cardiac hypertrophy have been more often assumed than demonstrated. Most studies dealing with coronary reserve have used pharmacological agents to induce coronary dilation. The conclusions of these studies may not be applicable to more physiological situations in which coronary vasodilation develops in response to a metabolic or ischemic stimulation. However, we recently found that the magnitude of pharmacologically and ischemia induced coronary vasodilator reserve, determined in the same animal, were comparable both in rats with normal cardiac mass and with cardiac hypertrophy secondary to renovascular hypertension [47]. In addition, differences in coronary reserve between normal and hypertrophied hearts were comparable, irrespective of the type of stimulus used (Figure 2). Finally, a significant ($r = 0.56$; $n = 22$; $p < 0.05$) linear correlation was found between pharmacologically and ischemia induced coronary reserve. These data suggest that pharmacologically induced coronary reserve provide a useful index of the coronary vasculature ability to respond to more physiological stimuli. Whether the conclusions of this study can be extended to other models of hypertensive cardiac hypertrophy or validate the use of pharmacological agents to assess the transmural differences in coronary reserve remains to be determined. In that connection, Grattam et al. recently reported in normal dogs that, although pharmacologically induced coronary dilation is larger than that elicited by metabolic or ischemic stimuli, the relative differences in flow reserve between subendocardial and subepicardial layers were remarkably similar irrespective of the types of stimuli used [48].

Besides the intrinsic dilatory capacities of the coronary vessels, myocardial

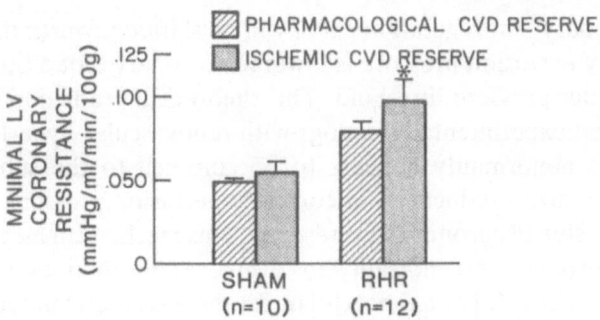

Figure 2. Comparison of pharmacologically and ischemia-induced coronary vasodilator (CVD) reserve in rats with renovascular hypertension (RHR) and their sham operated controls (SHAM). Pharmacological coronary reserve was determined after carbochrome using radioactive microspheres. Ischemic coronary reserve was measured during the hyperemic response following a transient coronary occlusion, using a combination of a microsphere and a Doppler technique. The magnitude of pharmacological and ischemic coronary reserve is comparable in both groups. Furthermore, the differences in reserve between the two groups are similar, irrespective of the type of stimulus applied. * $p < 0.05$ vs. SHAM.

flow supply is obviously influenced by the perfusion pressure. In hypertensive cardiac hypertrophy, coronary blood flow/unit mass – and presumably maximal myocardial oxygen delivery – is usually within normal limits (Tables 1–2), since the rise in perfusion pressure compensates for the elevated coronary resistance. A closer analysis of coronary flow reserve and its determinants indicates that a normal flow reserve is actually maintained because of an appropriate relationship between pressure, LV mass and total coronary resistance [19]. Since minimal coronary resistance for the entire LV is unchanged, coronary perfusion pressure will set maximal total flow and the ratio between perfusion pressure and LV mass will thus determine coronary flow reserve, i.e. total flow/LV mass. Hence, in hypertensive LVH, coronary flow reserve remains normal because, in most of the experimental models so far studied, cardiac hypertrophy is usually appropriate to the increased load and the pressure/mass ratio is normal. The role of an appropriate balance between arterial pressure and LV mass in determining coronary flow reserve has been substantiated by studies from our group in which blood pressure was dissociated from left ventricular mass either by therapeutic manipulations in renal hypertensive rats or by using strains with divergent degrees of cardiac hypertrophy and hypertension [15, 19]. A significant correlation was found between the pressure/LV mass ratio and pharmacologically induced coronary flow reserve either in renal hypertensive rats or in rats with genetically determined pressure/mass ratios [15]. The dependency of coronary flow reserve on a higher coronary perfusion pressure may have two important consequences.

First, the coronary autoregulation curve will be shifted towards the right, and when coronary perfusion pressure is lowered, coronary blood flow will begin to fall at a higher pressure threshold. This theoretical prediction has recently been confirmed experimentally in dogs with renovascular hypertension [49]. However, this abnormality appears to be confined to the subendocardial layers. Second, acute reductions in coronary perfusion pressure will cause a marked depression in coronary flow reserve. This mechanism may account for the higher morbidity and mortality from myocardial infarction reported in hypertensive patients [3] or animals [4] or for the increased infarct size in dogs with hypertensive left ventricular hypertrophy [50]. However, the consequences of a reduction in coronary perfusion pressure are more subtle than a simple hemodynamic relationship between flow and pressure would imply. Systemic blood pressure is one component of ventricular stress, and thus indirectly determines myocardial oxygen needs. It can be speculated that, in some situations, the fall in perfusion pressure will be associated with a parallel decrease in flow reserve and in myocardial oxygen requirements, thus maintaining a normal or near normal balance between supply and demand. The need to take into account both terms of the supply-demand equation is exemplified by a recent study by Inou et al. [51] showing that, in dogs with hypertensive left ventricular hypertrophy, acute reductions in arterial pressure to normal levels prevent the increase in mortality and normalize the infarct size following acute coronary occlusion. One explanation to account for these paradoxical beneficial effects is that the acute decrease in pressure leads to a dimition in myocardial oxygen needs – particularly in the subendocardial layers – and thus minimizes the adverse consequences of coronary occlusion and hypertensive cardiac hypertrophy.

2. Effects of antihypertensive treatment on coronary reserve

The demonstration that LVH can be reversed with antihypertensive measures and the potential role of myocardial perfusion abnormalities in the development of hypertensive cardiovascular complications has prompted various investigators to evaluate the effects of antihypertensive treatment in this situation.

2.1 *Pharmacologic treatment*

Table 3 summarizes various studies that have evaluated coronary reserve following chronic treatment with antihypertensive drugs and reversal of LVH. All these studies were conducted in rodents and various classes of antihypertensive medications alone or in combination, similar to those used in human hypertension, were administered. Reversal of LVH was always associated with an improvement or a normalization in the coronary reserve. The magnitude of this amelioration appears to parallel more the regression of cardiac hypertrophy than the type of antihypertensive medication used. A direct coronary vasodilatory effect of some of these agents cannot be excluded. This mechanism appears unlikely with captopril because adequate blood pressure control following nephrectomy in 1-clip 2-kidney Goldblatt renal hypertensive rats results in similar improvements in coronary reserve [19]. However, in a study using hydralazine, Tomanek et al. reported an amelioration in coronary reserve both in treated control and hypertensive rats suggesting that hydralazine may also exert a direct effect on the coronary vessels [17]. Of importance is that, in none of the studies reported so far, antihypertensive treatment resulted in a further depression in coronary flow reserve. The maintenance of an appropriate or nearly appropriate pressure to mass ratio may account for this finding. Based on the theoretical analysis provided earlier, drugs that have divergent effects of blood pressure and cardiac mass may cause a reduction in flow reserve, if blood pressure reduction is obtained without a simultaneous decrease in cardiac mass. However, in the absence in studies that have specifically addressed these questions, particularly in humans, it is premature to draw any definite conclusion at the present time.

2.2 *Nonpharmacological treatment: Effects of exercise*

Since nonpharmacological measures are currently advocated as the first line of treatment in most patients with hypertension, recent studies have evaluated the effects of physical exercise on the coronary circulation of hypertensive heart disease. The modest but significant antihypertensive effects of exercise in patients with hypertension [54] and the improvement in myocardial vascularity observed in animals following training programs [55] have raised hopes that exercise could prevent or correct the coronary circulation abnormalities of hypertensive heart disease. Physical conditioning initiated before the onset of hypertension and the development of LVH did not prevent the limitation in coronary reserve [20]. A trend towards a further reduction in coronary reserve was even noted in trained hypertensive rats, but the differences were marginally significant [20]. Studies in which exercise was begun during the established phase of hypertensive hypertrophy have yielded similar results (P. Wicker et al., unpublished observation).

These initial results should not detract from the other beneficial effects of exercise in hypertension [54]. In addition, the type and intensity of exercise may modulate the response of the coronary circulation and the possibility that more intense or more prolonged training programs may still be helpful remains to be investigated.

3. Coronary microcirculation in hypertensive cardiac hypertrophy

Tissue oxygenation depends not only on the total amount of blood delivered to the heart but also on an adequate flow distribution in the coronary microcirculation and on oxygen diffusion between capillaries and tissue. Microcirculatory flow and oxygen diffusion are determined by the structural and functional properties of the terminal coronary bed. Because of methodological limitations, most of our present knowledge in this area originates from anatomical investigations and very little is known about the functional characteristics of the coronary microcirculation in normal as well as in pathological conditions, including hypertensive heart disease.

Among the various parameters that can be measured to characterize the terminal coronary bed, capillary density and intercapillary distance have been the most widely investigated, since they determine tissue oxygenation according to the Krogh model [55]. The mean anatomical capillary density, which is defined as the number of capillaries/mm^2 of tissue cross-sectional area, has been found to be either reduced, particularly in the subendocardial layers [17, 18, 57–60] or unchanged [18, 57, 59, 61]. Accordingly, the mean distance between capillaries is either increased [34, 59] or normal [34, 61]. Studies in SHR suggest that the duration of hypertrophy and/or the age of the animal are

Table 3. Coronary reserve in hypertensive left ventricular hypertrophy: Effects of pharmacological treatment.

Author [Ref]	Rat/Model	Drug	Blood pressure	LV mass	Coronary vasodilator reserve	Coronary flow reserve
Wicker [19]	Rat/1C–2K	CEI	↓N	↓N	↑N	↔
Kobayashi [14]	Rat/1C–2K	CAEB	↓	↓	Not reported	↔
Tomanek [17]	Rat/SHR	Hydralazine	↓N		↑N	↔
Friberg [52]	Rat/SHR	Beta Blocker + CAEB	↓N	↓	↑	--
Gosse [53]	Rat/1C–2K	CEI	↓N	↓N	↑N	↔

CEI: converting enzyme inhibitor.
CAEB: calcium entry blocker.
↑, ↓: significant decrease or increase (as compared to untreated hypertensive rats) with (N) or without normalization.

important factors in modulating the response of the capillary bed to hypertension. In young SHR, epicardial capillarity remains normal [59, 61]. With the development of hypertrophy, capillary density significantly declines until cardiac mass reaches a plateau [58–60]. In one study, epicardial capillary density was reported to increase and then normalize following a long period of stable hypertrophy in SHR [59]. Other investigators, however, could not confirm this favorable course of events, in the same model [34, 35]. Apart from these divergences, most studies agree that capillary growth is not commensurate to cardiac growth, particularly in the subendocardial layers, during the stable phase of hypertrophy either in SHR or in other models of hypertension [17, 18, 34, 57–60]. The lack of capillary proliferation in pressure overload hypertrophy has been demonstrated by studies using autoradiographic techniques [62] or by the fact that the capillary-to-fiber ratio remains unchanged [57]. The heterogeneity of capillary spacing is another potential important variable governing tissue oxygenation [63]. Cellular hypoxia develops when peri-mitochondrial PO_2 reaches 0 mmHg and such a low PO_2 will be observed in those areas most remote from the capillary vessels [63]. Thus, the relative proportion of capillaries with long intercapillary distances will have a greater influence on the presence and magnitude of hypoxia than the average mean intercapillary distance [63]. Assuming a log-normal distribution for intercapillary distance, Rakusan et al. reported that the variability of intercapillary spacing was significantly higher in SHR, particularly in older animals [34]. If confirmed by further studies, these initial observations provide an attractive explanation for the frequent occurrence of areas of focal necrosis in hypertrophied hearts [64].

Very few data are available on the coronary microcirculation following pharmacological antihypertensive therapy. Studies by Tomanek et al. in young adult SHR indicate that mean capillary density was either improved or prevented from deteriorating during the developmental phase of hypertrophy by a treatment with alphamethyldopa [58] or a combination of hydralazine, reserpine, and hydrochlorothiazide [65]. Hydralazine alone, however, failed to influence mean capillary density [17]. In contrast to flow studies, results of investigations concerned with the effects of exercise on myocardial capillarity have not been consistent. A normalization in capillary density has been reported in SHR conditioned by running [53]. However, we [66] and others [67] could not demonstrate any beneficial effects of either a swimming [66] or a running [67] program on capillary density [66, 67] and capillary spacing heterogeneity [66]. In addition, one of these studies suggests that, when hypertension and cardiac hypertrophy are severe, exercise may be detrimental to the coronary circulation, as evidenced by a significant decrement in subendocardial capillary density [67].

Conclusions

Results from the studies analyzed in this review form a coherent picture of the response of the coronary circulation to hypertension and provide a plausible explanation for the frequent occurrence of ischemic manifestation or for the greater incidence of cardiovascular complications in patients with hypertensive heart disease. There are, however, several areas that require further clarification or have been virtually unexplored. Most of our current knowledge originates from animal studies and these experimental observations must be extended to clinical situations. The development of reliable and noninvasive methodologies for measuring coronary blood flow in man holds promise in that matter [6], but technical limitations still need to be overcome before these techniques can be applied on a larger scale. The mechanisms mediating the depression of coronary reserve still remain elusive. A better understanding of these mechanisms will undoubtedly open new therapeutic avenues, such as the possibility of slowing or even reversing the progression of these circulation abnormalities. Because they are directly relevant to tissue oxygenation, studies of the anatomical and functional characteristics of the coronary microcirculation need to be developed, but are also hampered by methodological difficulties. Answers to these questions will improve our understanding of hypertensive heart disease and translate into improved patient care.

References

1. Opherk D, Mall G, Zebe H, Schwarz F, Weihe E, Manthey J, Kubler W (1984): Reduction of coronary reserve: A mechanism for angina pectoris in patients with arterial hypertension and normal coronary arteries. *Circulation* 69: 1–7.
2. Harris CN, Aronow WS, Parker DP, Kapaln MA (1973): Treadmill stress test in left ventricular hypertrophy. *Chest* 63: 353–357.
3. Kannel WB, Sorlie P, Castelli WP, McGee D (1980): Blood pressure and survival after myocardial infarction (The Framingham Study) *Am J Cardiol* 45: 326–330.
4. Koyanagi S, Eastham C, Marcus ML (1982): Effects of chronic hypertension and left ventricular hypertrophy on the incidence of sudden cardiac death after coronary artery occlusion in conscious dogs. *Circulation* 65: 1192–1197.
5. Hoffman JIE (1984): Maximal coronary flow and the concept of coronary vascular reserve. *Circulation* 70: 153–159.
6. Marcus ML, Wilson RF, White CW (1987): Methods of measurement of myocardial blood flow in patients: A critical review. *Circulation* 76: 245.
7. Marcus ML, Harrison DG, Chilian WM, Koyanagi S, Inou T, Tomanek RJ, Martins JB, Eastham CL, Hiratzka LF (1987): Alterations in the coronary circulation in hypertrophied ventricles. *Circulation* 75 (suppl I): I-19.
8. Wicker P, Tarazi RC (1982): Coronary blood flow in left ventricular hypertrophy: A review of experimental data. *Eur Heart J* 3 (suppl A): 111–118.
9. Wicker PA, Tarazi RC (1987): The coronary circulation in hypertensive left ventricular

hypertrophy, in Safar ME (ed), *Arterial and Venous Systems in Essential Hypertension,* pp 167–180. Dordrecht-Boston: Martinus Nijhoff Publishers (DICM-series, Vol 63).

10. Strauer BE (1979): Ventricular function and coronary hemodynamics in hypertensive heart disease. *Am J Cardiol* 44: 999–1006.
11. Mueller TM, Marcus ML, Kerber RE, Young JA, Barnes RW, Abboud FM (1978): Effect of renal hypertension and left ventricular hypertrophy on the coronary circulation in dogs. *Circ Res* 42: 543–549.
12. Marcus ML, Mueller TM, Eastham CL (1981): Effects of short- and long-term left ventricular hypertrophy on coronary circulation. *Am J Physiol* 241: H358–H362.
13. Wangler RD, Peters KG, Marcus ML, Tomanek RJ (1982): Effects of duration and severity of arterial hypertension and cardiac hypertrophy on coronary vasodilator reserve. *Circ Res* 51: 10–18.
14. Kobayashi K, Tarazi RC (1983): Effect of nitrendipine on coronary flow and ventricular hypertrophy in hypertension. *Hypertension* 5 (suppl II): II-45–51.
15. Kobayashi K, Tarazi RC, Lovenberg W, Rakusan K (1984): Coronary blood flow in genetic cardiac hypertrophy. *Am J Cardiol* 53: 1360–1364.
16. Yamamoto J, Tsuchiya M, Saito M, Ikeda M (1985): Cardiac contractile and coronary flow reserves in dioxycorticosterone acetate-salt hypertensive rats. *Hypertension* 7: 569–577.
17. Tomanek RJ, Wangler RD, Bauer CA (1985): Prevention of coronary vasodilator reserve decrement in spontaneously hypertensive rats. *Hypertension* 7: 533–540.
18. Tomanek RJ, Palmer PJ, Pfeiffer GL, Schreiber KL, Eastham CL, Marcus ML (1986): Morphometry of canine coronary arteries, arterioles, and capillaries during hypertension and left ventricular hypertrophy. *Circ Res* 58: 38–46.
19. Wicker P, Tarazi RC, Kobayashi K (1983): Coronary blood flow with reversal of cardiac hypertrophy. *Am J Cardiol* 51: 1744–1749.
20. Wicker P, Tarazi RC (1987): Effects of exercise on the coronary circulation in conscious rats with renovascular hypertension. *Hypertension* 10: 74–81.
21. Peters KG, Wangler RD, Tomanek RJ, Marcus ML (1984): Effects of long-term cardiac hypertrophy on coronary vasodilator reserve in SHR rats. *Am J Cardiol* 54: 1342–1348.
22. Atkins JM, Mitchell HC, Pettinger WA (1977): Increased pulmonary vascular resistance with systemic hypertension. *Am J Cardiol* 39: 802.
23. Ferlinz J (1980): Right ventricular performance in essential hypertension. *Circulation* 61: 156.
24. Guazzi MD, Polese A, Bartorelli A, Loaldi A, Fiorentini C (1982): Evidence of a shared mechanism of vasoconstriction in pulmonary and systemic circulation in hypertension: A possible role of intracellular calcium. *Circulation* 66: 881.
25. Wicker P, Tarazi RC (1985): Right ventricular coronary flow in arterial hypertension. *Am Heart J* 110: 845–850.
26. Pool PE, Piggott WJ, Seagren SC, Skelton CL (1976): Augmented right ventricular function in systemic hypertension-induced hypertrophy. *Cardiovasc Res* 10: 124.
27. Nunez B, Messerli FH, Amodeo C, Garavaglia G, Schmieder R, Frohlich ED (1986): The right ventricle (RV) is thicker in hypertensive patients with left ventricular hypertrophy (LVH). *J Am Coll Cardiol* 7: 111A (abstract).
28. Olivari MT, Fiorentini C, Polese A, Guazzi MD (1978): Pulmonary hemodynamics and right ventricular function in hypertension. *Circulation* 57: 1185.
29. Opherk D, Zebe H, Weihe E, Mall AG, Durr Ch, Gravert B, Mehmel HC, Schwarz F, Kubler W (1981): Reduced coronary dilatory capacity and ultrastructural changes of the myocardium in patients with angina pectoris but normal coronary arteriograms. *Circulation* 63: 817.
30. Cannon RO, Bonow RO, Bacharach SL, Green MV, Rosing DR, Leon MB, Watson RM,

Epstein SE (1985): Left ventricular dysfunction in patients with angina pectoris, normal epicardial coronary arteries, and abnormal vasodilator reserve. *Circulation* 71: 218–226.

31. Savage DD, Drayer JIM, Henry WL, Mathews EC Jr, Ware JH, Gardin JM, Cohen ER, Epstein SE, Laragh JH (1979): Echocardiographic assessment of cardiac anatomy and function in hypertensive subjects. *Circulation* 59: 623–632.

32. Friberg P, Nordlander M, Lundin S, Folkow B (1985): Effects of aging on cardiac performance and coronary flow in spontaneously hypertensive and normotensive rats. *Acta Physiol Scand* 125: 1–11.

33. Wicker P, Vitullo J, Healy B (1988): Coronary reserve in normal and hypertrophied hearts during cardiac maturation and aging. *J Am Coll Cardiol* 2: 190A (abstract).

34. Rakusan K, Hrdina PW, Turek Z, Lakatta EG, Spurgeon HA, Wolford GD (1984): Cell size and capillary supply of the hypertensive rat heart: quantitative study. *Basic Res Cardiol* 79: 389–395.

35. Engelmann GE, Vitullo JC, Gerrity RG (1987): Morphometric analysis of cardiac hypertrophy during development, maturation, and senescence in spontaneously hypertensive rats. *Circ Res* 60: 487–494.

36. Marcus ML: Effects of cardiac hypertrophy on the coronary circulation, in: *The Coronary Circulation in Health and Disease,* pp 285–306. New York: McGraw-Hill.

37. Culpepper WS (1983): Cardiac anatomy and function in juvenile hypertension: current understanding and future concerns. *Am J Med* 75 (suppl 3A): 57–61.

38. Folkow B (1978): Cardiovascular structural adaptation: Its role in the initiation and maintenance of primary hypertension. *Clin Sci Mol Med* 55: 3s–22s.

39. Chilian WM, Eastham CL, Marcus ML (1986): Microvascular distribution of coronary vascular resistance in beating left ventricle. *Am J Physiol* 251: H779–788.

40. Rakusan K, Cheng M, Wicker P, Healy B (1987): Morphometry of coronary arterioles in normal and hypertrophic rat heart, in: *Microcirculation: An Update,* Vol 2. Proceedings of the Fourth World Congress for Microcirculation, Tokyo, Japan, 1987.

41. Tomanek RJ, Schalk KA, Nadle T, Harrison DG (1987): Coronary vascular growth in dogs with long-term hypertension. *Circulation* 76 (suppl IV): IV–328 (abstract).

42. Nabel EG, Gibbons GH, Dzau VJ (1985): Pathophysiology of experimental renovascular hypertension. *Am J Kidney Dis* 5: A111–119.

43. Abboud FM (1982): The sympathetic system in hypertension. State-of-the-Art review. *Hypertension* 4 (suppl II): II-208–225.

44. Vlahakes GJ, Baer RW, Uhlig PN, Verrier EI, Bristow JD, Hoffman JIE (1982): Adrenergic influence in the coronary circulation of conscious dogs during maximal vasodilation with adenosine. *Circ Res* 51: 371–384.

45. Gavras H, Liang C-S, Brunner HR (1978): Redistribution of regional blood flow after inhibition of the angiotensin-converting enzyme. *Circ Res* 43 (suppl I): I-59–63.

46. Dzau VJ (1987): Renin angiotensin system and arterial wall in hypertension, in: Safar ME (ed), *Arterial and Venous Systems in Essential Hypertension.* Dordrecht-Boston: Martinus Nijhoff Publishers (DICM-series, Vol 63).

47. Wicker P, Samad M (1987): Pharmacological coronary reserve predicts the response of the coronary bed to ischemia hypertensive cardiac hypertrophy. *Fed Proc* 46: 1408 (abstract).

48. Grattan MT, Hanley FL, Stevens MB, Hoffman JIE (1986): Transmural coronary flow reserve patterns in dogs. *Am J Physiol* 250: H276–283.

49. Harrison DG, Marcus ML, Florentine MS, Cooper SM, Brooks LA (1987): Coronary autoregulation in hypertension and left ventricular hypertrophy. *Fed Proc* 46: 1240 (abstract).

50. Koyanagi S, Eastham CL, Harrison DB, Marcus ML (1982): Increased size of myocardial infarction in dogs with chronic hypertension and left ventricular hypertrophy. *Circ Res* 50: 55–62.

51. Inou T, Lamberth WC Jr, Koyanagi S, Harrison DG, Eastham CL, Marcus ML (1987): Relative importance of hypertension after coronary occlusion in chronic hypertensive dogs with LVH. *Am J Physiol* 253: H1148–H1158.

52. Friberg P, Nordlander M (1986): Influence of long-term antihypertensive therapy on cardiac function, coronary flow and myocardial oxygen consumption in spontaneously hypertensive rats. *J Hypertens* 4: 165–173.

53. Gosse P, Grellet J, Bonoron S, Tariosse L, Besse P, Dallocchio M (1987): Effects du perindopril sur l'hypertrophie ventriculaire gauche, la reserve coronaire et les proprietes mechaniques du muscle papillaire du rat avec hypertension arterielle renovasculaire. *Arch Mal Caeur* 80: 905–910.

54. Jennings G, Nelson L, Nestel P, Esler M, Korner P, Burton D, Bazelmans J (1986): The effects of changes in physical activity on major cardiovascular risk factors, hemodynamics, sympathetic function, and glucose utilization in man: A controlled study of four levels of activity. *Circulation* 73: 30–40.

55. Schaible TF, Scheuer J (1985): Cardiac adaptations to chronic exercise. *Prog Cardiovasc Dis* 27: 297–324.

56. Kreuzer F (1982): Oxygen supply to tissues: The Krogh model and its assumptions. *Experientia* 38: 1415–1426.

57. Anversa P, Loud AV, Giacomelli F, Wiener J (1978): Absolute morphometric study of myocardial hypertrophy in experimental hypertension, II: Ultrastructure of myocytes and interstitium. *Lab Invest* 38: 597–609.

58. Tomanek RJ, Davis JW, Anderson SC (1979): The effects of alpha-methyldopa on cardiac hypertrophy in spontaneously hypertensive rats: Ultrastructural, stereological, and morphometric analysis. *Cardivasc Res* 13: 173–182.

59. Tomanek RJ, Searls JC, Lachenbruch PA (1982): Quantitative changes in capillary bed during developing, peak, and stabilized cardiac hypertrophy in the spontaneously hypertensive rat. *Circ Res* 51: 295–304.

60. Crisman RP, Rittman B, Tomanek RJ (1985): Exercise-induced myocardial capillary growth in the spontaneously hypertensive rat. *Microvasc Res* 30: 185–194.

61. Anversa P, Melissari M, Beghi C, Olivetti G (1984): Structural compensatory mechanisms in rat heart in early spontaneous hypertension. *Am J Physiol* 246: H739–H746.

62. Ljungqvist A, Unge G (1973): The proliferative activity of the myocardial tissue in various forms of experimental cardiac hypertrophy. *Acta Path Microbiol Scand,* Section A, 81: 233–240.

63. Turek Z, Rakusan K (1981): Lognormal distribution of intercapillary distance in normal and hypertrophic rat heart as estimated by the method of concentric circles: its effect on tissue oxygenation. *Pfluegers Arch* 391: 17–21.

64. Buchner F (1971): Qualitative morphology of heart failure. Light and electron microscopic characteristics of acute and chronic heart failure. *Methods Achiev Exp Pathol* 5: 60–120.

65. Tomanek RJ (1979): The role of prevention or relief of pressure overload on the myocardial cell of the spontaneously hypertensive rat: A morphometric and stereologic study. *Lab Invest* 40: 83–91.

66. Rakusan K, Wicker P, Abdul-Samad M, Healy B, Turek Z (1987): Failure of swimming exercise to improve capillarization in cardiac hypertrophy of renal hypertensive rats. *Circ Res* 61: 641–647.

67. Marcus KD, Tipton CM (1985): Exercise and its effects with renal hypertensive rats. *J Appl Physiol* 59: 1410–1415.

24. Hypertension and coronary atherosclerosis

ARAM V. CHOBANIAN

Introduction

Hypertension is a major contributor to the development of coronary arterial disease and its major complications. Patients with hypertension have at least a two-fold increase in risk for myocardial infarction, angina pectoris, and sudden death [1, 2]. Even mild elevations in blood pressure appear to accelerate the development of these problems. Despite the high prevalence rate of hypertension in the general population and the well-known epidemiologic observations regarding its effects on cardiovascular complications, remarkably little information is available regarding the influence of hypertension on the coronary vasculature.

Robertson and Strong [3] have provided interesting data regarding the nature and extent of coronary arterial disease in relatively young normotensive and hypertensive men who died of noncardiovascular causes. This very large International Atherosclerosis Project involved approximately 23,000 autopsied cases from 14 different countries. The percentage of coronary artery surface affected by fatty streaks and raised lesions was assessed in normotensive and hypertensive men. As shown in Figure 1, which summarizes the data in 25- to 34-year old individuals, the mean extent of atherosclerotic disease was considerably greater in hypertensive than normotensive subjects in almost every country included in the study. Fatty streaks, fibrous plaques, and advanced lesions with calcification all were seen more frequently in the hypertensive group as was the prevalence of coronary disease causing significant lumenal stenosis. Such findings have been supported by published data from other post-mortem studies as well [4, 5].

M.E. Safar & F. Fouad-Tarazi (eds.), The heart in hypertension.
© *1989 Kluwer Academic Publishers, Dordrecht –*

Influence of hemodynamic factors on the arterial wall

The focal nature of atherosclerosis and the particular vulnerability of certain areas of the vasculature to lesion development have served to focus attention on the role of hemodynamic stresses or mechanical factors in atherogenesis. The artery may be considered as a relatively incompressible tube whose diameter changes only minimally within physiologic ranges of blood pressure [6]. Circulating blood exerts both circumferential and tangential stresses on the vessel wall. The circumferential tension appears to be absorbed predominantly by the arterial media. As a general rule, medial tension is kept constant over a wide range of mammalian species and vessel sizes by regulation of the number of medial lamellar units and thereby, the thickness of the media [7]. When intravascular pressure rises, the stress on the media should also increase and, with chronic hypertension, the artery appears to adapt appropriately by increasing its smooth muscle cell (SMC) mass and its collagen and elastin content [8, 9]. However, hypertension may also stimulate medial SMC to migrate into the arterial intima and proliferate there. Resultant intimal changes could become a focus for intimal lesion development. The arterial endothelium normally represents an important barrier to entry of macromolecules into the arterial wall [10]. This barrier appears to be altered in the rabbit by hypertension [11] as well as by cholesterol feeding [10], causing marked increase in intimal permeability. No data relevant to the coronary circulation are available as yet.

Localization of arterial lesions

Studies in the cholesterol-fed rabbit have demonstrated that the initial arterial lesions in the aorta occur primarily distal to the orifices or flow dividers of the major branch vessels where shear stress would be expected to be maximal [12]. However, in the coronary arteries, the lesions have a different distribution and tend to surround completely the ostia.

In human subjects, aortic atherosclerosis tends to occur more proximal than distal to the branchings [13]. Coronary atherosclerosis in both young and middle-aged adults is most commonly located in the proximal regions of the major coronary arteries and decreases in frequency with increasing distance from the ostia [14, 15]. The region representing the flow divider between the left anterior descending and left circumflex coronary arteries tends to be spared. Studies by Stary [16] in children have indicated that intimal thickening and early manifestations of intimal lipid accumulation in the coronary circulation appear most often at the bifurcation of the main coronary artery and along the lateral borders.

The effects of hypertension on the distribution of arterial plaques has been

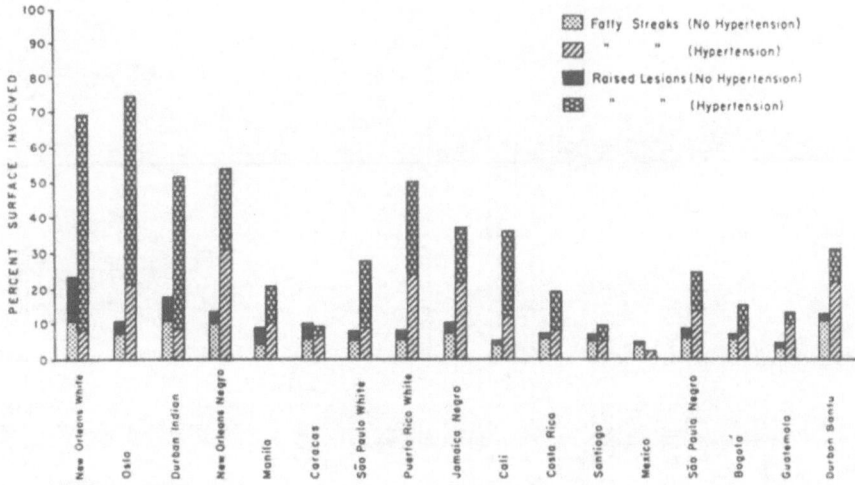

Figure 1. Mean extent of atherosclerotic lesions in coronary arteries of men, aged 25 to 34 years by presence and absence of hypertension and by location-race group. Adapted from Robertson and Strong [3].

unclear. We recently have investigated the influence of one-kidney, one-clip renovascular hypertension on atherosclerosis in the Watanabe rabbit which exhibits an increase in low-density and intermediate-density lipoproteins due to a genetic defect in the cellular receptor for low-density lipoproteins. Plasma cholesterol levels in the animals we have studied have generally been in the 300–600 mg/dl range. Renovascular surgery has been performed at three months of age and the animals are being followed for periods of one to 12 months after initiation of hypertension. A marked increase in aortic atherosclerosis has been observed in the hypertensive as compared with the normotensive Watanabe rabbit [17]. The arterial lesions are much more diffuse in distribution and not merely localized to the areas distal to the ostia of the major branch vessels (Figures 2 and 3). Whether the latter findings are related to differences in distribution of lesions as a result of hypertension is unknown since they may reflect the acceleration of atherogenesis and the greater severity of the disease in the hypertensive animals. Our preliminary data would suggest that coronary atherosclerosis is also accelerated in these hypertensive rabbits but further studies are required to confirm these initial findings.

Experimental studies on the effects of hypertension on the arterial wall

Elevation of blood pressure in experimental animals will induce a multiplicity of

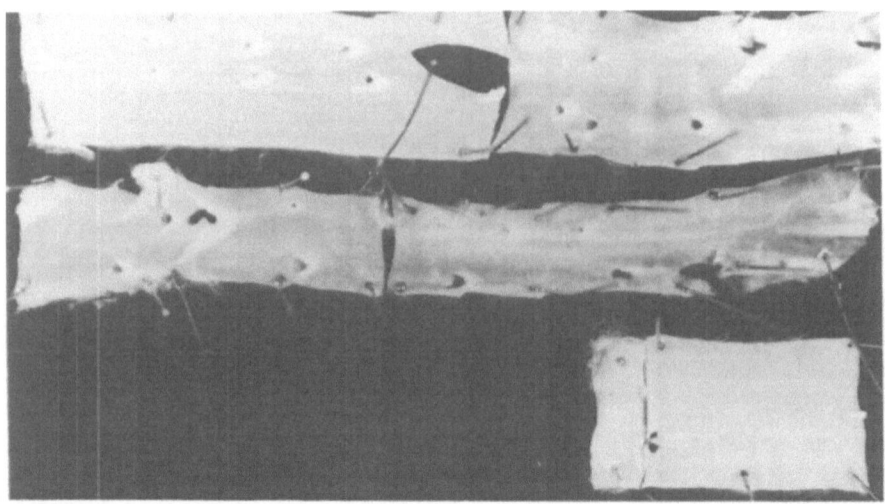

Figure 2. Photograph of the intimal surface of aorta in a 9-month old male Watanabe hyper-cholesterolemic rabbit which had sham surgery performed at three months of age. Systolic blood pressure averaged 105 mmHg. The upper portion of the descending thoracic aorta is shown in segment A and the lower thoracic and upper abdominal aorta in segment B. The aortic arch is shown in segment C. Note the atherosclerotic lesions around the ostia of the intercostal vessels and over scattered areas of thoracic and abdominal aorta. The aortic arch has extensive atherosclerosis over much of its surface. Adapted from Chobanian [47].

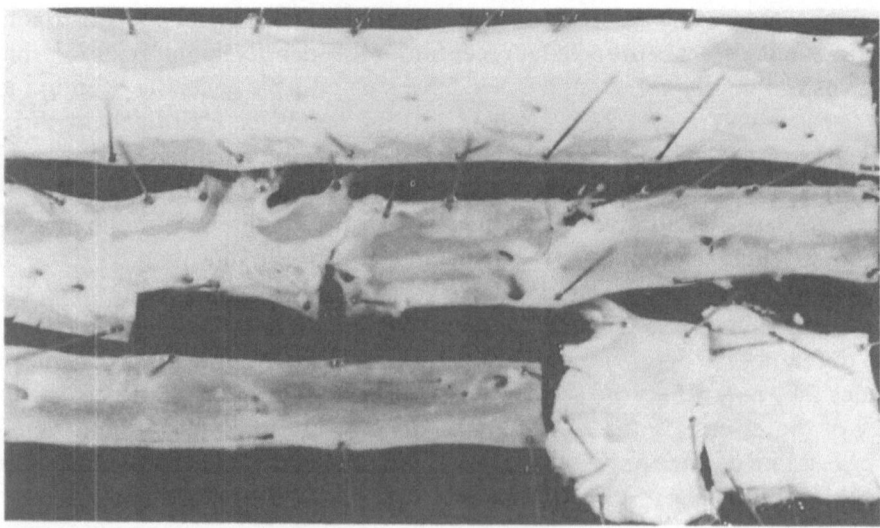

Figure 3. Photograph of the intimal surface of aorta in a 9-month old Watanabe hypercholesterole-mic rabbit which had renovascular surgery performed at three months of age. Systolic blood pressure averaged 146 mmHg. Segments A, B and C represent areas relatively similar to those shown in Figure 2. Note the diffuse distribution of atherosclerosis over most of the aortic surface as well as the massive involvement of the aortic arch. Adapted from Chobanian [47].

changes within the arterial wall. As noted earlier, there is an increase in SMC mass which may be secondary either to an increase in SMC number [18] or an increase in cell size with or without the development of nuclear hyperploidy [19, 20]. SMC hyperploidy involves an increase in cellular DNA content as a result of an apparent failure of cells that have completed mitosis to divide. Why hypertension may promote this process is unknown but the effect has primarily in chronic models of hypertension in the rat. In man, polyploid cells have been noted in the arterial wall and their prevalence may increase with age [21], but the role of hypertension in this regard is uncertain.

Hypertension may stimulate both the migration of SMC from the media to the intima as well as the proliferation of these cells. We have demonstrated increases in intimal SMC in both the deoxycorticosterone-salt (DOC-salt) and the spontaneous models of hypertension in the rat [22]. Aortic explants from both models studied in tissue culture have demonstrated increased rates of SMC proliferation [23, 24]. Intimal SMC accumulation and proliferation are also hallmarks of atherosclerosis and are considered important in lesion development, particularly in the build-up of connective tissue components which are synthesized by these cells.

The stimulus for increased arterial SMC growth in hypertension is unknown. Denudation of the arterial endothelium and platelet aggregation have not been a consistent feature of the models of hypertension that we have studied and it is unlikely that the growth factor for SMC present in platelets is involved. However, with the increased permeability of the arterial wall caused by hypertension, other circulating growth factors might be present in higher concentrations in the intima. Also, since macrophage infiltration into the artery appears to be promoted by increased blood pressure [22], growth factors of macrophage origin [25] could conceivably be involved. Futhermore, vascular endothelial cells and SMC themselves also appear to produce growth factors [26], and the expression of such endogenous substances might perhaps be promoted by hypertension.

The endothelium also can be altered markedly by hypertension. Changes in size and shape of the cells have been observed [27] and as noted above, the increased permeability of the arterial wall in hypertension appears to be secondary to functional alterations in this cell layer. In addition, our studies in rats have indicated that the adherence of white blood cells to the endothelial surface is enhanced by blood pressure elevation [22]. Such adherent cells appear to penetrate into the intima and might contribute to the genesis of the atherosclerotic lesion. The proposed sequence of changes occurring in the arterial wall following blood pressure elevation is shown in Figure 4.

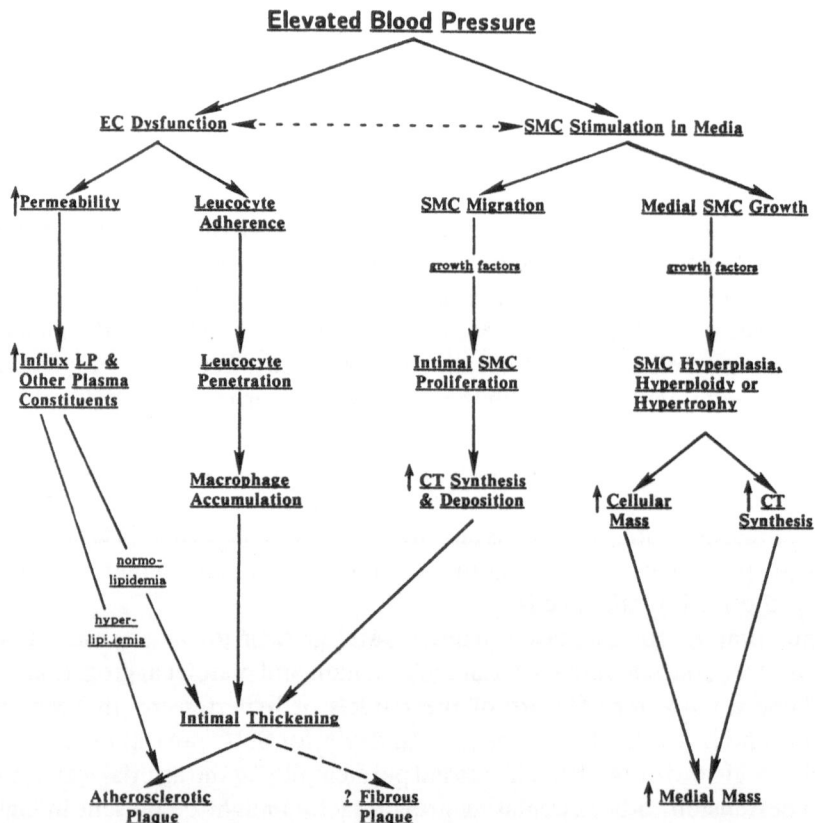

Figure 4. Proposed effects of hypertension on the arterial intima and media. EC, endothelial cell; SMC, smooth muscle cell; CT, connective tissue; and LP, lipoprotein. Adapted from Chobanian [48].

Effects of hypertension on atherogenesis

Marked similarities are present between the effects of hypercholesterolemia and hypertension on the arterial intima. The major differences appear to be related to the presence of endothelial denudation, platelet adherence, lipid accumulation, and atherosclerotic plaque formation with hypercholesterolemia but not with hypertension. Hypertension does not appear to promote the latter changes on its own when plasma lipids and lipoproteins are present in low concentration [11]. However, as we have observed in the Watanabe hypercholesterolemic rabbit and as McGill and co-workers [28] have shown in the cholesterol-fed baboon, increased blood pressure promotes atherogenesis when serum cholesterol is increased.

Hypertension and microvascular changes in the coronary circulation

With cardiac systole, the small intramyocardial vessels are compressed by the contractile muscle. It has been proposed that because of the compression, such arteries are not exposed to high intravascular pressure levels and are thereby protected from the effects of hypertension. However, studies in hypertensive animals and in man by Weiner and Giacomelli [29] have indicated that increased wall thickening and enhanced vascular permeability may be present, similar to the microvascular changes occurring in other organs. Such changes may be of clinical importance as suggested by the studies of Strauer [30], who observed a reduction of coronary reserve and an increase in coronary resistance in hypertensive patients, even when the large coronary arteries are unaffected by disease. How much of the changes are due to structural rather than functional alterations is unclear. The microvascular changes may be particularly relevant clinically when left ventricular hypertrophy is present in the hypertensive individual. This issue is discussed in detail in other sections of this book and will not be considered further here.

Antihypertensive therapy and atherogenesis

The arterial changes induced by hypertension, once established, appear to be difficult to reverse. Our previous studies have indicated that the accumulation of connective tissue components will persist for prolonged periods, even after relatively brief periods of hypertension [9]. In addition, the nuclear polyploidy which develops in rats as a result of hypertension may remain unchanged despite normalization of blood pressure [20].

Considerable interest has developed recently regarding the effects of antihypertensive drugs on the atherosclerotic process. Calcium antagonists and beta adrenergic blockers have been most actively studied in this regard. The vast majority of studies have used the hypercholesterolemic rabbit as the experimental animal model.

The studies with calcium antagonists are based in part on the observations that arterial calcification is increased with age and is accentuated in the presence of atherosclerotic disease. Several agents which have been shown to affect tissue calcium deposition may inhibit atherosclerosis in the rabbit in response to cholesterol feeding. These have included diphosphonates and lanthanum chloride [31, 32]. Nifedipine, verapamil, and diltiazem have been reported to inhibit development of cholesterol-induced atherosclerosis [33–35] although some other studies [36], including one with Watanabe rabbits treated with nifedipine [37], have failed to support a protective action. Calcium antagonists may inhibit SMC growth, both in vitro and in tissue culture [38] as well as in vivo following balloon-catheter-induced endothelial denudation [39]. Calcium antagonists can also influence several aspects of lipid and lipoprotein metabolism in SMC and endothelial cells maintained in tissue culture [40], but the relationship of such actions to atherogenesis is unclear.

Beta blockers are also of interest with respect to possible inhibitory effects on atherogenesis in the cholesterol-fed rabbit model. We and others have shown a marked inhibition of aortic atherosclerosis with propranolol [41, 42] and metoprolol [43]. Our studies have also demonstrated a modest effect with d-propranolol as well as the racemic mixture, suggesting that properties of the drug unrelated to its beta-receptor-blocking action might contribute to the effect. In addition, we have recently observed that the increased arterial permeability induced by cholesterol feeding may be somewhat inhibited with propranolol [44], suggesting the possibility of a membrane-mediated action of the drug. Several interesting in vitro effects of propranolol on lipid metabolism also have been demonstrated, but as with the calcium antagonists, the clinical significance of such actions remains uncertain.

Other antihypertensive drugs, such as reserpine [45] and guanethidine [46], also may retard the development of atherosclerosis in the rabbit. These observations, when combined with the data involving calcium antagonists and beta blockers, suggest that blood pressure lowering itself may be important and may help protect the arterial wall against the injurious effect of hypercholesterolemia.

Acknowledgement

Supported in part by NIH grant HL 18318 (Hypertension NRDC).

References

1. Kannel WB, Sorlie P (1975): Hypertension in Framingham, in: Paul O (ed), *Epidemiology and Control of Hypertension,* p 553 ff. New York: Stratton Intercontinental Medical Books.
2. Society of Actuaries Build and Blood Pressure Study (1959): Chicago, Chicago Society of Actuaries 1: 367.
3. Robertson WB, Strong JP (1968): Atherosclerosis in persons with hypertension and diabetes mellitus. *Lab Invest* 18: 538–551.
4. Bell ET, Clawson BJ (1928): Primary (essential) hypertension: A study of four hundred and twenty cases. *Arch Pathol* 5: 939–1002.
5. Winter MD Jr, Sayre GP, Millikan CH, Barker NW (1958): Relationship of degree of atherosclerosis of internal carotid system in the brain of women to age and coronary atherosclerosis. *Circulation* 18: 7–18.
6. Patel DJ, Vaishnav RN, Gow BS, Kot PA (1984): Hemodynamics. *Ann Rev Physiol* 36: 125–154.

7. Wolinsky H, Glagov (1967): A lamellar unit of aortic medial structure and function in mammals. *Circ Res* 20: 99–111.
8. Chobanian AV (1987): The arterial smooth muscle cell in systemic hypertension. *Am J Cardiol* 60: I-90–98.
9. Brecher P, Chan CT, Franzblau C, Chobanian AV (1978):Effects of hypertension and its reversal on aortic metabolism in the rat. *Circ Res* 43: 561–569.
10. Chobanian AV, Menzoian JO, Shipman J, Heath K, Haudenschild CC (1983): Effects of endothelial denudation and cholesterol feeding on in vivo transport of albumin, glucose, and carotid artery. *Circ Res* 53: 805–814.
11. Chobanian AV, Brecher PI, Haudenschild CC (1986): Effects of hypertension and of anti-hypertensive therapy on atherosclerosis. *Hypertension* 8 (suppl I): I-15–21.
12. Cornhill JF, Roach MR (1976): A quantitative study of the localization of atherosclerotic lesions in the rabbit aorta. *Atherosclerosis* 23: 489–501.
13. Caro CG, Fitz-Gerald JM, Schroter RC (1971): Atheroma and arterial wall shear: Observation, correlation, and proposal of a shear-dependent mass transfer mechanism for atherogenesis. *Proc R Soc Lond (Biol)* 177: 109–159.
14. Montenegro MR, Eggen DA (1968): Topography of atherosclerosis in the coronary arteries. *Lab Invest* 18: 586–593.
15. Seed WA, Fox B (1980): Location of early atheroma in the human coronary arteries, in: Nerem RM, Guyton JR (eds), *Hemodynamics and the Arterial Wall*, p 90 ff. Houston: University of Houston Press.
16. Stary HC (1978): The ultrastructure of nonatherosclerotic intimal thickening in the coronary arteries of primates and in man, in: Nerem RM, Cornhill JF (eds), *The Role of Fluid Mechanisms in Atherogenesis*. Columbus: Ohio State University Press.
17. Chobanian AV, Lichtenstein AH, Nilhake V, Haudenschild CC, Drago R, Nickerson C (1989): Influence of hypertension on aortic atherosclerosis in the Watanabe rabbit. *Hypertension* 14 (in press).
18. Rorive GL, Carlier PJ, Foidart JM (1980): Hyperplasia of rat artery smooth muscle cells associated with development and reversal of renal hypertension. *Clin Sci* 59: 335s–339s.
19. Owens GK, Schwartz SM (1982): Alterations in vascular smooth muscle mass in the spontaneous hypertensive rat: Role in cellular hypertrophy, hyperploidy and hyperplasia. *Circ Res* 51: 280–289.
20. Lichtenstein AH, Brecher P, Chobanian AV (1986): Effects of deoxycorticosterone-salt hypertension on cell ploidy in the rat aorta. *Hypertension* 8 (suppl II): II-50–54.
21. Barrett TB, Sampson P, Owens GK, Schwartz SM, Benditt EP (1983): Polyploid nuclei in human arterial wall smooth muscle cells. *Proc Natl Acad Sci (USA)* 80: 882–885.
22. Haudenschild CC, Prescott MF, Chobanian AV (1980): Effects of hypertension and its reversal on aortic intimal lesions of the rat. *Hypertension* 2: 33–44.
23. Haudenschild CC, Grunwald J, Chobanian AV (1985): Effects of hypertension on migration and proliferation of smooth muscle in culture. *Hypertension* 7 (suppl I): I-101–104.
24. Grunwald J, Chobanian AV, Haudenschild CC (1987): Smooth muscle cell migration and proliferation: Atherogenic mechanisms in hypertension. *Atherosclerosis* 67: 215–222.
25. Nathan CF (1987): Secretory products of macrophages. *J Clin Invest* 79: 319–326.
26. Schwartz SM, Campbell GR, Campbell JH (1986): Replication of smooth muscle cells in vascular disease. *Circ Res* 58: 427–444.
27. Haudenschild CC, Prescott MF, Chobanian AV (1981): Aortic endothelial and subendothelial cells in experimental hypertension and aging. *Hypertension* 3 (suppl I): I-148–153.
28. McGill HC Jr, Carey KD, McMahan CA, Marinez YN, Cooper TE, Mott GE, Schwartz CJ (1985): Effects of two forms of hypertension on atherosclerosis in hyperlipidemic baboon. *Arteriosclerosis* 5: 481–493.

29. Weiner J, Giacomelli F (1982): Hypertension and the coronary artery, in: Kalsner S (ed), *The Coronary Artery,* pp 448–473. New York: Oxford University Press.
30. Strauer B (1984): The coronary circulation in hypertensive heart disease. *Hypertension* 6 (suppl III): III-74–80.
31. Kramsch DM, Aspen AJ, Rozier LJ (1981): Atherosclerosis: Prevention by agents not affecting abnormal levels of blood lipids. *Science* 213: 1511–1512.
32. Kramsch DM, Aspen AJ, Apstein CS (1980): Suppression of experimental atherosclerosis by the Ca^{2+}-antagonist lanthanum. *J Clin Invest* 65: 967–981.
33. Henry PD, Bentley KL (1981): Suppression of atherogenesis in cholesterol-fed rabbit treated with nifedipine. *J Clin Invest* 68: 1366–1369.
34. Rouleau JL, Parmley WW, Stevens J, Wikman-Coffelt J, Sievers R, Mahley RW, Havel RJ (1983): Verapamil suppresses atherosclerosis in cholesterol-fed rabbits. *J Am Coll Cardiol* 1: 1453–1460.
35. Ginsberg R, Davis K, Bristow MR, McKennet K, Kodsi SR, Billingham ME, Schroeder JS (1983): Calcium antagonists suppress atherogenesis in aorta but not in the intramural coronary arteries of cholesterol-fed rabbit. *Lab Invest* 49: 154–158.
36. Stender S, Stender I, Nordestgaard B, Kjeldsen K (1984): No effect of nifedipine on atherogenesis in cholesterol-fed rabbit. *Arteriosclerosis* 4: 389–394.
37. Van Niekerk JLM, Hendriks T, De Boer HHM, Van 't Laar A (1984): Does nifedipine suppress atherogenesis in WHHL rabbits? *Atherosclerosis* 53: 91–98.
38. Nilsson J, Sjolund M, Palmberg L, von Euler AM, Jonzon B, Thyberg J (1985): The calcium antagonist nifedipine inhibits arterial smooth muscle cell proliferation. *Atherosclerosis* 58: 109–122.
39. Handley DA, Van Valen RG, Melden MK, Saunders RN (1986): Suppression of rat carotid lesion development by the calcium channel blocker PN 200–100. *Am J Pathol* 124: 88–93.
40. Chobanian AV (1987): Effects of calcium channel antagonists and other antihypertensive drugs on atherogenesis. *J Hypert* 5: S43–S48.
41. Chobanian AV, Brecher P, Chan C (1985): Effects of propranolol on atherogenesis in the cholesterol-fed rabbit. *Circ Res* 56: 755–762.
42. Whittington-Coleman PJ, Carrier O Jr, Douglas BH (1973): The effects of propranolol on cholesterol-induced atheromatous lesions. *Atherosclerosis* 18: 337–345.
43. Ostlund-Lindqvist AM, Lindqvist P, Brautigam J, Olsson G, Bondgers G, Nordborg C (1988): The effect of metoprolol on diet-induced atherosclerosis in rabbit. *Arteriosclerosis* 8: 40–45.
44. Sasaki K, La Morte WW, Nickerson CJ, Fuller RM, Chobanian AV, Menzoian JO (1987): Inhibition of cholesterol-induced increases in arterial wall permeability by propranolol. *J Surg Res* 43: 565–570.
45. Smith THG, Rossi GV (1962): The effect of reserpine and mecamylamine on experimental atheromatosis in the normotensive and hypertensive rat. *J Pharmacol Exp Ther* 135: 367–373.
46. Whittington-Coleman PJ, Carrier O Jr (1970): Effects of agents altering vascular calcium in experimental atherosclerosis. *Atherosclerosis* 12: 15–24.
47. Chobanian AV (1988): Comparison between the arterial effects of hypertension and hypercholesterolemia and their influence on atherogenesis. *Jap J Hypert* 10: 69–76.
48. Chobanian AV: Recent observations on the role of hypertension in atherogenesis, in: Meyer P, Marche P (eds), *Blood Cells and Arteries in Hypertension and Atherosclerosis.* New York: Raven Press.

25. Clinical trials, coronary insufficiency, and large arteries in hypertension

MICHEL E. SAFAR

Although hypertension is an important cardiovascular risk factor, clinical trials [1–8] have shown that the blood pressure reduction induced by antihypertensive drugs is not followed by an equivalent improvement in the incidence and severity of coronary insufficiency. This fact, one of the hardest to understand in the treatment of hypertension, raises several questions. First, it is possible that the entry criteria in the different therapeutic trials played a role in the incidence of coronary insufficiency in hypertensive patients. Second, coronary ischemia is undoubtedly related to alterations in large coronary arteries. This finding is partly unexpected since it is commonly believed that hypertensive vascular disease is exclusively due to a reduction in the caliber of small arteries, and does not involve modifications of large vessels.

In this review, it will be shown that alteration in the function of large arteries is one of the most common hemodynamic features of patients with hypertension. Such abnormalities could interfere with the interpretation the results of clinical trials, independently of any association with an atherosclerotic process. They might also partly explain the unexpected frequency of coronary ischemic events in patients treated for hypertension.

Clinical trials and coronary insufficiency in hypertension: A reappraisal

It is well accepted that antihypertensive treatment is effective in preventing cardiovascular complications in severe and moderate hypertension. However, several limitations to this general assumption have been demonstrated [1–8]. First, the results of several clinical trials are contradictory with respect to the protection afforded to patients with a diastolic blood pressure of 90 to 94 mmHg. Second, although the reduction in the incidence of stroke is consistent even in mild hypertension, the improvement afforded by primary preven-

M.E. Safar & F. Fouad-Tarazi (eds.), The heart in hypertension.
© 1989 Kluwer Academic Publishers, Dordrecht –

tion has not exceeded 50% in any clinical trial. Third, one of the most important questions in patients with mild hypertension is the effectiveness of treatment in preventing ischemic cardiac disease. Whether antihypertensive drug treatment is effective in preventing myocardial infarction remains unresolved.

The improvement due to drug therapy mainly involves complications related directly to the mechanical effect of the elevated blood pressure such as cerebral hemorrhage, congestive heart failure and abdominal aneurysms [2]. In contrast, the incidence of ischemic vascular accidents, as observed in the coronary and carotido-cerebral circulations, remains elevated despite adequate treatment. The latter observation suggests that alterations of large arteries, considered either as an associated factor (atherosclerosis) or as a consequence of the elevated blood pressure, play an independent role in cardiovascular morbidity and mortality, even in patients adequately treated for hypertension]9–11].

An important question to resolve is the possibility that the choice of diastolic pressure as the criterion for evaluating severity of hypertension in clinical trials has led to the role of large arteries in hypertension being overlooked. According to WHO definitions, sustained hypertension is defined as a systolic pressure above 160 mmHg and/or a diastolic pressure above 95 mmHg, or both [12]. Despite this definition, in most clinical trials [1–8] diastolic blood pressure was the only inclusion criterion used in primary prevention studies. In this review, it will be strongly suggested that this approach may greatly modify interpretation of the results of therapeutic trials, particularly in cases of patients with mild hypertension.

Table 1 illustrates the blood pressure characteristics of hypertensive patients on entry into the Hypertension and Detection Follow-up program [3]. Patients were classified into three subgroups, exclusively on the basis of the level of diastolic blood pressure [13]. In Stratum I, in which the diastolic pressure range lay between 90–104 mmHg, it is clear that systolic and pulse pressures were relatively much more elevated than the diastolic pressure itself, especially in older subjects. Table 1 shows that pulse pressure was quite similar in Stratum I and Stratum III when analyzed in term of absolute values. However, for the level of diastolic pressure, the role of the elevated pulse and systolic pressures in the manometric definition of hypertension is clearly more important in Stratum I than in Stratum III (Table 1). Such an observation raises crucial questions with regard to analysis of the blood pressure curve, as previously described by MacDonald, Milnor and O'Rourke [10, 14, 15].

The blood pressure curve may be divided into two components (Figure 1): a steady component, i.e. mean arterial pressure, which reflects steady flow, and a pulsatile component, i.e. pulse pressure – the difference between systolic and diastolic pressure – which reflects pulsatile flow. Whereas mean arterial pressure is influenced only by cardiac output and vascular resistance, pulse pressure is determined by independent hemodynamic mechanisms such as the pattern of ventricular ejection, the timing of reflected waves and the reduction of arterial compliance and distensibility. Therefore, at any given value of cardiac output and ventricular ejection, blood pressure is influenced by two principal factors: (1) the level of vascular resistance, i.e. the caliber of small arteries, which determines mean arterial pressure, and (2) the level of arterial distensibility and compliance, i.e. the status of large arteries, which determines pulse pressure. Thus, for a given mean arterial pressure and ventricular ejection, individual subjects may have various levels of pulse and systolic pressure, depending on the reduction of arterial compliance and distensibility and consequently on the status of large arteries. Furthermore, in the case of large vessels, another pathophysiological factor, of paramount importance, must be considered: experimental studies have shown that reduced arterial compliance and distensibility do not only produce an increase in systolic pressure but also a decrease in diastolic pressure [16]. Indeed, the level of diastolic pressure is expected to be lower since the reduction in arterial compliance impairs the diastolic perfusion of arterioles.

Table 1. Systolic and pulse pressure according to the level of diastolic pressure in different age ranges, according to the Hypertension Detection Follow-up Program study [13] (with permission of American Heart Association).

Subgroups	Age (years)	Stratum I (90–104 mmHg)		Stratum II (90–114 mmHg)		Stratum III (115 + mmHg)	
		Medication		Medication		Medication	
		Yes	No	Yes	No	Yes	No
Diastolic	30–39	95.0	93.4	102.3	102.6	113.0	116.8
blood	40–49	94.7	94.2	102.9	102.0	113.4	116.7
pressure	50–59	94.1	94.3	103.4	102.9	114.1	113.8
(mmHg)	60–69	94.4	93.8	102.8	102.3	113.4	113.4
Systolic	30–39	139.1	136.8	148.0	148.7	163.6	172.0
blood	40–49	144.0	141.4	156.6	153.2	171.0	176.4
pressure	50–59	149.5	149.1	164.1	163.0	181.6	181.4
(mmHg)	60–69	158.4	158.2	171.0	172.0	189.1	193.3
Pulse	30–39	44.1	43.4	45.7	46.1	56.6	55.2
pressure	40–49	49.3	47.2	52.7	51.1	57.6	59.7
(mmHg)	50–59	55.5	54.8	60.7	60.2	66.5	67.6
	60–69	64.0	64.4	68.2	69.7	75.7	79.9

Note that, at any level of diastolic pressure, a disproportionate increase in systolic pressure is more frequent above than below 50 years, in particular in Stratum I. For the sake of simplicity, only mean values in each population are given.

From these different observations, it is evident that large vessels participate in the mechanisms of elevated blood pressure and it seems likely that the use of diastolic pressure as the exclusive criterion of the severity of hypertension has been prejudicial to the interpretation of therapeutic trials. First, elevated systolic and mean arterial pressures may be associated with a decreased diastolic pressure, and this may lead to exclusion of some hypertensive patients at risk in therapeutic trials. Second, the level of systolic and pulse pressure is not taken into account in the cardiovascular risk, although it is a more important independent factor than diastolic pressure in patients aged over 50 years [17–18]. Third, since systolic pressure is a marker of large vessels changes, the problem of the status of large arteries is often ignored, even though antihypertensive drug treatment has been shown to have little influence on the incidence of ischemic arterial disease, especially in the coronary circulation.

Basis for the demonstration of intrinsic alterations of peripheral large arteries in hypertensive humans

The possibility that the large arteries might be modified in essential hypertension was dismissed for a long time, since only their conduit function was taken into consideration. However, large arteries have also a buffering function related to the visco-elastic properties of the arterial wall [10]. Indeed, they are able to dampen the pulsatile systolic output of the ventricle (Windkessel effect) into a continuous flow at the peripheral level. As shown in Chapter 12 of this book, it is usual to investigate the visco-elastic properties of the vessel wall by evaluating the slope of the pressure-volume relationship within a given artery (Figure 2) [10, 14, 15]. The change in volume divided by the change in pressure (or arterial compliance) represents the slope of the pressure-volume relationship and is used as a quantitative index describing the elasticity of the system. Non invasive models for the determination of arterial compliance and distensibility have been proposed and validated in the literature [10, 14, 15, 19–21] and have been described in other parts of this book (Chapter 12).

Forearm arterial compliance has been evaluated using models derived from the Moens-Korteweg equation (Figure 2) in patients with untreated hypertension, compared with age- and sex-matched normal subjects [23, 24]. In older subjects with isolated systolic hypertension, whereas distensibility and diameter were not significantly different in patients and in controls, arterial compliance was significantly reduced in hypertensives. In patients with sustained systolo-diastolic essential hypertension of middle age, similar results were observed. Thus, it is clear that, in patients with untreated hypertension, the reduction in arterial compliance occurs at the same mean arterial pressure

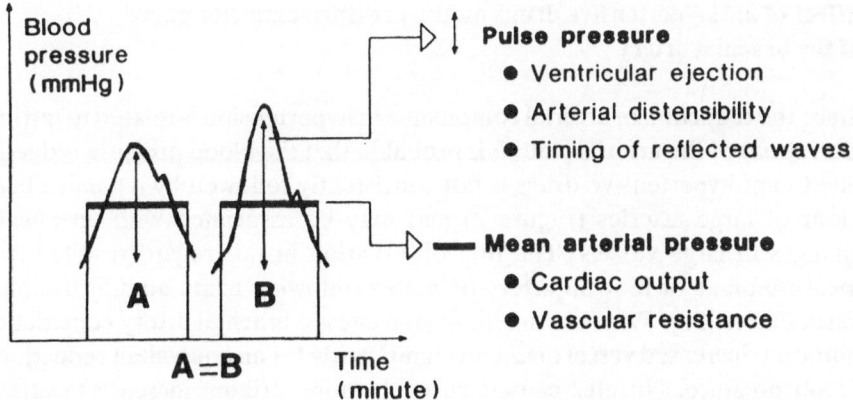

Figure 1. Blood pressure: mean arterial pressure versus pulse pressure (see text). Notice that, for the same mean arterial pressure (i.e. the same surface of the blood pressure curve), two subjects (A and B) may have different values of pulse pressure, depending on ventricular ejection, arterial compliance and timing of reflected waves. The differences in pulse pressure affect not only systolic pressure (which is higher in B than in A) but also diastolic pressure (which is lower in B than in A) when arterial compliance is reduced.

as in controls and therefore reflects intrinsic alterations of the arterial wall [22]. Of course, such alterations may be due either to acceleration of the normal ageing process in the presence of elevated blood pressure, or to a complication of atherosclerosis or to a combination of both factors. Although important, this problem will not be discussed in detail in this review. However, it is clear that, whatever the mechanisms may be, abnormalities of large arteries may play an important role in cardiovascular morbidity and mortality in patients treated for hypertension.

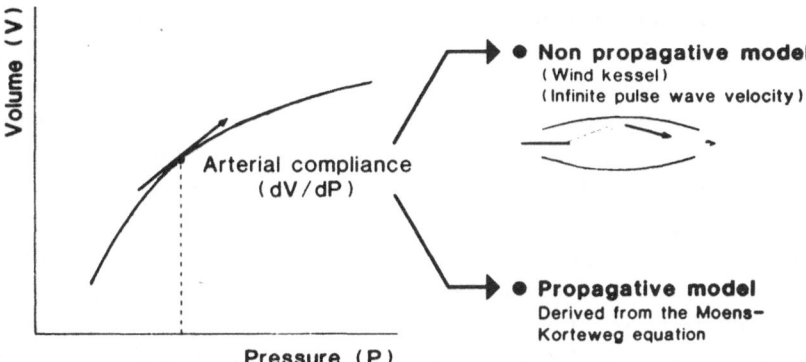

Figure 2. Definition of arterial compliance on the basis of a given pressure-volume (or pressure-diameter) curve. Methods for the determination of arterial compliance are described in Chapter 12. On the right is a schematic representation of the Windkessel effect (see Chapter 12).

Effect of antihypertensive drugs on the pressure-diameter curve
of the brachial artery

Since the reduction of arterial compliance in hypertension is related to intrinsic alterations of the arterial wall, it is probable that the blood pressure reduction due to antihypertensive drugs is not consistently followed by a passive behaviour of large arteries (Figure 2) and may be associated with unexpected changes in large vessels. The first observation in this regard resulted from measurements of brachia artery diameter following acute administration of vasodilators [25]. Whereas dihydralazine caused brachial artery constriction, diltiazem increased vessel diameter significantly for an equivalent reduction in blood pressure. Nitrates caused an even more striking increase in arterial caliber [26].

Studies with antihypertensive drugs have shown that the reduction in blood pressure may be associated with different changes in brachial artery diameter (Figure 3). Such studies are important to consider even if they can be extended with difficulty to the problem of systemic (anti) compliance. Whereas the brachial artery diameter is increased after administration of nitrates [26, 27], converting enzyme inhibitors [27], calcium blockers [25, 27, 28] and some beta-blocking drugs, such as pindolol [29], no significant change was observed following propranolol [29, 30], alpha- and alpha-beta-blocking drugs [31, 32], and some diuretics [33]. Whether the diameter is unchanged or decreased, the results clearly indicate that a shift of the pressure-diameter curve toward lower values of blood pressure occurs following antihypertensive drug treatment (Figure 3). This shift demonstrates that antihypertensive drugs act on the arterial wall independently on the mechanical effect of the blood pressure reduction. The only possible exception to this rule involves dihydralazine and its derivatives which reduce arterial diameter [25, 34].

The concept of unexpected changes in the diameter of large arteries following antihypertensive drug treatment has been further extended to the study of modifications in aortic and brachial arterial compliance and distensibility, i.e. to the changes in the slope of the pressure-diameter curve (Figure 4). Whereas dihydralazine and derivatives [34], propranolol [30], urapidil [31] and possibly diuretics [33] are unable to modify arterial compliance and distensibility, calcium blockers (nifedipine, nicardipine, nitrendipine) [27, 28, 35], nitrate compounds [26, 27, 35], converting enzyme inhibitors (captopril, enalapril) [27, 30] and the alpha-beta blocking drugs labetolol and medroxalol [32, 36] significantly increase it for an equivalent blood pressure reduction [27]. Such changes have been attributed to non-equivalent relaxant effects of the different antihypertensive drugs on the arterial wall [28]. Calcium blockers and converting enzyme inhibitors have been shown to have a more potent relaxant

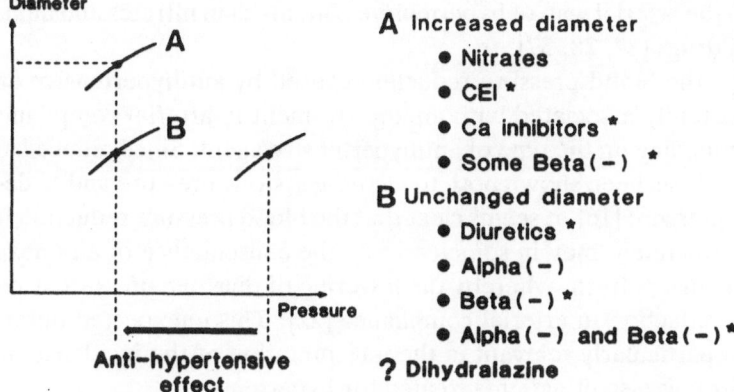

Figure 3. Effect of antihypertensive drugs on brachial artery diameter: practically all antihypertensive agents cause both a blood pressure reduction and a reset of the pressure diameter curve. References for the drugs are indicated in the text.

(* Long term) means that the results have been obtained not only in acute but also in long-term situations. (–) means blocker.

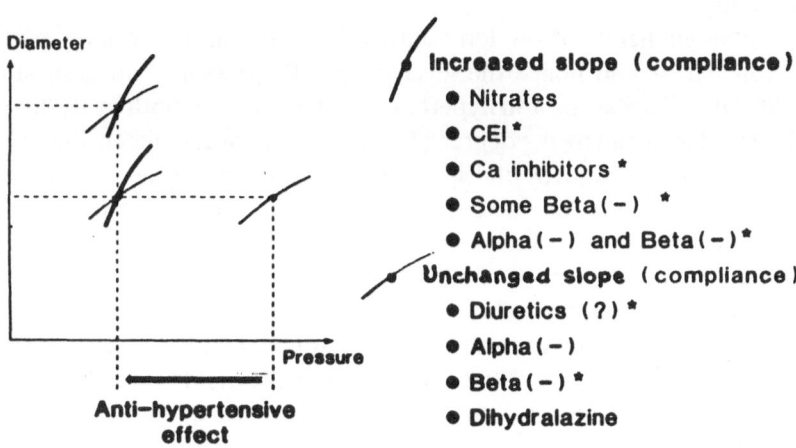

Figure 4. Expected effects of anti-hypertensive drugs on the slope (i.e. arterial compliance) of the pressure-diameter curve. References for the drugs are indicated in the text.

(* Long term) means that the results have been obtained not only in acute but also in long-term situations. (–) means blocker.

effect on the arterial wall of hypertensive patients than nitrates and alpha-beta blocking drugs [27, 28, 37].

Finally, the blood pressure reduction caused by antihypertensive drugs is not consistently associated with an improvement in arterial compliance, the effect depending on the type of antihypertensive agent. Since reduced arterial compliance has been shown both to increase systolic pressure and to decrease diastolic pressure [16], it seems clear that the blood pressure reduction following drug treatment may in some cases be the consequence of an unexpected hemodynamic pattern, whereby the lowering of diastolic pressure is possibly due to a reduction in arterial compliance [22]. This unexpected observation might be particularly relevant in the interpretation of the incidence of coronary artery disease in patients treated for hypertension.

Relevance of the intrinsic alterations of large arteries to the coronary circulation of hypertensive patients

Many factors may contribute to the incidence of coronary insufficiency in patients treated for essential hypertension. In this section, it is emphasized that, independently of the atherosclerotic process, decreased arterial compliance may have deleterious effects on the coronary circulation through modifications in arterial compliance and the oxygen supply-demand ratio of the myocardium.

The metabolic needs of the left ventricle are determined in large part by end-systolic stress and hence the level of systolic pressure and arterial distensibility [10]. Cardiac mass in hypertensives is influenced both by the level of vascular resistance and by the degree of reduction of arterial distensibility [35]. The latter factor acts in favor of disproportionate increase in systolic pressure, and a further increase in end-systolic stress [35]. Thus, decreased aortic distensibility influences in turn the oxygen need of the heart and the myocardial blood requirement, both of which are involved in cardiac hypertrophy and, ultimately, in congestive heart failure.

Metabolic blood supply depends less on systolic than on diastolic pressure, which is the driving pressure of the coronary circulation. At first sight, diastolic pressure seems to be little influenced by the elasticity of large arteries and much more by the caliber of small arteries (see Figure 1). However, animal experiments have shown that decreased arterial compliance causes both an increase in systolic pressure and a decrease in diastolic pressure, and this with practically no change in mean arterial pressure and cardiac output [10, 14–16]. In this regard, it has been shown that, in hypertensive patients, older subjects have a higher systolic pressure and a lower diastolic pessure than younger subjects for the same mean arterial pressure [38]. The same finding has been observed in patients with systolic hypertension and arteriosclerosis obliterans of the lower limbs [24, 35] (Table 2). Since mean blood pressure remains the same, and diastolic pressure is lower when compliance is decreased, coronary driving pressure may then fall, whereas the driving pressure (which is mean arterial pressure) in the other circulations remain maintained. If oxygen requirements remain the same or rise under various circumstances such as the development of cardiac hypertrophy, the supply-demand ratio may be altered [16]. For this reason alone, reduced systemic compliance may be itself detrimental to the heart, and not to the perfusion of other organs. Furthermore, there is an additional possibility that the large arteries may alter the coronary circulation of the hypertensive hypertrophied heart. Under normal conditions, the large epicardial coronary arteries are susceptible to have a significant Windkessel effect [39]. Although this has been poorly investigated in man, blood supply to the endocardium might suffer through this mechanism even when overall coronary blood flow is normal.

It was believed for a long time that only the small coronary arteries were altered in the hypertrophied hypertensive heart, thus causing a decrease in coronary reserve [40]. The present observations suggest that the large coronary arteries may also participate to the functional alterations of the coronary circulation. In this respect, it is important to note that the actions of antihypertensive drugs on peripheral and coronary large arteries are often similar in terms of the modifications in vessel caliber produced [41]. Furthermore, the magnitude of drug-induced vasomotor change on intraluminal diameter is comparable even between normal and stenotic coronary segments. Drugs such as nitrates, which predominantly dilate large coronary arteries, and do not interfere with the metabolic autoregulation of myocardial perfusion, have the

Table 2. Systolic pressure in patients with arteriosclerosis obliterans of the lower limbs [24, 35] (with permission of American Heart Association).

	Normal subjects (n = 18)	Arteriosclerosis obliterans (n = 25)
Age (years)	52 ± 13	54 ± 15
Systolic blood pressure (mmHg)	124 ± 13	148 ± 15***
Diastolic blood pressure (mmHg)	70 ± 4	64 ± 10*
Mean blood pressure (mmHg)	88 ± 9	91 ± 15
Heart rate (b/min)	76 ± 9	67 ± 15*
'Systolic pressure-heart rate' product (arbitrary unit)	9.3 ± 2.9	9.5 ± 2.1

$\pm$ standard deviation.
  * $p < 0.05$.
*** $p < 0.001$.

greatest potential for direct coronary-mediated protection against ischemia [10, 15, 26, 35]. The calcium-channel antagonist drugs such as diltiazem, verapamil and nifedipine cause only slight epicardial dilatation [41]. Drugs such as hydralazine, which dilate only at the arteriolar level and even reduce large artery diameter [25, 41], may improve cardiac performance through a reduction in vascular resistance and afterload reduction but also have the potential to provoke ischemia by enhancing the maldistribution of transmural perfusion observed in coronary occlusive disease.

In conclusion, the present review has emphasized that it is not sufficient to reduce blood pressure in patients treated for hypertension. It is also important to improve the status of the arterial wall. This suggests that hypertensive patients should be treated with compounds which have no adverse effect on the arterial wall, and which even have ancillary properties enabling the status of large arteries to be improved [42]. Obviously, such approaches require new developments in cardiovascular pharmacology in the future.

References

1. Veterans Administration Cooperative Study Group on Antihypertensive Agents (1970): Effects of treatment on morbidity in hypertension, II: Results in patients with diastolic blood pressure averaging 90 through 114 mmHg. *JAMA* 213: 1143–1152.
2. Freis ED (1986): Borderline mild systemic hypertension: Should it be treated? *Am J Cardiol* 58: 642–645.
3. Hypertension Detection and Follow-up Cooperative Group (1979): Five year findings of the hypertension detection and follow-up program, I: Reduction in mortality of persons with high blood pressure, including mild hypertension. *JAMA* 242: 2562–2571.
4. The Multiple Risk Factor Intervention Trial Research Group (1982): Multiple risk factor intervention trial, risk factor changes and mortality results. *JAMA* 248: 1465–1477.
5. The Management Committee (1980): The Australian therapeutic trial in mild hypertension. *Lancet* 1980/1: 1261–1267.
6. Miall WE (1986): The mild hypertension dilemma: results of the British MRC trial. *J Clin Hypertension* 3: 12s–21s.
7. European Working Party on High Blood Pressure in the Elderly (1985): Mortality and morbidity results from European Working Party on High Blood Pressure in Elderly trial. *Lancet* 1985/1: 1349–1354.
8. The IPPPSH Collaborative Group (1985): Cardiovascular risk and risk factors in a randomized trial of treatment based on the beta-blocker Oxprenolol; The international prospective primary prevention study in hypertension (IPPPSH). *J of Hypertension* 3: 379–392.
9. Safar ME (1985): Focus on the large arteries in hypertension. *J Cardiovasc Pharmacol* 7 (suppl 2): S 1–4.
10. O'Rourke MF (1982): *Arterial Function in Health and Disease* pp 14–125. Edinburgh-London-New York: Churchill Livingstone.
11. Epstein FH (1980): In: *Prevention and Treatment of Coronary Disease and Its Implications*, pp 1–11. Amsterdam: Excerpta Medica.
12. The Joint National Committee on Detection, Evaluation and Treatment of High Blood

Pressure (1984): The 1984 report of the Joint National Committee on Detection, Evaluation and Treatment of High Blood Pressure. *Arch Intern Med* 144: 1045–1057.

13. Polk FB, Cutter G, Daugherty RM, Gosch F, Heyden S, Shulman N, Tyroler HA (1983): Hypertension detection and follow up program: Baseline physical examination characteristics of the hypertensive participants. *Hypertension* 5: IV–92.

14. McDonald DA (1974): Arterial impedance, in: *Blood Flow in Arteries*, 2nd ed, p 351. Baltimore: Williams and Wilkins.

15. Milnor WR (1982): *Hemodynamics*, pp 49–134. Baltimore/London: Williams and Wilkins.

16. Randall OS, Van den Bos GC, Westerhof N (1984): Systemic compliance: Does it play a role in the genesis of essential hypertension? *Cardiovasc Res* 18: 455–462.

17. Kannel WB, Dawber TR (1973): Hypertensive cardiovascular disease (The Framingham Study), in: Onesti G, Kim KE, Moyer JH (eds), *Hypertension – Mechanisms and Management*, pp 93–110. New York: Grune and Stratton.

18. Darrè B, Girerd X, Safar M, Cambien F, Guize L (1988): Pulsatile versus steady component of blood pressure. A cross-sectional analysis and a prospective analysis on cardiovascular mortality. *Hypertension* 13: 392–400.

19. Safar ME, Peronneau J, Levenson J, Simon A (1981): Pulsed Doppler: Diameter, velocity and blood flow of brachial artery in sustained essential hypertension. *Circulation* 63: 393–400.

20. Gribbin B, Pickering TG, Sleight P (1979): Arterial distensibility in normal and hypertensive man. *Clin Sci* 56: 413–419.

21. Smulyan H, Vardan S, Griffiths A, Gribbin B (1984): Forearm arterial distensibility in systolic hypertension. *J Am Coll Cardiol* 3: 387–396.

22. Safar ME, Simon ACh (1986): Hemodynamics in systolic hypertension, in: Zanchetti A, Tarazi RC (eds), *Handbook of Hypertension*, Vol 7: *Pathophysiology of Hypertension, Cardiovascular aspects*, pp 225–241. Amsterdam: Elsevier.

23. Safar ME, Simon ACh, Levenson JA (1984): Structural changes of large arteries in sustained essential hypertension. *Hypertension* 6 (suppl III): 117–121.

24. Safar ME, Laurent St, Asmar RE, Safavian A, London GM (1987): Systolic hypertension in patients with arteriosclerosis obliterans of the lower limbs. *Angiology* 38: 287–295.

25. Safar ME, Simon ACh, Levenson JA, Cazor JL (1983): Hemodynamic effects of Diltiazem in hypertension. *Circ Res* 52 (suppl 1): 169–173.

26. Simon ACh, Levenson JA, Levy BY, Bouthier JE, Peronneau PP, Safar ME (1982): Effect of nitroglycerin in peripheral large arteries in hypertension. *Br J Clin Pharm* 14: 241–246.

27. Safar ME, Bouthier JA, Levenson JA, Simon ACh (1983): Peripheral large arteries and the response to antihypertensive treatment. *Hypertension* 5 (suppl III): 63–68.

28. Safar ME, London GM, Asmar RG, Hugues CJ, Laurent SA (1986): An indirect approach for the study of the elastic modulus of the brachial artery in patients with essential hypertension. *Cardiovasc Res* 20: 563–567.

29. Maarek BL, Bouthier JA, Simon ACh, Levenson JA, Safar ME (1986): Comparative effects of propranolol and pindolol on small and large arteries and veins of the forearm circulation in hypertensive man. *J Cardiovasc Pharmacol* 8 (suppl 4): S61–66.

30. Simon ACh, Levenson J, Bouthier JD, Safar ME (1985): Effects of chronic administration of Enalapril and Propranolol on the large arteries in essential hypertension. *J Cardiovasc Pharmacol* 7: 856–861.

31. Levenson JA, Simon AC, Bouthier JC, Benetos A, Safar ME (1984): Post-synaptic Alpha-blockade and brachial artery compliance in essential hypertension. *J of Hypertension* 2: 37–41.

32. Levenson JA, Simon ACh, Benetos A, Achimastos A, Iannascoli F, Safar ME (1986): Vasodilatator effect of a new adrenergic receptor drug, Medroxalol, on hypertensive forearm vessels. *Hypertension* 8: 174–179.

33. Safar ME, Laurent St, Safavian A, Pannier B, Asmar R (1988): Sodium and large arteries in hypertension: Effect of indapamide. *Am J Med* 84 (suppl 1B): 15–19.
34. Bouthier JA, Safar ME, Curien ND, London GM, Levenson JA, Simon ACh (1986): Effect of Cadralazine on brachial artery hemodynamics and forearm venous tone in essential hypertension. *Clin Pharmacol Ther* 39: 82–88.
35. Safar ME, Toto-Moukouo JT, Bouthier JA, Asmar RE, Levenson JA, Simon ACh (1987): Arterial dynamics, cardiac hypertrophy and anti-hypertensive treatment. *Circulation* 75 (suppl I): I 156–161.
36. Pithois Merli IM, Cournot AX, Georges DR, Pappo M, Safar ME (1987): Acute effect of Labetalol on hypertensive brachial artery. *J Clin Hypertension* 3: 479–496.
37. Safar ME, Laurent S, Bouthier JA, London GM (1986): Comparative effects of captopril and isosorbide dinitrate on the arterial wall of hypertensive human brachial arteries. *J Cardiovasc Pharm* 8: 1257–1261.
38. Messerli FH, Glade LB, Dreslinski GR, Dunn FG, Reisin E, McPhee AA, Frohlich E (1981): Hypertension in the elderly: Hemodynamic, fluid volume and endocrine findings. *Clin Sci* 61: 393–395.
39. Eng C, Jentzer JH, Kirk ES (1982): The effects of the coronary capacitance on the interpretation of diastolic pressure flow relationships. *Circ Res* 50: 334–341.
40. Hoffman JIE (1987): A critical view of coronary reserve. *Circulation* 75 (suppl 1): 1–6.
41. Brown BG (1985): Response of normal and diseased epicardial coronary arteries to vasoactive drugs: Quantitative arteriographic studies. *Am J Cardiol* 56: 23E–29E.
42. Safar ME (1988): Therapeutic trials and large arterics in hypertension. *Am Heart J* 115: 702–710.

PART FOUR

Reversion of cardiac hypertrophy

26. Left ventricular hypertrophy and its reversion in hypertension

FETNAT M. FOUAD-TARAZI

In studying the mechanism of cardiac hypertrophy and function in response to an increased load, Meerson [1] suggested that the initial response to increased load is a stage of cardiac hyperfunction which results in an increased activation of nucleic acid and protein synthesis. It was also suggested that this initial phase of 'hyperadaptation' is followed by a stage of 'adaptive' cardiac hypertrophy during which ATP consumption per unit mass decreases and the concentration of high energy phosphate compounds returns to normal. Functionally, the main consequence of the adaptive changes would be to normalize cardiac work [1] by spreading the increased function of the organ to a greater mass, so that the term 'intensity of the functioning of structures' (IFS) was proposed to define the quantity of function generated per unit mass of an organ per unit time [1]. Indeed, indices of systolic cardiac function in hypertension have been reported repeatedly to be generally normal [2–8]. On the other hand, when the stage of nucleic acid activation and protein synthesis was inhibited by administering actinomysin D, animals subjected to acute pressure overload died of heart failure [1].

Despite these seemingly beneficial effects of the hypertrophy process, the Framingham study has reported that the development of left ventricular hypertrophy in hypertensive patients is usually associated with a high incidence of morbidity and mortality [9]. Also, Pfeffer et al. [10] have shown that in the spontaneously hypertensive rat, impairment of cardiac performance occurs as age advances and is associated with dilation of the hypertrophied ventricle. The rate of this transition from a compensated to a decompensated stage of hypertrophy is conceivably different among various hearts and could be related to the mechanisms by which LV functional reserve decreases in the hypertrophied heart following the initial hyperadaptation and adaptation phases. Although these mechanisms have not been fully defined, they could be related to an unbalanced growth of the myocardium relative to its vascular

M.E. Safar & F. Fouad-Tarazi (eds.), The heart in hypertension.
© *1989 Kluwer Academic Publishers, Dordrecht –*

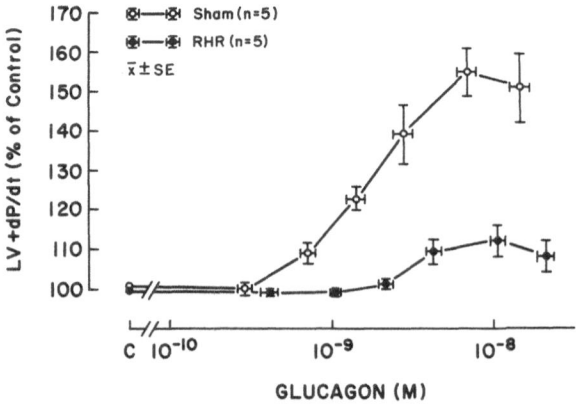

Figure 1. Left ventricular dP/dt – glucagon dose response curve (at perfusion pressure 80 mmHg) in 2 groups of hearts: hypertrophied hearts from renovascular hypertensive rats and age matched sham operated controls. The response was blunted in the hypertrophied hearts. Permission from Fouad et al. [15].

supply, neural support and possibly to alterations in the enzymatic processes related to left ventricular diastolic relaxation or to other cellular changes. In this context, the hypertrophied heart was shown, in the rat model, to respond less effectively to adrenergic beta and alpha agonists [11–14]. Moreover, the inotropic reserve of the hypertensive hypertrophied rat heart was also blunted in response to other stimuli of adenylate cyclase system such as glucagon and the vasoactive intestinal peptide VIP [15]. These changes suggested that at the organ level, the unbalanced growth of the hypertrophied heart has resulted in a much greater increase in the mass of the heart compared to its sympathetic innervation and has resulted in deprivation of the heart from a major positive inotropic support, the adrenergic nervous system. Similarly, at the level of the coronary microcirculation, this unbalanced growth of the heart was shown to be associated with a lag of vascular growth [16] and a reduction of capillary density [17]. Accordingly, the diffusion distances of oxygen is increased and areas of relative hypoxia may develop. Indeed, diffuse fibrotic changes have been frequently described in the subendocardium of hypertrophied ventricles [18] which were attributed to inadequacy of coronary perfusion. Moreover, Zak and Fischman have shown in 1971 [19] that at the cellular level, energy provision for the hypertrophied heart is reduced because of the decrease in the mass of the mitochondria. Also, alterations in the primary structure of myosin has been described in pressure-overloaded hearts with a reduction in alpha heavy chains, HC alpha [20, 21] with associated decrease in muscle shortening velocity [20].

As far as the diastolic function of the heart is concerned, it was demonstrated as early as 1971 by Meerson and co-workers [22, 23], that a decrease in the area of the sarcolemma relative to the cellular mass occurs in compensatory hypertrophy and is associated with similar changes at the level of the sarcoplasmic reticular membrane. In this respect, Chidsey [24] has shown that in the hypertrophied heart of rabbits with induced aortic stenosis, the reduced ability of the sarcoplasmic reticulum to take up the calcium ion, is accompanied by an increase in the amount of calcium ion in the mitochondria at the expense of energy provision and a decrease in ATP synthesis. Along these lines, it was demonstrated that significant depression in several measures of sarcoplasmic reticular function were reported in severe ventricular hypertrophy due to mechanically induced increase in afterload [25–27] or to spontaneous hypertension [28]. As a result, reduction in ion transport mechanism occurs leading to impaired ability of the hypertrophied myocardium to remove calcium from the sarcoplasm and impairment of the relaxation process; this 'incomplete diastole syndrome' may be taken as an initial link in the pathogenetic chain by which ventricular hypertrophy leads to cardiac insufficiency [1].

On the whole, whereas compensatory hypertrophy prevents acute cardiac insufficiency, the unbalanced nature of the hypertrophy process interferes with the structural organization of the heart at multiple levels, and may form the basis for a transition from adapation to chronic insufficiency [1]. Reversal of hypertensive ventricular hypertrophy, therefore, appeared to be desirable. Simple reduction of pressure load, however, did not prove to be always associated with regression of left ventricular hypertrophy. This lack of a strong correlation was shown in both the spontaneously hypertensive rat and in man [29–32]. These results suggested that other factors beside pressure overload play a role in the reversal – and possibly the development – of left ventricular hypertrophy in hypertension. The reversibility of left ventricular hypertrophy in hypertensive humans has been demonstrated by many centers (for review see ref. 33). In general, reduction of left ventricular mass became evident after at least 8–12 weeks of antihypertensive therapy. It is to be noted, however, that regression of left ventricular hypertrophy and its extent varied according to the pharmocological agents used and the interplay of associated modulating factors. Sympatholytics including methyldopa and reserpine were reported to induce significant regression of left ventricular hypertrophy. Converting enzyme inhibititors such as captopril and enalapril, and calcium entry blockers also led to significant reduction of left ventricular mass in the hypertrophied heart of both hypertensive patients and hypertensive experimental animals. Although data regarding the effectiveness of diuretics and of beta blockers were controversial in that respect, more recent studies showed that sustained control of blood pressure may be of importance to achieve regression of left ventricular hypertrophy with these two classes of drugs. Direct arteriolar vasodilators, on the other hand, such as hydralazine and trimazosin failed to reduce left ventricular mass in the hypertensive hypertrophied hearts except when associated with beta blockade or methyldopa therapy. In general, the spectrum of response of ventricular mass to antihypertensive therapy supported the concept that factors other than blood pressure level also influence regression of left ventricular hypertrophy [31].

Concern rose regarding the functional aspect of regression of left ventricular hypertrophy. Since RNA per unit myocardial tissue was shown to decrease [34] while myocardial collagen does not [35], these changes in myocardial composition were thought to carry potentially important implications as regard cardiac performance [36, 37]. In humans, however, most studies reported that left ventricular ejection fraction and frational shortening were unchanged after reduction of left ventricular mass by antihypertensive therapy even when evaluated in relation to changes in left ventricular stress [30, 38]. More studies are needed, however, to assess the ability of a regressed heart to meet sudden overloads induced by exercise or escape from blood pressure control. Efforts to reduce vascular hypertrophy simultaneously [39] may prove to be of marked value in this regard.

In conclusion, the recent interest in the role of the 'heart in hypertension', has enriched our knowledge concerning the mechanisms of cardiac hypertrophy and function in hypertension. Moreover, the methodological advances allowing acurate quantification of left ventricular mass and function have helped expansion of this field of research from animal models to human hypertensive subjects as well as to siblings of hypertensive patients [40]. Their non-invasive nature permitted sequential follow-up of patients during treatment. Thus, data generated from both human and animal studies, led to the identification of a spectrum of cardiac effects of antihypertensive therapy apart from their hemodynamic effects, and opened the way to further investigation regarding the relationship between cardiac and vascular alterations in hypertension.

References

1. Meerson FZ (1983): in Katz AM (ed), *The Failing Heart: Adaptation and Deadaptation,* pp 323. New York: Raven Press.
2. Grossman W, et al. (1964): Cardiac hypertrophy: Useful adaptation or pathologic process? *Am J Med* 14: 133.
3. Pfeffer MA, Pfeffer JM (1983): Cardiac hypertrophy in the spontaneously hypertensive rat: Adaptation or primary myopathy? in: Tarazi RC, Dunbar JB (eds), *Perspectives in Cardiovascular Research,* Vol 8, p 193. New York: Raven Press.
4. Fouad FM, Tarazi RC, Gallagher JH, MacIntyre WJ, Cook SA (1980): Abnormal left ventricular relaxation in hypertensive patients. *Clin Sci* 59: 411s.
5. Inouye I, Massie B, Loge D, Topic N, Silverstein D, Simpson P, Tubau J (1983): Abnormal

left ventricular filling: an early finding in mild to moderate systemic hypertension. *Am J Cardiol* 53: 120.

6. Burger SB, Strauer BE (1981): Left ventricular hypertrophy in chronic pressure load due to spontaneous essential hypertension, I: Left ventricular function, left ventricular geometry, and wall stress, in: Strauer BE (ed), *The Heart in Hypertension,* p 13. Berlin–Heidelberg–New York: Springer Verlag.

7. Karliner JS, Williams D, Gorwit J, Crawford MH, O'Rourke RA (1977): Left ventricular performance in patients with left ventricular hypertrophy due to systemic arterial hypertension. *Br Heart J* 39: 1239.

8. Abi Samra F, Fouad FM, Tarazi RC (1983): Determinance of left ventricular hypertrophy and function in hypertension. *Am J Med* 75 (3A): 16–33.

9. Kannel WB, Gordon T, Offit D (1969): Left ventricular hypertrophy by electrocardiogram: Prevalence, incidence and mortality in the Framingham study. *Ann Intern Med* 71: 89.

10. Pfeffer JM, Pfeffer MA, Fishbein MC, Frohlich ED (1979): Cardiac function and morphology with aging in the spontaneously hypertensive rat. *Am J Physiol* 237: H-461–468.

11. Saragoca M, Tarazi RC (1981): Left ventricular hypertrophy in rats with renovascular hypertension. Alterations in cardiac function and adrenergic response. *Hypertension* 3(6): 782–789.

12. Ayobe HM, Tarazi RC (1983): Beta-receptors and contractile reserve in left ventricular hypertrophy. *Hypertension* 5 (suppl II): II-92–97.

13. Woodcock EA, Johnson CL (1979): Decreased cardiac beta-adrenergic receptors in renal hypertension in the rat. *Circ Res* 45: 560–565.

14. Fouad FM, Shimamatsu K, Hanna MM, Khairallah PA, Tarazi RC (1985): Impaired inotropic responses to alpha-adrenergic stimulation in experimental left ventricular hypertrophy. *Circulation* 71: 1023–1028.

15. Fouad FM, Shimamatsu K, Said SI, Tarazi RC (1986): Inotropic responsiveness in hypertensive left ventricular hypertrophy: Impaired inotropic response to glucagon and vasoactive intestinal peptide in renal hypertensive rats. *J Cardiovasc Pharmacol* 8: 398–405.

16. Wicker P, Vitullo J, Healy B (1988): Coronary reserve in normal and hypertrophied hearts during cardiac maturation and aging. *J Am Coll Cardiol* 11: 190A.

17. Marcus ML, Koyanagi S, Harrison DG, Hiratzka LF, Wright CD, Doty DB, Eastham CL (1983): Abnormalities in coronary circulation secondary to cardiac hypertrophy, in: Tarazi RC, Dunbar JB (eds), *Perspectives in Cardiovascular Research,* Vol 8, p 273. New York: Raven Press.

18. Buchner F (1971): Qualitative morphology of heart failure: Light and electron microscopic characteristics of acute and chronic heart failure (Review). *Methods Achiev Exp Pathol* 5: 20–120.

19. Zak R, Fischman DA (1971): Studies on protein synthesis in heart muscles during development and in experimentally produced hypertrophy, in: Alpert NR (ed), *Cardiac Hypertrophy.* New York: Academic Press.

20. Lompres AM, Schwartz K, d'Albis A, Lacombe G, Van Thiem N, Swynghedauw B (1979): Myosin isoenzyme redistriction in chronic heart overload. *Nature* (London) 282: 105–107.

21. Sen S, Young DR (1986): Role of sodium in modulation of myocardial hypertrophy in renal hypertensive rats. *Hypertension* 8: 918–924.

22. Meerson FZ, Kapelko VI, Nurmatov AA (1971): Physiological evaluation of the capacity of the diastole mechanism. *Acta Cardiol* 26: 547–567.

23. Meerson FZ, Kapelko VI (1975): The significance of the interrelationship between the intensity of the contractile state and the velocity of relaxation in adapting cardiac muscle to function at high work loads. *J Mol Cell Cardiol* 7: 793–806.

24. Chidsey CA (1974): Calcium metabolism in the normal and failing heart, in: Braunwald E (ed), *The Myocardium: Failure and Infarction.* New York: H.P. Publishing.

25. Suko J, Vogel JHK, Chidsey CA (1970): Intracellular calcium and myocardial contractility, 3: Reduced calcium uptake and ATPase of the sarcoplasmic reticular fraction prepared from chronically failing calf hearts. *Circ Res* 27: 235–247.

26. Sordahl LA, McCollum WB, Wood WG, Schwartz A (1973): Mitochondria and sarcoplasmic reticulum function in cardiac hypertrophy and failure. *Am J Physiol* 224: 497–502.

27. Lamers JMJ, Stinis JT (1979): Defective calcium pump in the sarcoplasmic reticulum of the hypertrophied rabbit heart. *Life Science* 24: 2313–2320.

28. Limas CJ, Cohn JN (1977): Defective calcium transport by cardiac sarcoplasmic reticulum in spontaneously hypertensive rats. *Circ Res* 40: 162–169.

29. Tarazi RC (1979): Reversal of cardiac hypertrophy: possibility and clinical implications, in: Robertson JIS, Calwell ADS (eds), *Left Ventricular Hypertrophy in Hypertension,* p 55. London: Academic Press/London: Royal Society of Medicine. Royal Soc of Med Int'l Cong and Symp Series, Vol 9.

30. Tarazi RC, Fouad FM (1985): Reversal of cardiac hypertrophy by medical treatment. *Ann Rev Med* 36: 407–414.

31. Tarazi RC, Sen S, Fouad FM (1982): Regression of myocardial hypertrophy, in: Braunwald E, Mock MB, Watson J (eds), *Congestive Heart Failure: Current Research and Clinical Applications,* pp 151–163. New York: Grune & Stratton.

32. Tarazi RC, Frohlich ED (1987): Is reversal of cardiac hypertrophy a desirable goal of antihypertensive therapy? *Circulation* 75 (suppl I): I–113–117.

33. Fouad-Tarazi FM, Liebson PR (1987): Echocardiographic studies of regression of left ventricular hypertrophy in hypertension. *Hypertension* 9 (suppl II): II–65–68.

34. Rabinowitz M, Zak R (1972): Biochemical and cellular changes in cardiac hypertrophy. *Ann Rev Med* 23: 245.

35. Cutilletta AF (1980): Regression of myocardial hypertrophy, II: RNA synthesis and RNA polymerase activity. *J Mol and Cell Cardiol* 12: 827.

36. Tarazi RC (1977): The heart in hypertension, in: Davis JO, Laragh JH, Selwyn A (eds), *Hypertension: Mechanisms, Diagnosis and Management,* p 135. New York: H.P. Publishing.

37. Tarazi RC, Levy MN (1982): Cardiac responses to increased afterload. State-of-the Art review. *Hypertension* 4 (suppl II): II–8–18.

38. Nakashima Y, Fouad FM, Tarazi RC (1984): Regression of left ventricular hypertrophy from systemic hypertension by enalapril. *Am J Cardiol* 53: 1044–1049.

39. Fouad-Tarazi FM (1987): Structural cardiac and vascular changes in hypertension: response to treatment. *Current Opinion in Cardiology* 2: 782–786.

40. Savage DD, Abbott RD, Padgett S, Anderson SJ, Garrison RJ (1983): Epidemiologic features of left ventricular hypertrophy in normotensive and hypertensive subjects, in: Ter Keurs HEDJ, Schipperheyn JJ (eds), *Cardiac Left Ventricular Hypertrophy,* pp 2–15. Boston – The Hague – Dordrecht – Lancaster: Martinus Nijhoff Publishers (DICM-Series, Vol 33).

27. Regression of cardiac hypertrophy: Experimental animal model
A review

SUBHA SEN

Introduction

Cardiac hypertrophy in hypertension has usually been regarded as a secondary response to increase in pressure load to the heart. Recent studies [1–4], however, have shown that factors other than blood pressure control are responsible for both development and regression of myocardial hypertrophy.

During the past decade, several laboratories have established that during hypertrophy in hypertension, a significant alteration in the myocardial biochemical composition and architecture takes place. As a consequence, a reduced compliance and diminished performance occurs as well. In this article, I have summarized the progress that has been made to date to demonstrate the mechanism of regression of hypertrophy, especially its biochemical changes.

Changes in total protein

Zak et el. [5] have shown that the level of intracellular proteins are determined by a balance between their rates of synthesis and degradation. During the development and regression of hypertrophy, both of these rates can be expected to change. The possible control sites of synthesis and degradation are: (1) cardiac mitochondrial cytochromes that accumulate early after imposition of pressure overload, as a result of an increased rate of synthesis and decreased rate of degradation, and (2) the half-life of myosin heavy chains in the steady state as determined from incorporation kinetics, using leucyl tRNA as a precursor, to be 5–6 days, and (3) the existence of a pool of newly synthesized myofilaments which are not fully incorporated into the core of myofibrils is indicated by the incorporation data.

M.E. Safar & F. Fouad-Tarazi (eds.), The heart in hypertension.
© *1989 Kluwer Academic Publishers, Dordrecht –*

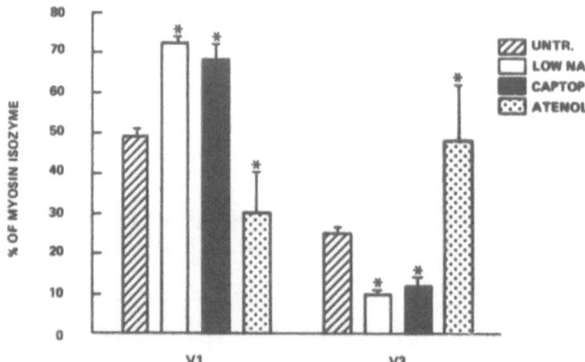

Figure 1. Effect of various treatment on distribution of myosin isozymes in renal hypertensive rats. *p<0.05.

Note: A significant increase in shifting of V_3 to V_1 after captopril and low sodium therapy whereas atenolol increased V_3.

Changes in contractile protein and collagen

The two important protein components of the myocardium which are believed to be responsible for functional consequences to the heart are myosin and collagen. There are suggestive evidences that even a qualitative change with or without a quantitative change in the distribution of these two types of protein may cause a significant alteration in the functional ability of the heart.

Myosin isoforms

Persistence of myocardial hypertrophy has been shown to be associated with a gradual decline in the maximum velocity of cardiac muscle shortening that usually correlates with the decreased calcium ATPase activity of myosin [6]. Recently it has been demonstrated that during persistent cardiac hypertrophy, cardiac myosin isoforms shift from type V_1, a faster migrating type, to type V_3, a form that migrates more slowly [7–9]. Furthermore, it has been demonstrated that the change in myosin isozymes is a result of cellular regulation of myosin biosynthesis depending on two separate genes that code for two types of heavy chains. V_1 and V_3 are the two homodimer phenotypes of the genes, whereas V_2 is the mixed heterodimer phenotypes involving both genes [10–12]. Recently, Sen and Young [13] have shown that in renal hypertensive rats there is a significant shift of myosin isoforms from type V_1 to type V_3, which can be corrected or reversed by either antihypertensive therapy with captopril or sodium deprivation from V_3 to V_1. On the other hand, a treatment with the β-blocker atenolol increases V_3 myosin phenotypes. This observation was confirmed by Dussaule et al. [14]; they demonstrated in two-kidney, one-clip hypertensive rats that treatment with captopril regressed hypertrophy and also showed that up-regulation of myosin isoform from V_3 to V_1 occurs. Sen and Young [15] further continued this study and confirmed the similar shifting of myosin isoform in spontaneously hypertensive rats and demonstrated that type of myosin isozyme distribution pattern can be corrected by either captopril therapy or by sodium deprivation. Dussaule et al. [14] concluded that the cardiac effect most probably relates to normalization of blood pressure in the absence of any stimulation of the sympathetic nervous system. However, data from Sen and Young [15] showed that the changes in myosin isozyme distribution can occur independent of muscle mass and heart rate, blood pressure and sympathetic outflow. Therefore, the factor(s) responsible for signaling of myosin V_1 or V_3 biosynthesis is still not clear.

Change of collagen

Alteration in collagen component of the myocardium also occurs during development of hypertrophy in hypertension. Sen [16] has shown that an increase in rate of collagen synthesis paralleled an increase in content of myocardial collagen in spontaneously hypertensive rats. Not only did the total collagen change but the collagen phenotypes of type III and type V also changed during development of hypertension and hypertrophy. These changes can be corrected by normalization of blood pressure. Recently, Weber et al. [17] demonstrated that in pressure overload hypertrophied myocardium, clinical and experimental evidence indicates that the proportion of collagen relative to muscle is increased. Factors that appear to influence collagen growth during the hypertrophy process include age, species, rapidity with which the overload occurs, the nature of lesion leading to pressure overload and the severity and duration of overload. Morphologically, the heart's collagen matrix consists of a complex weave with tendinous insertions that surround myocytes, grouping them into myofibers, strands of collagen that connect adjoining myofibers, and collagenase struts that join myocytes to other myocytes and capillaries. In a primate preparation [17] of perinephritis with systemic hypertension, it was observed that the tendinous elements of the weave and the strands of collagen lying between the myofibers were increased in number and physical dimension. The functional consequences of a remodeling of collagen matrix that accompanies myocardial hypertrophy remain to be elucidated. A better understanding of the dynamic behavior of collagen matrix may offer new insights into the pathogenesis of ventricular dysfunction that accompanies chronic pressure overloaded state.

Determinants of cardiac hypertrophy in hypertension

Regression of cardiac hypertrophy. We have shown that cardiac hypertrophy in spontaneously hypertensive rats can be prevented or reversed by antihypertensive treatment [18–20]. This has been confirmed by other investigators both in experimental and human subjects [21–23]. One of the significant observations that came out of our laboratory is the diversity among various antihypertensive drugs in regression of myocardial hypertrophy. Despite normalization of blood pressure, all drugs do not regress hypertrophy. α-methyldopa regressed hypertrophy with moderate control of blood pressure, whereas captopril controlled hypertrophy with normalization of blood pressure. On the other hand, vasodilators such as hydralazine and minoxidil both control blood pressure effectively, but hydralazine did not alter myocardial mass, whereas minoxidil actually increased it. This demonstrated a dissociation between regression of hypertrophy and blood pressure control in this model.

The biochemical composition of the myocardium also changes with regression of hypertrophy. We have shown [13, 15] that SHR treated either with captopril or by exposure to low sodium developed a normal myosin isozyme distribution pattern, whereas the restoration in biochemical composition in myocardium did not correlate with the arterial pressure or the myocardial mass, suggesting again that factors other than blood pressure control affects the regression of myocardial hypertrophy or its biochemical composition. The collagen phenotypic pattern also can be restored by proper antihypertensive therapy.

Role of adrenergic system. The suggestion [24] that neurohormonal factors may play an important role in initiating hypertrophy was based not only on the discrepancies observed between blood pressure control and ventricular mass but also on the observation that in experimental conditions there is an increased sympatholytic activity which induces an increase in myocardial mass. We have shown [25] that catecholamines may be involved in initiation and regression of myocardial hypertrophy. A good correlation was observed between levels of catecholamines and cardiac mass both during development and regression of myocardial hypertrophy by using various antihypertensive drugs. Vasodilators like hydralazine and minoxidil, which are known to have an effect on increased sympathetic outflow, increased cardiac hypertrophy or did not regress cardiac hypertrophy, whereas sympatholytic drugs that reduce catecholamines result in a regression of myocardial hypertrophy. Furthermore, we have also shown that treatment with propranolol alone neither reduced myocardial hypertrophy nor lowered blood pressure. Upon addition of a small amount of hydralazine, thereby reducing blood pressure, induced regression of hypertrophy. This study demonstrated that although some degree of blood pressure control is necessary, the involvement of the β-adrenergic system in the reduction of myocardial hypertrophy is an important factor.

During the past decade significant work has been done to evaluate the involvement of adenylate cyclase activity during development and regression of hypertrophy. Kumano and Khairallah [26] have shown that in different models of cardiac hypertrophy the decreased inotropic responsiveness to isoproterenol is associated with different biochemical defects in β-adrenergic receptor responses coupling pathway, and that reversal in function occurs when there is no apparent change in the catalytic subunit of adenylate complex. Upsher and Khairallah [27] have reported that in renal hypertensive rats a significant increase in binding sites of β-adrenergic receptors at acute stages of hypertension and almost normal at the chronic phase. The hypothesis they put forward is that the different models of hypertensive hypertrophy are associated with varying changes in β-adrenergic receptors, suggesting that any consequential changes in myocardial function may be the result of other post-receptor mechanisms.

Local factors

The development and regression of cardiac hypertrophy cannot be fully explained by blood pressure control alone. Studies from our laboratory [28] have shown that a local factor produced by the myocardial cell may be responsible for initiation of hypertrophy in hypertension. We have demonstrated the existence of a factor in the myocardium of spontaneously hypertensive rats that stimulates protein synthesis in type V_1 in vitro. We have shown that it not only increases incorporation of tritiated leucine or ^{14}C phenylalanine on myocyte protein but also increases specific activity of the leucyl tRNA. The factor was found to be present predominantly in the hypertrophied heart and a trace quantity in the normal heart. On the basis of this observation, we hypothesize that the factor(s) responsible for initiation of myocardial hypertrophy reside within the myocardial cell, and when the heart is exposed to stress, in this case hypertension, local factors are released which in turn trigger protein synthesis. However, further studies are necessary to demonstrate the relationship between hypertension and hypertrophy and release of the factors of the myocardium.

We have shown that sodium also can play a modulatory role in alteration of myocardial composition and structure. Lindpaintner and Sen [29] have shown that dietary sodium can play an important role in renal hypertensive rats. Sodium restriction did not reverse hypertension in renal hypertensive rats, but led to a significant reduction in heart weight/body weight ratio in those rats compared to rats on normal diet. The hypertrophied hearts from animals on regular diets show depressed levels of tissue catecholamine, whereas those from animals on sodium-deficient diets showed normal catecholamine. Here we have demonstrated a dissociation of blood pressure on cardiac hypertrophy on two-kidney, one-clip model similar to previous findings in other models like SHR [20, 29]. This study supports the concept that factors other than blood pressure control contribute to the mechanism for development or regression of cardiac hypertrophy. Dietary sodium appears to be one such factor.

Conclusion

The structural cardiovascular responses to hypertension are not homogeneous. Important differences are found in the biochemical composition of the myocardium both during development and regression of hypertrophy. Antihypertensive therapy with various types of drugs with known pharmacologic action showed that normalization of blood pressure by all the drugs does not necessarily demonstrate similar type of changes in the biochemical composition of the heart. Consequently, the functional capability of such hearts may vary according to the composition, whether it consists of high collagen or normal collagen or high V_3 type myosin or nomal V_3. The development or regression of hypertrophy does not depend on mechanical load alone, but seems to be modulated at many levels by (a) increased pressure load, (b) the level of cardioadrenergic system, and (c) local growth factors.

Acknowledgment

I wish to thank David Young and Carolee Petscher for their technical assistance and JoAnne Holl for her skilled typing assistance. Statistical analysis was done by using the PROPHET Computer System which is supported in part by the National Institute of Health, Division of Research Resources. Supported in part by grant HL 27838.

References

1. Sen S, Tarazi RC, Khairallah PA, Bumpus FM (1974): Cardiac hypertrophy in spontaneously hypertensive rats. *Circ Res* 35: 775–781.
2. Sen S, Tarazi RC, Bumpus FM (1976): Biochemical changes associated with development and reversal of cardiac hypertrophy in spontaneously hypertensive rats. *Cardiovasc Res* 10: 254–261.
3. Grant RP (1953): Aspects of cardiac hypertrophy. *Am Heart J* 46: 154–158.
4. Ehrstrom MC (1948): Enlargement of heart in hypertension. *Acta Med Scand* 103 (suppl 206): 86–93.
5. Zak R, Martin AF, Reddy MK, Rabinowitz M (1976): Control of protein balance in hypertrophied cardiac muscle. *Circ Res* 38 (suppl I): I–145–150.
6. Hamrell BB, Low RB (1978): The relationship of mechanical V_{max} to myosin ATPase activity in rabbit and marmot ventricular muscle. *Phlugers Archive* 337: 119–124.
7. Lompre AM, Mercadier JJ, Wisnewsky C, et al. (1981): Species and age-dependent changes in the relative amounts of cardiac myosin isozymes in mammals. *Dev Biol* 84: 286–290.
8. Mercadier JJ, Lompre AM, Wisnewsky C, et al. (1981): Myosin isozymic changes in several models of rat cardiac hypertrophy. *Circ Res* 49: 525–532.
9. Gorza L, Pauletto P, Pessin SC, Sartore S, Schiaffino S (1981): Myosin distribution in normal and pressure overloaded rat ventricular myocardium. *Circ Res* 49: 1003–1009.
10. Sinha AM, Umeda PK, Kavinsky CJ, et al. (1982): Molecular cloning of mRNA sequence for cardiac α and β myosin heavy chains: Expression in ventricles of normal, hypertrophied and thyroxic rabbits. *Proc Soc Natl Acad Sci* (USA): 79: 5847–5851.
11. Mahdavi V, Chambers AP, Nadal-Ginard B (1984): Cardiac α and β myosin heavy chain genes are organized in tandem. *Proc Soc Natl Acad Sci* (USA): 2626–2630.
12. Hoh JFY, Yeoh GPS, Thomas MAW, Higginbottom L (1979): Structural differences in the heavy chains of rat ventricular myosin isozymes. *Febs Let* 97: 330–334.
13. Sen S, Young DR (1986): Role of Na^+ in modulation of myocardial hypertrophy in renal hypertensive rats. *Hypertension* 8: 918–923.
14. Dussaule JC, Michel JB, Auzan C, Schwartz K, Corvol P, Menard J (1986): Effect of antihypertensive treatment on the left ventricular isomyosin profile in one-clip, two-kidney hypertensive rats. *J Pharmacol Exp Ther* 236: 512–518.
15. Sen S, Young DR: Effect of antihypertensive therapy on myosin isozyme distribution pattern in SHR. *Fred Proc* (in press).
16. Sen S (1982): Alteration in myocardial phenotypes in SHR (abstract). *J Moll Cell Cardiol* 14: 60.
17. Weber KT, Janicki JS, Pick R, et al. (1987): Collagen in the hypertrophied, pressure overloaded myocardium. *Circulation* 75: I–40–47.
18. Sen S, Tarazi RC, Bumpus FM (1976): Biochemical changes associated with development and reversal of cardiac hypertrophy in spontaneously hypertensive rats. *Cardiovasc Res* 10: 154–161.
19. Sen S, Tarazi RC, Bumpus FM (1977): Cardiac hypertrophy and antihypertensive therapy. *Cardiovasc Res* 11: 427–433.
20. Sen S (1983): Regression of cardiac hypertrophy: Experimental animal model. *Am J Med* 95: 87–93.
21. Yamori Y, Morichuzo, Nishio T (1979): Cardiac hypertrophy in early hypertension. *Am J Cardiol* 44: 9642–9649.
22. Ishi S, Pegram BL, Frohlich ED (1980): Disparate effects of methyldopa and clonidine on cardiac myocytes and hemodynamics in rats. *Clin Sci* 59: 449s–452s.

23. Tomanek RJ, Davis JR, Anderson SC (1979): The effect of α-methyldopa on cardiac hypertrophy in SHR. *Cardiovasc Res* 13: 172–182.

24. Tarazi RC, Sen S (1979): Catecholamines and cardiac hypertrophy, in: Caldwell ADS (ed), *Catecholamines of the Heart*, pp 47–57. London: Academic Press / London: Royal Society of Medicine (Royal Soc of Med Int'l Cong and Symp Series, Vol 19)

25. Sen S, Tarazi RC (1983): Myocardial catecholamines in ventricular hypertrophy, in Katz A (ed), *Perspectives in Cardiovascular Research*, Vol 8, pp 309–318. New York: Raven Press.

26. Kumano K, Khairallah PA (1985): Adenylate cyclase activity during development and reversal of cardiac hypertrophy. *J Mol Cell Cardiol* 17: 537–548.

27. Upsher MA, Khairallah PA (1985): Beta-adrenergic receptors in rat myocardium during the development and reversal of hypertrophy and following chronic infusions of angiotensin II and epinephrine. *Arch Int Pharmacodyn Ther* 274: 65–79.

28. Sen S, Petscher C, Ratliff NR (1987): A factor that initiates myocardial hypertrophy in hypertension. *Hypertension* 9: 261–267.

29. Lindpaintner K, Sen S (1985): Role of sodium in hypertensive cardiac hypertrophy. *Circ Res* 57: 610–617.

28. Cardiac structure and function after treatment with adrenergic blocking agents

M. MOHSEN IBRAHIM

Introduction

Cardiac hypertrophy and left ventricular dysfunction constitute the main forms of cardiac involvement secondary to elevation of arterial pressure. Impairment of coronary vasodilator reserve and cardiac arrhythmias are also related to hypertension though less well recognized problems. Such changes in cardiac anatomy and funcion in hypertensive patients are not only due to increase in pressure overload but also to other modulating mechanisms. The sympathetic nervous system plays a central role among these mechanisms. Adrenergic blocking agents by both relieving the pressure overload and interfering with sympathetic functions can thus produce important changes in cardiac structure and function. Regression of cardiac hypertrophy, alterations in ventricular systolic and diastolic functions and improvement of coronary vasodilator reserve were all reported following adrenergic blockade therapy [1, 13]. Regression of ischemic changes and left ventricular strain pattern in the electrocardiogram can be demonstrated after the use of many of these drugs [14].

Adrenergic blocking agents were among the first antihypertensive drugs. The list includes central alpha agonists (e.g. alpha-methyl dopa, clonidine, guanfacine, and guanabenz), beta receptor blockers (e.g. propranolol, atenolol, sotalol), alpha receptor blockers (e.g. prazosin), and peripheral neuronal inhibitor agents (e.g. reserpine, guanethidine and bethanidine). Although these drugs share the common effects of reducing arterial pressure and interfering with sympathetic function differences do exist depending upon the type of agent, species and sex. Differences are also present between agents in the same subgroup of drugs.

M.E. Safar & F. Fouad-Tarazi (eds.), The heart in hypertension.
© *1989 Kluwer Academic Publishers, Dordrecht –*

Changes in cardiac structure

Adrenergic mechanisms and cardiac hypertrophy

The early development of structural cardiovascular changes in hypertension is a matter of adaptation to the increased pressure load, although the process may well also be genetically reinforced [15]. A prevailing genetic predisposition and/or trophic influences mediated via sympathetic nerves and beta adrenergic receptors may modulate the hypertrophic response to increase in arterial pressure. Catecholamines were shown to facilitate the incorporation of amino acids into myocardial and vascular proteins [16]. The permissive or aggravating role of adrenergic influences on cardiac hypertrophy was suggested many years ago and is supported by experiments in spontaneous hypertensive rats [17]. Exogenous catecholamines were found to provoke a hypertrophic response, whereas administration of guanethidine did prevent myocardial hypertrophy in rats in response to exercise [18]. Both propranolol and practolol administration have been shown to decrease ventricular weight in the rabbit and implicate the beta adrenergic receptors in hypertrophy. We found a positive correlation between left ventricular mass index and the extent of increase in heart rate after maximal exercise in hypertensive patients [3], however, there was no relationship between urinary catecholamine excretion and left ventricular hypertrophy.

Regression of cardiac hypertrophy

Adrenergic blocking agents induce regression in ventricular mass in experimental animals and treated hypertensive patients. In an early study we examined serial electrocardiographic records of 50 hypertensive patients that were followed for an average period of nine years [2]. Regression in ECG voltage was present in more than half of the patients receiving different antihyperten-

Table 1. Effects of adrenergic blocking agents: Changes in cardiac structure.

1. Anatomic: Regression of hypertrophy
   a) Wall thickness: vent septum and free wall
   b) LV mass
   c) Microscopic changes
2. Biochemical: Myocardial composition
   a) Myosin content
   b) Myosin isozyme distribution
   c) Collagen content

sive agents including adrenergic blocking drugs. Alterations in ECG voltage were thought to reflect regression in left ventricular mass. These early observations were confirmed by a large number of studies using echocardiography [3–7]. Recently we were able to demonstrate that regrssion of cardiac hypertrophy can occur as early as six weeks of atenolol [3] and ten weeks of guanfacine [10] antihypertensive therapy. Wollam et al. [19] found that the decrease in ECG voltage tended to lag behind the echocardiographic indices and did not attain statistical significance until three to six months after blood pressure was controlled. In a short term study of beta adrenergic blockade therapy [3] we found that changes in left ventricular wall thickness involved only the septum with minimal effect on posterior wall and that changes in left ventricular mass index correlated with a decrease in peak systolic stress.

Electron microscopic studies have also indicated that prolonged treatment with adrenergic blocking agents can decrease cell size [20]. In spontaneously hypertensive rats treated with methyldopa for 12 weeks, mean cell area in both subepicardium and subendocardium was significantly decreased when compared with that in untreated spontaneously hypertensive rats. These changes occured without significant reduction in systolic arterial pressure.

Regression of left ventricular hypertrophy correlates with arterial pressure control [4, 5, 21] and reduction in systolic wall stress [3]. Fouad et al. [22], however, reported reversal of left ventricular hypertrophy with methyl dopa without an associated blood pressure control, attributing these changes to a direct effect of sympathetic inhibition. Strauer et al. [23] addressed the question whether an antihypertensive agent lowering plasma catecholamines can induce regression of hypertrophy more effectively than an antihypertensive agent which does not affect or even augments plasma catecholamines. Both prazosin and clonidine induced a significant regression of echocardiographic indices of left ventricular hypertrophy. Patients treated with clonidine showed a somewhat greater reegression of hypertrophy for a given reduction in blood pressure, but the difference was not statistically significant. In six of the eight patients treated wih clonidine plasma catecholamine concentrations markedly dropped with decrease in cardiac hypertrophy, while the remaining two patients did not show any decrease in catecholamine concentrations and had little regression in left ventricular hypertrophy. Whether specific antihypertensive drugs are more effective in producing regression of left ventricular hypertrophy by direct effects or by actual control of blood pressure remains to be determined. In spontaneously hypertensive rats vasodilator therapy – hydralazine and minoxidil – failed to induce regression of cardiac hypertrophy inspite of adequate control of arterial pressure [24]. The varied effects of different drugs on cardiac hypertrophy may be related to several factors including effects on catecholamines, hemodynamic changes, cardiac output, heart rate, reflex sympathetic stimulation and biochemical alterations of cardiac muscle.

Changes in myocardial composition

Antiadrenergic agents have different effects on myocardiac composition of myosin and collagen. Myosin the contractile element of heart muscle exists in three different forms of isozymes: V_1, V_2 and V_3 designated according to their electrophoretic mobility, V_1 being the fastest in an electric field and V_3 the slowest. Isozyme shifts in response to hypertension have been demonstrated in many animal species. The myosin isozyme distribution pattern during development and reversal of hypertension in rats has been studied by Sen [25]. A significant shift of V_1 (high ATPase, high contractile myosin type) to V_3 (low ATPase, slow contractile myosin type) was found after six weeks of persistence of hypertension. The modifications in the patterns of isomyosins during antihypertensive therapy could be due to removal of the overload per se or to a direct effect of the drugs. This latter hypothesis is supported by the recent observations that some antihypertensive drugs are capable of inducing a shift in the pattern of the ventricular isomyosins. Atenolol therapy produced significant increase in V_3 without any change in arterial pressure [25]. Similarly propranolol [26] leads to a shift towards slow isomyosin in experimental rats. Reserpine in combination of hydrochlorthiazide and hydralazine normalized blood pressure and reversed myocardial hypertrophy but did not change myosin isozyme pattern [27].

Collagen is the other important structural component of the myocardium. In the pressure-overloaded, hypertrophied myocardium, clinical and experimental evidence indicates that the proportion of collagen relative to muscle is increased. Collagen is the most abundant and would appear to be the most important of the extracellular structural proteins [28]. In patients with essential or renovascular hypertension, collagen has been found to occupy a larger than normal proportion of the hypertrophied myocardium [28]. Myocardial collagen synthesis may be stimulated by the elevated systolic wall stress of the myocardium. It has been suggested that collagen once formed and extruded into the interstitial space is not accessible to removal [29], however, recent studies proved the reversibility of cardiac collagen tissue. Animal studies showed that the reversibility of collagen depends upon the agent used, duration of therapy, age of animal studied and duration of hypertension before the institution of therapy. Treatment with alpha-methyl dopa and Captopril reversed hypertrophy to the same extent in spontaneously hypertensive rats, but the biochemical profile of the myocardium was quite different. Treatment with alpha-methyl dopa resulted in an increase in collagen, where as treatment with Captopril actually reduced the collagen content of the heart. Sen et al. [30] found that six weeks of therapy with alpha-methyl dopa caused a reversal of hypertrophy in SHRs and an increase in myocardial collagen concentration. Beta adrenergic blocking drugs were found to have similar effects (S. Sen, 1987, personal communication).

Left ventricular function

Systolic function and myocardial contractility

Adrenergic blockade whether central or peripheral can (a) reduce arteriolar tone, (b) interfere with venconstriction and limit venous return, and (c) decrease myocardial contractility and heart rate [31]. Effects on LV systolic function depends on factors such as: type of the drug used, method of administration, duration of therapy, basal contractile state of the left ventricle, extent of reduction in afterload, the degree of sympathetic adrenegeric tone, and alterations in myocardial composition after therapy. Furthermore, the effects of antihypertensive therapy on myocardial contractility are difficult to assess when the traditional tests of ejection performance are used, since reduction in afterload can mask depression in muscle contractility.

Inspite of their inhibitory effect on sympathetic function many of the adrenergic blocking agents had no direct depressant action on myocardial contractility under basal conditions. In the basal resting state the sympathetic adrenergic system has little influence on cardiac performance, therefore, adrenergic blocking drugs will influence cardiac contractility to a very small extent and in the absence of a direct cardiac depressant action it is not surprising that these agents do not have a negative inotropic effect. In most instances reduction of sympathetic drive does not reduce cardiac output specifically in patients with compensated hearts. In conditions where cardiac output decreases following some forms of antiadrenergic therapy, peripheral factors rather than a direct cardiac action are the responsible mechanisms in many cases.

Beta-adrenergic receptor blocking drugs (β-blockers)

The individual β-blockers vary in their potency, duration of action and properties such as cardioselectivity, intrinsic sympathomimetic activity (ISA) and membrane stabilizing activity (MSA), but in general they have a similar antihypertensive effect and they slow the heart rate and tend to reduce the cardiac output, at least in the short term [32]. However, they differ in regard to their effect on cardiac output after long term therapy. The initial observations that long term reduction of arterial pressure with propranolol attributable to chronic lowering of cardiac output with little or no change in peripheral resistance [33] were different from the long term hemodynamic effects of pindolol – a β-blocker with ISA – in patients with hypertension where reduction of arterial blood pressure could be ascribed to a long term lowering of total peripheral resistance whereas the cardiac output remained unchanged [34]. β-blockers without ISA specially propranolol reduce cardiac output. This effect is seen specially when patients are studied under conditions associated with high sympathetic drive to the heart e.g. during muscular exercise. Reybrouck et al. [35] in a chronic study using a cardio selective β-blocker found that maximal exercise heart rate was reduced by 34% and this was compensated by 31% enhancement in stroke index. Consequently cardiac index decreased by only 14% while mean pulmonary artery pressure increased by 20%. It was concluded that the compensatory action of the stroke volume, resulted from the interaction of an increased preload and decreased impedance. In acute studies, however, no change occured in stroke volume although β-blockers produced a significant negative chronotropic effect and an increase in preload.

The mechanisms of reduction in cardiac output after beta-adrenergic blockade therapy are: (1) slowing of the heart rate, (2) depression of myocardial contractility, and (3) reduction in venous filling [36]. Decrease in venous return may be secondary to contraction of blood volume or redistribution of intravascular volume. Reduction in plasma volume may be in part a sequence of a reduction in renin output [37].

When examining their effects on myocardial contractility considerable differences were observed between different β-blockers, it seems that cardioselective drugs or those with ISA may have less cardiac depressant action. We found that reduction in cardiac index following atenolol therapy (a cardioselective β-blocker) in hypertensive patients was due to both cardiac slowing and decrease in stroke volume index [8]. The left ventricular end diastolic volume (EDV) did not change after atenolol treatment despite cardiac slowing. We also found that oral atenolol therapy produced no significant change in the ejection phase indices of myocardial performance viz: fractional shortening, ejection fraction and VCF and it did not depress myocardial contractility. The reduction in stroke volume was probably due to a decrease in venous filling and thus EDV would not increase with cardiac slowing as would be expected if venous return remained unchanged [38]. Redistribution of intravascular volume away from the heart secondary to an increase in venous distensibility that favours a diminution in venous return can cause a fall in stroke volume.

A decrease in venous tone after beta-adrenergic blockade with pindolol has been reported in hypertensive patients [39]. Although myocardial contractility plays a role in systolic pump function changes in venous filling are apparently overriding. Studies in animals have shown that atenolol has no negative inotropic effect [40]. However, acute i.v. studies in man showed a depression of isovolumic indices of myocardial performance in both normal subjects and in patients with coronary artery disease [41]. Ejection phase indices were depressed significantly in coronary patients.

The lack of depressant effect on myocardial contractility in hypertensive patients has significant clinical importance, because a negative inotropic effect is not welcomed in patients with cardiac insufficiency or in borderline impairment of left ventricular function. In another study [42] we gave atenolol to hypertensive patients with cardiomegaly and incipient heart failure. The drug was safe and symptoms of cardiac decompensation improved inspite of beta-adrenergic blockade. However, in patients with coronary artery disease and cardiac decompensation and particularly in conditions when systolic heart function is maintained through increased sympatho-adrenal drive, administration of β-blockers will carry a great risk since withdrawal of adrenergic support can seriously compromise left ventricular function and can lead to pulmonary edema and severe heart failure.

Propranolol, in contrast to atenolol, causes a reduction in the indexes of left ventricular contractility such as peak LV dp/dt max and velocity of fiber shortening. Studies in anesthesized dogs showed that oxprenolol (having ISA) depressed the left ventricular function curve considerably less than propranolol [43]. In both conscious and anesthetized dogs, the contractile force of the left ventricle was slightly augmented by oxprenolol and reduced by propranolol. These dissimilarities could be due both to the ISA displayed by oxypropranolol and to the more marked direct cardiodepressant action of propranolol. Sundberg and Gordin [44] compared the effects of 3 β-blockers with different profiles on left ventricular function in healthy volunteers: pindolol (nonselective with strong ISA), nadolol (nonselective without ISA), and acebutolol (cardioselective with weak ISA). Unlike the other β-blockers pindolol did not depress left ventricular function at rest, while during exercise all 3 β-blockers had equal adverse effects.

The effect of beta-adrenergic blocking drugs on cardiac contractility cannot be explained simply in terms of establishment of beta-adrenoceptor blockade and the associated withdrawal of sympathetic support. The mechanisms whereby these drugs alter cardiac contractility are complex. It has been shown [45, 46] that at least some of the β-blockers interact with the plasma membrane in such a way that its capacity to store calcium ions for subsequent release is impaired and also reduce the capacity of the sarcoplasmic reticulum to accumulate calcium ions for subsequent release, hence, less calcium ions is made available for contraction. Furthermore, there are recent evidences that β-blockers can alter the myosin isozyme distribution pattern in hypertensive rats. Sen et al. [25] found that β-blockers even without lowering blood pressure resulted in a shift of V_1 to V_3. It has been demonstrated that the V_3 type of myosin is associated with a reduction in myocardial contractility and V_1 is associated with increased contractility of the heart [47, 48].

Central alpha-adrenergic agonists

Methyldopa, clinidine, guanfacine and guanabenz are the prototypes of centrally acting antihypertensive drugs which are known to act primarily via alpha-adrenergic receptors in the brain. Tiamenidine, lofexidine, and azepexol are experimental compounds with a similar mode of action, but their therapeutic values have not been established in detail [49]. The central mechanisms of reserpine probably involve the stimulation of central alpha-adrenergic receptors by endogenous norepinephrine released from presynoptic storage sites, however, its major hypotensive mechanism is the depletion of norepinephrine from peripheral storage sites in postganglionic sympathetic nerve endings.

Central inhibition of sympathetic tone has important hemodynamic and pathophysiological consequences. Blood pressure lowering is brought about by reduction in peripheral vascular resistance and cardiac output without significant reflex increases in heart rate. Blood flow to vital organs is maintained. Attenuation of effect may occur as a result of volume expansion. Central alpha-adrenergic agonists differ, however, regarding their predominant effect whether on cardiac output or on peripheral resistance. Methyl dopa apparently lowers arterial pressure by reducing vascular resistance rather than by lowering cardiac output [50]. Clonidine, on the other hand, reduces blood pressure through reduction in cardiac output with no change in peripheral vascular resistance [51]. The hemodynamic effects will vary, however, depending on individual conditions before treatment and on physiological reactions to treatment. In patients on long term methyldopa therapy cardiac index may also be reduced [52]. The reduction in cardiac output following clonidine therapy was partly due to bradycardia, a direct cardiac depressant action was not observed in heart lung preparations except with very high doses [53]. Hemodynamic measurements after both acute and chronic treatment with guanfacine showed that the cardiac output remained unchanged, the calculated total peripheral resistance decreased, and the stroke volume increased.

Sympatholytic therapy may influence cardiac contractility in hypertensive patients. Studies on cardiac performance, assessed by simultaneous echo,-phono-, and electrocardiography, revealed no functional depression after guanabenz at single oral doses as high as 16 mg [54]. No significant changes was reported in left ventricular stroke volume, cardiac output or ejection fraction with either methyldopa or guanabenz after one and six months of therapy [55]. We examined the effects of guanfacine on myocardial contractility [10]. Since reduction in afterload can mask depression in muscle contractility we used the left ventricular end-systolic stress-end systolic dimension relation which is highly sensitive to contractile state as it incorporates afterload and is independ-

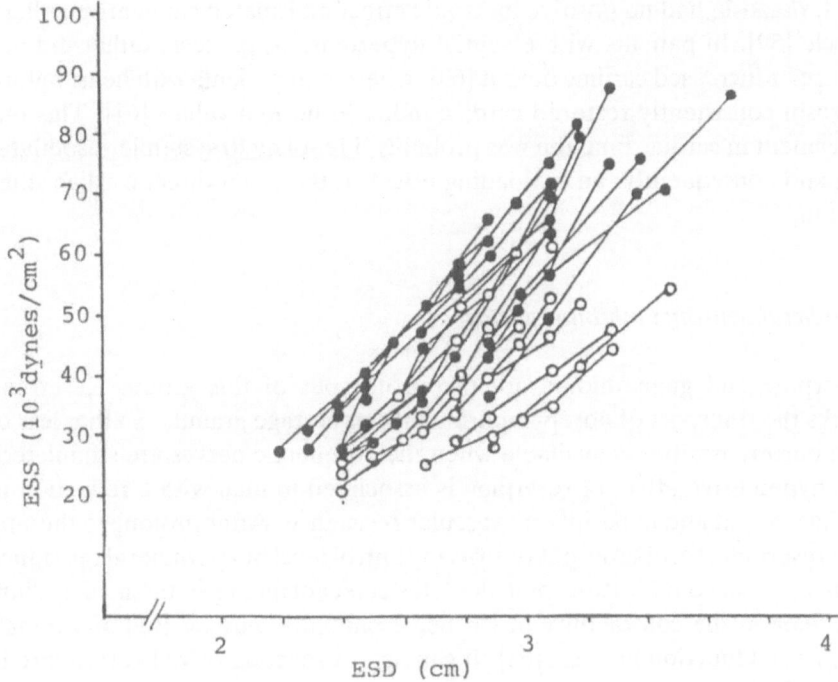

*Figure 1.*End-systolic stress-dimension relation (ESS-ESD) for 14 hypertensive patients before (closed circles) and after guanfacine therapy (open circles). Each line represents an individual patient. The slope (E max) dit not change after treatment.

ent of preload. The slope of this relation (E max) can be used to determine contractile performance under the influence of antihypertensive therapy. The E max did not change significantly after guanfacine therapy (Fig. 1). We concluded that reduction in central sympathetic nerve activity by guanfacine given in therapeutic hypotensive doses does not depress myocardial contractility in hypertensive patients.

Alpha-adrenergic receptor blockers

Prazosin is an alpha-adrenergic blocking agent which leaves prejunctional alpha receptors at the sympathetic nerve terminals unblocked and the feedback regulation of neurotransmitters intact. It produces sustained reduction in blood pressure through direct arteriolar and venous dilatation without reflex increase in heart rate, renin release, or a vasoreceptor mediated compensatory rise in cardiac output [56, 57]. The myocardial contractility as measured by left ventricular dp/dt max was increased by prazosin in dogs [58]. On the other hand, prazosin had no positive inotropic effect on isolated cat heart papillary muscle [59]. In patients with essential hypertension, prazosin either did not change or increased cardiac output [60], whereas in patients with heart failure prazosin consistently restored cardiac index to normal values [61]. This improvement in cardiac function was probably due solely to systemic vasodilatation and consequently, an 'unloading effect' rather than direct cardiac stimulation.

Peripheral neuronal inhibitor agents

Reserpine and guanethidine are the prototypes of this group. Reserpine blocks the transport of norepinephrine into its storage granules so that less of the neurotransmitter is available when the adrenergic nerves are stimulated. The hypotensive effect of reserpine is associated in man with a reduction in cardiac output and in peripheral vascular resistance. After prolonged therapy with reserpine, cardiac output returns to control level but peripheral resistance remains reduced [62]. Reserpine depletes catecholamines in the myocardium and depress the contractility of cat heart papillary muscles [63] and impair myocardial function in dogs. [64]. It can aggravate congestive heart failure in man [65].

Guanethidine depletes the reserve pool of the neurotransmitter and decreasing the amount released when the nerve is stimulated. Myocardial catecholamine stores are partially depleted which is presumably responsible for a decrease in heart rate, stroke volume and cardiac output, contributing to the hypotensive action of the drug. In long-term therapy cardiac output was not lowered in either the recumbent or the standing position and systemic vascular resistance and heart rate were reduced [66].

Diastolic function and left ventricular filling

Abnormalities in diastolic function and left ventricular filling occur very early in hypertensive patients before impairment in systolic function and they are more severe in patients with left ventricular hypertrophy. Possible explanations include increased chamber stiffness due to left ventricular hypertrophy without changes in muscle properties and impaired left ventricular compliance due to either myocardial diastolic dysfunction or fibrosis [67, 68]. Furthermore, experimental studies showed that relaxation is delayed with increased afterload [69] and that filling is greatly influenced by relaxation [70]. These abnormalities in left ventricular diastolic function are reflected clinically in shortness of breath and congestive lung symptoms in the presence of normal systolic function and without heart failure, the development of left atrial enlargement, auricular fibrillation and atrial arrhythmias. The ability to reverse these abnormalities might be a beneficial attribute for any therapeutic agent.

The effects of β-adenoceptor blocking drugs on left ventricular diastolic function have been reported in a number of studies. Fouad et al. [11] described an improvement in left ventricular diastolic filling in the subset of hypertensive patients whose pressure was controlled by β-blockers (metoprolol or nadolol), although there were no significant changes in the treatment group as a whole. On the other hand, Inouye et al. [71] did not find any significant changes in the diastolic filling indexes during short-term propranolol therapy inspite of significant reduction in blood pressure. We recently examined the effects of Sotalol (a noncardioselective, β-blocker devoid of ISA or membrane stabilizing effects) therapy on diastolic function and left ventricular mass. We found that Sotalol can reverse diastolic filling abnormalities and that improvement was not related to a decrease in left ventricular mass [12]. The favourable effect of β-blockade therapy seemed to be attenuated in patients with regression in left ventricular hypertrophy. A possible explanation is that the thick ventricles secondary to pressure overload contain more collagen that normal and regression of hypertrophy would leave behind increased concentration of collagen. This will result in increased muscle stiffness and reduced diastolic compliance. Improvement in diastolic function seen in treated patients is possibly an indirect effect of antihypertensive action of Sotalol. Reduced afterload could, by restoring oxygen supply/demand balance and augmenting adenosine triphosphate supply, enhance relaxation [72]. Fouad et al. [11] found that patients who had remained hypertensive inspite of β-blockade therapy had slowing in their filling rate and filling fraction. A reduction in heart rate is associated with a decreased peak filling rate, thus any tendency of β-blockade therapy to improve left ventricular filling might be counterbalanced by the reduced heart rate. Furthermore, β-blockers may also impair relaxation facilitated by catecholamines.

References

1. Poblete PF, Kyle MC, Pipberger HV, Freis ED (1973): Effect of treatment on morbidity in hypertension. Veterans Administration Cooperative Study on Antihypertensive Agents: Effect on the electrocardiogram. *Circulation* 48: 481–490.
2. Ibrahim MM, Tarazi RC, Dustan HP, Gifford RW (1977): Electrocardiogram in evaluation of resistance to antihypertensive therapy. *Archives on Internal Medicine* 137: 1125–1129.
3. Ibrahim MM, Madkour MA, Mossallam R (1981): Factors influencing cardiac hypertrophy in hypertensive patients. *Clinical Science* 61: 1055–1085.
4. Sonotani N, Kubo S, Nishioka A, Takatsu T (1981): Electrocardiographic and echocar-

diographic changes after one to two-years treatment of hypertension: Analysis of voltages ($SV_1 + RV_5$), wall thickness, cavity, mass, and hemodynamics of the left ventricle. *Japanese Heart J* 22: 325–333.

5. Corea L, Bentivoglio M, Verdecchia P (1981): Reversal of left ventricular hypertrophy in essential hypertension by early and long-term treaatment with methyldopa. *Clinical Trials J* 18: 380–394.

6. Drayer JIM, Gardin JM, Weber MA, Aronow WS (1982): Changes in cardiac anatomy and function during therapy with alpha-methyldopa: An echocardiographic study. *Current Therapeutic Research* 32: 856–865.

7. Rowlands DB, Ireland MA, Glover DR, McLeay RAB, Stolland TJ, Littler WA (1981): The relationship between ambulatory blood pressure and echocardiographically assessed left ventricular hypertrophy. *Clinical Science* 61: 1015–1035.

8. Ibrahim MM Madkour MA, Mossallam R (1980): Effect of atenolol on left ventricular function in hypertensive patients. *Circulation* 62: 1036–1046.

9. Ibrahim MM, Madkour MA (1983): Effect of cardiac hypertrophy on left ventricular performance in hypertensive patients. *J Hypertension* 1: 275s–277s.

10. Ibrahim MM, Emile H, Madkour MA, Said GE (1985): Contractile performance following regression of left ventricular hypertrophy in hypertensive patients. *J Hypertension* 3: 461s–463s.

11. Fouad FM, Slominski MJ, Tarazi RC, Gallagher JH (1983): Alterations in left ventricular filling with beta-adrenergic blockade. *Am J Cardiol* 51: 161–164.

12. Ibrahim MM, Zaghloul SS, Helmi SM (1987): Effect of regression of left ventricular hypertrophy on diastolic function in hypertensive patients. *J Hypertension* 5: 411s.

13. Strauer BE (1980): *Hypertensive Heart Disease,* pp 84–85. Berlin-Heidelberg-New York: Springer Verlag.

14. Frohlich ED (1983): The heart in hypertension, in Generst J, Kuchel O, Hamet P, Cantin M (eds), *Hypertension, Physiopathology and Treatment,* 2nd edn, pp 791–810. New York: McGraw-Hill.

15. Folkow B (1982): Physiological aspects of primary hypertension. *Physiologic Rev* 62: 347–504.

16. Kallfelt BJ, Hjalmareson AC, Isaksson OG (1976): In vitro effects of catecholamines on protein synthesis in perfused rat heart. *J Molec & Cellular Cardiol* 8: 787–802.

17. Sen S, Tarazi RC, Kharallah PA, Bumpus FM (1974): Cardiac hypertrophy in spontaneously hypertensive rats. *Circulation Research* 35: 775–781.

18. Schwartz A (1971): Studies on mitochondria from normal, hypertrophied and falling myocardium, in: Albert NR (ed), *Cardiac Hypertrophy,* pp 522–536. New York: Academic Press.

19. Wollam GL, Hall WD, Porter VD, Douglas MB, Unger DJ, Blumenstein BA, Cotsonis GA, Knudtson ML, Felner JM, Schlant RC (1983): Time course of regression of left ventricular hypertrophy in treated hypertensive patients. American Journal of Medicine, *Proceedings of a Symposium: Left Ventricular Hypertrophy in Essential Hypertension,* pp 100–110.

20. Tamanek RJ, Davis JW, Anderson SC (1979): The effects of alpha methyldopa on cardiac hypertrophy in spontaneously hypertensive rats: Ultrastructural, sterological, and morphometric analysis. *Cardiovascular Research* 13: 173–182.

21. Rowlands DB, Glover DR, Ireland MA (1982): Assessment of left ventricular mass and its response to antihypertensive treatment. *Lancet* 1982/2: 467–470.

22. Fouad FM, Nakashima Y, Tarazi RC, Salcedo EE (1982): Reversal of left ventricular hypertrophy in hypertensive patients treated with methyldopa. Lack of association with blood pressure control. *Am J Cardiol* 49: 795–801.

23. Strauer BE, Bayer F, Brecht HM, Motz W (1985): The influence of sympathetic nervous activity on regression of cardiac hypertrophy. *J Hypertension* 3: 39s–44s.

24. Sen S, Tarazi RC, Bumpus FM (1977): Cardiac hypertrophy and antihypertensive therapy. *Cardiovascular Research*, 11: 427–433.
25. Sen S (1987): Factors regulating myocardial hypertrophy in hypertension. *Circulation* 75 (suppl I): I 81–84.
26. Pauletto P, Dalla Libera L, Vescovo G (1985): Propranolol induced changes in ventricular isomyosin composition in the rat. *Am Heart J* 109: 1269–1273.
27. Laura IK, Sen S (1984): Myosin isozyme distribution pattern and cardiac performance following antihypertensive therapy in spontaneously hypertensive rats (abstract). *Federation Proceedings* 43: 650.
28. Weber KT, Janicki JS, Pick R, Abrahams C, Shroff SG, Bashey RI, Chen RM (1987): Collagen in the hypertrophied, pressure-overloaded myocardium. *Circulation* 75 (suppl I): I 40–47.
29. Cutiletta AF, Dowell RT, Rudrick M, Archilla RA, Zak R (1979): Regression of myocardial hypertrophy (1). *J Molec & Cellular Cardiol* 7: 761–780.
30. Sen S (1983): Regression of cardiac hypertrophy. Experimental animal model. American Journal of Medicine, *Proceedings of a Symposium: Left Ventricular Hypertrophy in Essential Hypertension*, pp 87–93.
31. Tarazi RC (1978): Hemodynamic effect of aldomet, in Maxwell MH (ed), *Aldomet in the Management of Hypertension*, pp 73–75. West Point, Pa: Merck Sharp and Dohme.
32. Ulrych M, Frohlich ED, Dustan HP, Page IH (1968): Immediate hemodynamic effects of beta adrenergic blockade with propranolol in normotensive and hypertensive man. *Circulation* 37: 411–416.
33. Tarazi RC, Dustan HP (1972): Beta-adrenergic blockade in hypertension, practical and theoretical implications of long-term hemodynamic variations. *Am J Cardiol* 29: 633–640.
34. Hansson L (1986): Hemodynamics of metoprolol and pindolol in systemic hypertension with particular reference to reversal of structural vascular changes. *Am J Cardiol* 57: 29c–32c.
35. Reybrouck T, Amery A, Billiet L (1977): Hemodynamic response to graded exercise after chronic beta-adrenergic blockade. *J Applied Physiol* 42: 133–138.
36. Krauss XH, Schalekamp MADH, Kolsters G, Zaad GA, Birkhenhager WH (1972): Effects of chronic beta-adrenergic blockade on systemic and renal hemodynamic responses to hyperosmotic saline in hypertensive patients. *Clinical Science* 43: 385–391.
37. Julius S, Pascual AV, Abbrecht PT, London R (1972): Effect of beta-adrenergic blockade on plasma volume in human subjects. *Proceedings of the Society for Experimental Biology and Medicine* 140: 982–985.
38. DeMaria AN, Newmann A, Schubart PJ, Lee G, Mason DT (1979): Systemic correlation of cardiac chamber size and ventricular performance determined with echocardioggraphy and alterations in heart rate in normal persons. *Am J Cardiol* 43: 1–10.
39. Atterhog JH, Duner H, Pernow B (1976): Experience with pindolol, a beta receptor blocker, in treatment of hypertension. *Am J Medicine* 60: 872–880.
40. Hary JD, Knapp MF, Linden RJ (1974): The actions of a new beta-adrenergic blocking drug, ICI 66082, on the rabbit papillary muscle and on the dog heart. *Br J Pharmacol* 51: 169–174.
41. Lichtlen P, Amende I, Simon R, Engel JH, Hundeshagen H (1977): Left ventricular function and regional myocardial blood flow after atenolol in normals and patients with coronary artery disease. *Postgraduate Medical J* 53 (suppl 3): 85–93.
42. Ibrahim MM, Mossallam R (1981): Clinical evaluation of atenolol in hypertensive patients. *Circulation* 64: 368–374.
43. Nayler WG, McInnes I, Carson V, Swann J, Low TE (1969): The combined effect of atropine and B-adrenergic receptor antagonists on left ventricular function and coronary blood flow. *Am Heart J* 77: 246–258.
44. Sundberg S, Gordin A (1986): Influence of beta blockade and intrinsic sympathomimetic

activity on hemodynamics, inotropy and respiration at rest and during exercise. *Am J Cardiol* 57: 1394–1399.

45. Nayle WG (1970): The effect of beta-adrenergic blocking drugs on myocardial function; an explanation at the subcellular level. *Postgraduate Medical J* 46 (suppl): 90–96.

46. Scales B, McIntosh DAD (1968): Effect of propranolol and its optical isomers on the radio calcium uptake and the adenosine triphosphatase of skeletal and cardiac sarcoplasmic reticulum fractions (SRF). *J Pharmacol Exper Therapeutics* 160: 261–270.

47. Lompre A, Schwartz K, d'Aglis A, La Combe G, Thiem NU, Swyngedauis B (1979): Myosin isoenzyme redistribution in chronic heart overload. *Nature* 282: 105–112.

48. Mercadier JJ, Lompre C, Wisnewsky JL, Samuel J, Bervovici B, Swyngedauis B (1981): *Circulation Research* 49: 525–532.

49. Van Zwieten PA, Theolen MJC, Timmermans PMW (1984): The hypotensive activity and side effects of methyldopa, clonidine, and guanfacine. *Hypertension* 6 (suppl II): II 28–33.

50. Onesti G, Brest AN, Novack P, Kasparian H, Moyer JH (1964): Pharmacodynamic effects of alpha-methyldopa in hypertensive subjects. *Am Heart J* 67: 32–38.

51. Constantine JW, McShane WK (1968): Analysis of cardiovascular effects of 2-(2,6-dichlorophenylamine)-2-imidazoline hydrochloride (Catapres). *Europ J Pharmacol* 4: 109–123.

52. Lund-Johansen P (1972): Hemmodynamic changes in long term α-methyldopa therapy of essential hypertension. *Acta Med Scand* 192: 221–226.

53. Hoefke W (1980): Clonidine, in Scriabine A (ed), *Pharmacology of Antihypertensive Drugs*, pp 55–61. New York: Raven Press.

54. Shah RS, Walker BR, Vanov SK, Helfant RH (1976): Guanabenz effects on blood pressure and noninvasive parameters of cardiac performance in patients with hypertension. *Clin Pharmacol & Therap* 19: 732–737.

55. Walker BR, Shah RS, Ramanathan KB, Vanov SK, Helfant RH (1977): Guanabenz and methyldopa on hypertension and cardiac performance. *Clin Pharmacol & Therap* 22: 868–874.

56. Lund-Johansen P (1975): Hemodynamic changes at rest and during exercise in long-term prazosin therapy for essential hypertension. *Postgraduate Medicine* 58 (suppl): 45–52.

57. Stokes GS, Oates HF (1978): Prazosin: New alpha-adrenergic blocking agent in treatment of hypertension. *Cardiovasc Med* 3: 41–57.

58. Scriabine A (1980): Prazosin, in Scriabine A (ed), *Pharmacology of Antihypertensive Drugs*, pp 153. New York: Raven Press.

59. Riggs K, Mason DT, Lee G (1978): Direct inotropic effects of the afterload reducing agents, hydralazine and prazosin, evaluated in isolated cat papillary muscle preparation. *Am J Cardiol* 41: 366.

60. Koshy MC, Mickley D, Bourgoignie J, Blaufox MD (1977): Physiologic evaluation of a new antihypertensive agent: Prazosin HCl. *Circulation* 55: 533–537.

61. Mehta J, Iacona M, Feldman RL, Pepine CJ, Conti CR (1978): Comparative hemodynamic effects of intravenous nitroprusside and oral prazosin in refractory heart failure. *Am J Cardiol* 41: 925–930.

62. Kisin I, Yazhakov S (1976): Effects of reserpine, guanethidine and methyldopa on cardiac output and its distribution. *Europ J Pharmacol* 35: 253–260.

63. Lee WC, Shideman FE (1959): Role of myocardial catecholamines in cardiac contractility. *Science* 129: 967–968.

64. Wileken DEL, Brender RD, Shorey CD, McDonald GJ (1967): Reserpine: Effect on structure of heart muscle. *Science* 157: 1332–1334.

65. Braunwald E, Chidsey CA, Harrison DC, Gaffney TE, Kahler RI (1963): Studies on the function of the adrenergic nerve endings in the heart. *Circulation* 28: 958–969.

66. Chamberlain DA, Howard J (1964): Guanethidine and methyldopa: A hemodynamic study. *Br Heart J* 26: 528–536.
67. Gaasch WH, Levine HJ, Quinones MA, Alexander JK (1976): Left ventricular compliance: mechanisms and clinical implications. *Am J Cardiol* 38: 645–653.
68. Grossman W, McLaurin L (1976): Diastolic properties of the left ventricle. *Ann Internal Med* 84: 316–326.
69. Brutsaert DL, Housmans PR, Goethals MA (1980): Dual control of relaxation: Its role in the ventricular function in the mammalian heart. *Circulation Research* 47: 637–652.
70. Fioretti R, Brower R, Geert T, Meester T, Serruys P (1980): Interaction of left ventricular filling and filling during early diastole in human subjects. *Am J Cardiol* 46: 197–203.
71. Innouye IK, Massie BM, Loge D, Simpson P, Tubau JF (1984): Failure of antihypertensive therapy with diuretic, betablocking and calcium channel-blocking drugs to consistently reverse left ventricular diastolic filling abnormalities. *Am J Cardiol* 53: 1583–1587.
72. Shigakawa M, Dougherty JP, Katz AM (1978): Reaction mechanism of calcium dependent ATP hydrolysis by skeletal muscle sarcoplasmic reticulum in the absence of added alkali salts. *J Biological Chemistry* 253: 1442–1450.

29. Cardiac structure and function after vasodilating drugs (dihydralazine-minoxidil)

M. HANI AYOBE

The last decade had witnessed the comeback of hydralazine and the introduction of minoxidil into clinical practice. Both drugs are potent direct-acting arterial vasodilators, and have been used to treat patients with essential hypertension resistant to other drugs, and also to some extent in the treatment of congestive heart failure [1–3]. However, the clinical improvement on hydralazine and minoxidil is only temporary and cannot be maintained for long periods of time without some form of adjunctive therapy. The drop in blood pressure and vascular resistance induced by hydralazine and minoxidil is offset by a compensatory increase in cardiac output initiated by reflex sympathetic stimulation, high levels of circulating catecholamines, activated renin-angiotensin system and volume expansion [3, 4].

The excessive load imposed upon the heart by the operation of such compensatory mechanisms may contribute to the poor cardiac response to hydralazine and minoxidil therapy and may account for the failure or reversal or even exacerbation of hypertension-induced cardiac lesions [5].

The alterations in cardiac structure and function induced by hydralazine and minoxidil that may limit the favourable value of such important drugs are analyzed and evaluated in this discussion.

Effects on cardiac hypertrophy in experimental and clinical hypertension

Since the cardiac hypertrophy develops as a corollary to the stress imposed on the heart, reversal of hypertensive hypertrophy is therefore dependent on removal of the stressful stimulus by blood pressure reduction. However, discrepancies between control of hypertension and regression of hypertrophy were reported by Tarazi in both man and animals [6, 7]. The ventricular weight of spontaneously hypertensive rats (SHR) showed a widely divergent response

M.E. Safar & F. Fouad-Tarazi (eds.), The heart in hypertension.
© 1989 Kluwer Academic Publishers, Dordrecht –

to methyldopa, hydralazine and minoxidil although all three had adequately controlled the blood pressure. Only methyldopa reduced ventricular weight, although its degree of control of hypertension was probably not as good as that obtained with hydralazine and minoxidil. On the other hand, hydralazine had no effect on left ventricular (LV) weight while minoxidil even increased it further [8, 9].

Similarly, human studies revealed the same difference among various anti-hypertensive agents as regards their effect on cardiac hypertrophy. Hydralazine was ineffective in regression of hypertrophy while sympatholytics such as methyldopa and reserpine were associated with significant regression of LV hypertrophy [7, 10].

The dissociation between the hypotensive effect of hydralazine and minoxidil and their effects on cardiac hypertrophy suggests that hemodynamic, neuro-humoral or other factors may interfere with the regression of hypertrophy expected from reduction of pressure load alone [11]. Cardio-adrenergic stimulation may play an important role in that regard since the combination of hydralazine or minoxidil with a sympatholytic or a beta blocker was effective in regressing cardiac hypertrophy both clinically in hypertensive patients [7] and experimentally in SHR [9, 12].

Effects on cardiac catecholamines and relation to cardiac hypertrophy

According to Tarazi and his collaborators, cardiac catecholamines may have a special role in the development of cardiac hypertrophy of hypertension. Also such adrenergic factors seem to play an important role in modulating the response of cardiac hypertrophy to blood pressure reduction. The regression of cardiac hypertrophy was only obtained with antihypertensive therapy whenever ventricular catecholamines were reduced. Hydralazine which controlled blood pressure but did not reduce ventricular catecholamines or even increased its level, did not reverse hypertrophy; while its combination with reserpine or with propranolol, which controlled blood pressure and reduced ventricular catecholamine concentration, reversed hypertrophy [12, 13].

Effects on biochemical composition of hypertrophied myocardium

Biochemical alterations in hypertrophied myocardium of hypertensive rats treated with antihypertensive drugs reflect the effects of such agents on cardiac hypertrophy. With hydralazine, which dit not regress cardiac hypertrophy, the biochemical profile that accompany regression of myocardial hypertrophy was not seen, and the hypertrophy-related abnormalities persisted in the form of reduced DNA concentration and increased content and concentration of RNA and hydroxyproline. On the other hand, with minoxidil treatment which increased cardiac hypertrophy, the biochemical profile obtained was that of more hypertrophic changes with a significant increase in RNA and hydroxyproline concentrations [14]. Since collagen formation and by inference deposition of fibrous tissue are evaluated from changes in ventricular hydroxyproline, the hypertrophied myocardium associated with hydralazine or minoxidil therapy contain more collagen than normal and may influence the functional capacity of the heart [15]. Interference with hydroxyproline synthesis was reported to interfere with some, but not all, aspects of papillary muscle contractility [16].

Minoxidil-induced cardiac hypertrophy

In a recent study the induction of cardiac hypertrophy has been demonstrated in normotensive Sprague-Dawley rats given minoxidil (80 mg Litre^{-1} drinking water) for 4 weeks [17]. This minoxidil-induced cardiac hypertrophy was not prevented either by treatment with 6-hydroxydopamine (100 mg/kg, i.v., two injections with one week apart) or by prior bilateral adrenalectomy. Moreover, minoxidil-induced hypertrophy was not only confined to the left ventricle, but was generalized to the whole heart including atria, right ventricle as well as left ventricle (Table 1). This generalized hypertrophy was not simply due to retention of a higher water content in the hypertrophied myocardium since the dry weight/wet weight ratio of the different cardiac chambers was unchanged by minoxidil treatment [17, 18].

Hence, minoxidil-induced cardiac hypertrophy represents a peculiar model of generalized hypertrophy which is completely dissociated from hypertension and free from LV pressure overload, and contrary to our expectations was independent on catecholamines secreted by cardiac sympathetic nerves or released from the adrenal medulla. Although it is difficult to speculate for its

*Table 1.*Effects of minoxidil treatment on weights of whole heart and chambers (expressed as percent increase) in sham-operated, adrenalectomized and 6-hydroxydopamine-treated rats.

Experimental group	Percent increase in cardiac weight/body weight			
	Atria	Right ventricle	Left ventricle	Whole heart
Sham-operated	24*	26**	19**	20**
Adrenalectomized	42**	36**	12**	19**
6-hydroxydopamine	22**	16**	18**	16**

* p < 0.05; ** p < 0.01.

mechanism, yet it could be related to cardiac effects of prolonged minoxidil therapy such as excessive hemodynamic load [19] and myocardial ischemia [20].

Alterations in myocardial beta adrenoceptors

Hypertension has been shown to diminish the inotropic responsiveness to beta adrenergic stimulation, probably due to the associated reduction in the numbers of LV beta adrenoceptors reported in most animal models of hypertension [21]. Control of renovascular hypertension by nephrectomy of the ischemic kidney or by treatment with captopril which led to regression of cardiac hypertrophy 6 weeks from the start of treatment, was effective in improving the inotropic responsiveness to beta agonist stimulation and return of ventricular beta adrenoceptordensity toward normal [22]. On the other hand, control of hypertension by hydralazine or minoxidil, which did not regress cardiac hypertrophy, had failed to reverse the changes in myocardial beta adrenoceptors in SHR, and the receptor numbers remained similar to those of untreated SHR [23, 24].

The cardiac hypertrophy induced in normotensive Sprague-Dawly rats treated for a month with minoxidil ($80\,mg\;Litre^{-1}$ drinking water) was investigated by us for changes in myocardial beta adrenoceptors by binding to ^3H-dihydroalprenolol [17]. The results obtained have clearly shown that minoxidil had a significant effect in lowering the receptor concentrations in the hypertrophied left ventricles without change in the dissociation constant or in the number of total receptor sites (Table 2). A similar, but unexpected, fall in the receptor concentrations was also found in the hypertrophied LV of adrena-

*Table 2.*Effects of minoxidil treatment on beta-adrenoceptors in the left ventricles of sham-operated and adrenalectomized rats.

	Sham-operated		Adrenalectomized	
	Control	Minoxidil	Control	Minoxidil
Receptor density (fmol/mg protein)	29 ± 1.5	21.9 ± 1.6**	29.4 ± 1.7	23.9 ± 1.7*
Total receptor recovery (pmol/LV)	1.7 ± 0.1	1.7 ± 0.1	2.2 ± 0.2	1.9 ± 0.2
Dissociation constant (nM)	2.1 ± 0.3	3.1 ± 0.6	2.8 ± 0.2	2.9 ± 0.2

Values are means ± one standard error; * $p < 0.05$; ** $p < 0.01$.

lectomized rats maintained on saline while receiving the same minoxidil treatment (Table 2). These results suggest that the effects of minoxidil on myocardial beta adrenoceptors are not dependent on circulating catecholamines of adrencortical hormones. The basis of alterations in myocardial beta adrenoceptors in minoxidil-treated rats, might be attributed to the hypertrophic process *per se*. This could arise from the diluting effect of new myocardial tissue which changes the cell size and imposes a different surface-volume relationship, with consequent decrease in the number of receptors per unit area of cell membrane [17, 25].

Effects on coronary blood flow and cardiac lesions

According to Tarazi, the influence of antihypertensive agents on coronary blood flow depends on their effects on the balance between the afterload, the degree of LV hypertrophy and the driving head of pressure for coronary circulation [26]. Observations in patients with hypertensive heart disease have shown that hydralazine-induced afterload reduction and the associated fall in myocardial oxygen demands may help relieve coronary insufficiency and reduce anginal pains [26, 27]. However, experimental studies have shown that reduction in arterial blood pressure without change in LV mass was associated with a reduction in coronary vascular reserve [28]. Thus coronary flow reserve could be seriously altered by hydralazine and minoxidil therapy, which normalizes blood pressure but not the LV mass [6], and this may account for angina pectoris and other adverse cardiac effects reported in patients treated with hydralazine [29], or minoxidil [20].

Such disturbing symptoms of coronary insufficiency, could be accounted for by severe myocardial hypoxia induced by the tachycardia and the excessive hemodynamic effects of the drugs, and can be controlled by adequate beta adrenergic blockade or sympatholytic drugs [5, 20]. The severe hypoxia may also contribute to the drug-induced cardiomyopathy and/or myocardial necrosis reported in certain animal species, although not documented in man [30].

In conclusion, this discussion has presented considerable evidence for the cardiac effects of hydralazine and minoxidil. Of particular importance in this respect is failure of regression or even augmentation of hypertrophy and its functional consequences on contractility and responsiveness specially to adrenergic stimulation.

Moreover, since cardiac hypertrophy has been recently related to hypertrophy in resistance vessels [31], the possible relationship between the structural responses of the heart and of the vessels to antihypertensive therapy, and its functional and clinical implications could be of great importance.

Acknowledgements

The author gratefully acknowledge the help and cooperation of Dr. Fetnat M. Fouad, Cleveland Clinic Ohio. Also the efforts of Dr. Nagui Salama (Ciba-Geigy) and Dr. Kadria Al-Said (Upjohn), Cairo Scientific Offices, are appreciated.

References

1. Koch-Weser J (1978): The comeback of hydralazine. *Am Heart J* 95: 1–3.
2. Levine TB (1985): Role of vasodilators in the treatment of congestive heart failure. *Am J Cardiol* 55: 32A–35A.
3. Linas SL, Nies AS (1981): Minoxidil. *Ann Intern Med* 94: 61–65.
4. Markham RV Jr, Gilmore A, Pettinger WA, Brater DC, Corbett JR, Firth BG (1983): Central and regional hemodynamic effects and neurohumoral consequences of minoxidil in severe congestive heart failure and comparison to hydralazine and nitroprusside. *Am J Cardiol* 52: 774–781.
5. Fouad FM, Tarazi RC (1983): Cardiac factors in response to antihypertensive treatment. *Hypertension* 5 (suppl III): III 43–48.
6. Tarazi RC (1983): Regression of left ventricular hypertrophy by medical treatment: Present status and possible implications. *Am J Med* 26: 80–86.
7. Tarazi RC, Fouad FM (1985): Reversal of cardiac hypertrophy by medical treatment. *Ann Rev Med* 36: 407–414.
8. Sen S, Tarazi RC, Khairallah PA, Bumpus FM (1974): Cardiac hypertrophy in spontaneously hypertensive rats. *Circ Res* 35: 775–781.
9. Sen S, Tarazi RC, Bumpus FM (1977): Cardiac hypertrophy and antihypertensive therapy. *Cardiovasc Res* 11: 427–433.
10. Tarazi RC, Fouad FM (1984): Reversal of cardiac hypertrophy in man. *Hypertension* 6 (suppl III): III 140–146.
11. Tarazi RC, Sen S, Saragoca M, Khairallah P (1982): The multifactorial role of catecholamines in hypertensive cardiac hypertrophy. *Europ Heart J* 3 (suppl A): 103–110.
12. Tarazi RC, Sen S (1979): Catecholamines and cardiac hypertrophy, in Mezey KC, Caldwell ADS (eds), *Catecholamines and the Heart,* pp 57–67. London: Academic Press/London: Royal Society of Medicine (Royal Society of Medicine International Congress and Symposium Series No 8).
13. Sen S, Tarazi RC (1983): Regression of myocardial hypertrophy and influence of adrenergic system. *Am J Physiol* 244: H 97–101.
14. Sen S, Tarazi RC, Khairallah PA, Bumpus FM (1976): Cardiac hypertrophy and its reversal by antihypertensive drugs in spontaneously hypertensive rats (SHR). *Clin Exp Pharmacol Physiol* 3 (suppl): 173–177.
15. Sen S (1983): Regression of cardiac hypertrophy. *Am J Med* 26: 87–93.
16. Bing LHL, Fanburg BL, Brooks WW, Matsushita S (1978): The effect of the lathyrogen beta-aminopropionitrile (BAPN) on the mechanical properties of experimentally hypertrophied rat cardiac muscle. *Circ Res* 43: 632–637.
17. Ayobe MH, Bennett C, Tarazi RC, Khairallah PA (1984): Minoxidil-induced cardiac hypertrophy: Relation to adrenergic stimulation and effect on LV beta-receptors (abstract). *Fed Proc* 43: 3080.

18. Tarazi RC, Ayobe MH, Bennet C, Khairallah PA (1986): Minoxidil-induced cardiac hypertrophy in 6-hydroxydopamine-treated rats and in adrenalectomized rats. *Under publication*.
19. Tarazi RC, Ferrario CM, Dustan HP (1977): The heart in hypertension, in Genest J, Koiw E, Kuchol O (eds). *Hypertension, Physiopathology and Treatment*, pp 738–754. New York: McGraw-Hill.
20. Gilmore EG, Weil J, Chidsey C (11970): Treatment of essential hypertension with a new vasodilatr in combination with beta-adrenergic blockade. *New Engl J Med* 282: 521–537.
21. Ayobe MH, Tarazi RC (1983): Beta-receptors and contractile reserve in left ventricular hypertrophy (LVH), *Hypertension* 5 (suppl I): I 192–197.
22. Ayobe MH, Tarazi RC (1984): Reversal of changes in myocardial beta-receptors and inotropic responsiveness with regression of cardiac hypertrophy in renal hypertensive rats (RHR). *Circ Res* 54: 125–135.
23. Chatelain P, Waelbroeck M, Camus JC, De Neff P. Robberecht P, Roba J, Christophe J (1981): Comparative effects of α-*methyldopa*, propranolol and hydralazine therappy on cardiac adenylate cyclase activity in normal and spontaneously hypertensive rats. *Europ J Pharmacol* 72: 17–25.
24. Hanna MK, Engelmann GL, Gerrity RG, Khairallah PA (1985) Myocardial adrenergic receptors in long term antihypertensive therapy (abstract). *Fed Proc* 44: 1646.
25. Ayobe MH, Tarazi RC (1986): Alterations in myocardial beta adrenoceptor in minoxdil-induced cardiac hypertrophy. *Under publication*.
26. Tarazi RC, Levy MN (1982): Cardiac response to increased afterload. *Hypertension* 4 (suppl II) : II 8–18.
27. Strauer BE (1980): *Hypertensive Heart Disease*. New York: Springer Verlag.
28. Wicker P, Tarazi RC, Kobayashi K (1983): Coronary blood flow with reversal of cardiac hypertrophy. *Am J Cardiol* 51: 1744–1749.
29. Moyer JH (1953): Hydralazine (Apresoline) hydrochloride: Pharmacological observations and clinical results in the therapy of hypertension. *AMA Arch Intern Med* 91: 419–439.
30. Sobota JTT, Martin WB, Carlson RG, Feenstra ES (1980): Minoxidil: Right atrial cardiac pathology in animals and in man. *Circulation* 62: 376–387.
31. Sano T, Tarazi RC (1987): Differential structural responses of small resistance vessels to antihypertensive therapy. *Circulation* 75: 618–626.

30. The effect of converting enzyme inhibitors on the hemodynamic profile of hypertension

ROBERT J. CODY

Introduction

No class of drugs in the last decade has had as great an impact on the therapy of hypertension as the angiotensin converting enzyme inhibitors. In the course of a decade, since the use of oral converting enzyme inhibitors, a large amount of information has been generated to clearly profile this class of drugs. The hemodynamics of these drugs have been the subject of previous reviews [1–4], and will not be treated extensively here. The main purpose of this review is to summarize the salient features of the hemodynamic effects of converting enzyme inhibitors in terms of central and peripheral hemodynamics, and to discuss the long-term therapeutic implications of these drugs and the likely impact of newer converting enzyme inhibitors.

The hemodynamic profile of hypertensive patients

The hemodynamics of hypertension can be rather complex, depending on whether one evaluates animal models of hypertension, or studies patients with hypertension. The hemodynamics of human hypertension can also be complex depending on several factors. These include age, duration and severity of hypertension, and whether the hypertensive population under study consists of essential hypertension, or subsets of less common hypertension, such as renal vascular disease or endocrine etiologies. Isolated systolic hypertension will not be discussed in this context, as this typically is a further subset of disease, attributable to either degenerative changes in the arterial system, or labile hypertension. For the most part, an increase of blood pressure is due to an increase of peripheral resistance. Ventricular remodelling and adaptive changes of cardiac output may have additional impact on the hemodynamics of

M.E. Safar & F. Fouad-Tarazi (eds.), The heart in hypertension.
© *1989 Kluwer Academic Publishers, Dordrecht –*

hypertension. Both concentric and eccentric hypertrophy of the left ventricle have been identified [5], which may effect both systolic and diastolic performance of the ventricle. The pulmonary circulation has been less well studied in hypertension, because of the requirement for invasive approaches to methodology. Nonetheless, it does appear that pulmonary resistance and pressure are increased in patients with hypertension [6], and that exercise induces a further increase of pulmonary pressure and attenuated reduction of pulmonary resistance [7–10]. Even less well studied are the filling conditions of the right and left ventricle. That is, while right atrial pressure and pulmonary capillary wedge pressure are normal at rest, these pressures may increase dramatically during exercise [9, 10], consistent with increased ventricular wall stress, or an independent abnormality of the diastolic properties of the ventricle. It is against this background that the angiotensin converting enzyme inhibitors have been studied.

Resting hemodynamics

The first report of the hemodynamic response of hypertensive patients to captopril demonstrated a reduction of blood pressure, mediated by reduction of systemic vascular resistance [11]. This anti-hypertensive response was intensified by the co-administration of diuretics, inducing a state of sodium depletion and angiotensin-dependent vascular tone. The reduction of blood pressure and vascular resistance was associated with a reduction of pulmonary capillary wedge pressure, yet heart rate and cardiac output were unchanged. The reason for an absence of reflex tachycardia has never been fully identified. It has been postulated that an increase of vagal tone, rather than a withdrawal of sympathetic tone, may account for this observation [12, 13]. These data suggested that the converting enzyme inhibitors might be effective in patients with congestive heart failure, corroborating early reports of intravenous teprotide in heart failure [14]. This hemodynamic pattern was also identified with enalapril [1, 4, 15, 16, 17], confirming a similar mechanism of action, despite different pharmacologic properties.

Exercise hemodynamics

The importance of the hemodynamic response to exercise in hypertension merits more intensive study, and an overview of this subject is provided by Dr. Lund-Johansen in this text. In response to exercise, there is a marked increase of blood pressure, with an ineffective reduction of systemic vascular resistance, to accommodate the three-to-five fold increase of cardiac output that is typically observed. The influence of converting enzyme inhibitors on the exercise response have been evaluated [7, 18]. In patients with mild to moderate hypertension, captopril was associated with the improvement of not only resting hemodynamics, but also the hemodynamic response to exercise. This was characterized by a more appropriate relaxation of the arterial system to accommodate the increase of cardiac output, as judged by reduction of overall vascular resistance, and of the blood pressure response to exercise. There was also a tendency for pulmonary pressures to decrease. The importance of this observation cannot be overstated. Traditionally, hemodynamics have been determined in supine resting patients, where conditions do not necessarily reflect the cardiovascular stress that is generated during daily activities. The invasive nature of such hemodynamic studies limits the practical application of these techniques to large patient populations. However, a more extensive profile of the hemodynamic response to exercise is available with the use of non-invasive radionuclide methodologies [19, 20]. Studies performed with captopril and enalapril have demonstrated that systolic function, as judged by ejection fraction, is well maintained, or even improved, in the setting of blood pressure reduction. It is also clear that converting enzyme inhibitors have a very favorable effect on ventricular relaxation indices [18].

Ventricular morphology and coronary dynamics

The issues surrounding myocardial adaptation and remodelling in hypertension, while not fully resolved, have clarified the adaptive response of the ventricle. A detailed discussion of these findings is beyond the scope of this presentation. Several issues, however, should be highlighted. In hypertensive patients, it is typical to observe either concentric or eccentric ventricular hypertrophy [5, 21]. This may depend on the severity and duration of hypertension, and may even be influenced by sexual differences and ageing. More recent data suggests that hypertrophy itself, independent of blood pressure, may be associated with increased cardiovascular morbidity [22, 23]. Several reports have shown that converting enzyme inhibitors are associated with regression of left ventricular mass [17, 24–26]. While it may be argued that much of this mass reduction reflects ventricular volume and stroke volume, there is evidence that free wall thickness also decreases. It is conceivable that changes in coronary artery volume and flow may also effect these anatomic changes, as converting enzyme inhibitors improve coronary flow and myocardial energetics in hypertensive patients [27]. There is evidence to suggest that angiotensin II has an adverse effect on the myocardium of hypertensive patients [25], so that reducing circulating and tissue levels of angiotensin II with converting enzyme inhibitors is highly desirable.

Peripheral arterial responses to converting enzyme inhibitors

Resistance in the arterial bed has traditionally been calculated as the quotient of blood pressure and cardiac output. Since this is a calculated index and requires invasive methodology (particularly during exercise), it has been difficult to characterize arterial flow characteristics in large population studies. More recently, Doppler-based methodologies of blood flow in the resistance-sized vessels have provided a better characterization and a reasonable estimate of arterial compliance [28], and a means to test the concept of chronic arterial adaptation hypertension [29]. With this technique, the anti-hypertensive effects of converting enzyme inhibitors are associated with a favorable effect on arterial compliance [30, 31]. Since hormonal and structural changes in resistance arteries directly influence ventricular performance and morphologic remodelling by increasing afterload and wall stress, the long-term arterial response is of central importance. Thus, anti-hypertensive therapy with converting enzyme inhibitors may therefore favorably improve the peripheral and central maladaptive changes observed in patients with hypertension.

Effects on renal hemodynamics

It is important to at least briefly discuss this issue, since changes in renal hemodynamics could theoretically have a major impact on the long-term outcome of converting enzyme inhibitor therapy in hypertension. It is unusual to see a major increase of renal blood flow or glomerular filtration rate with anti-hypertensive therapy, as these indices are relatively normal in the baseline state. In general, converting enzyme inhibitors do not have an adverse effect on renal hemodynamics, and the reduction of blood pressure is usually associated with a reduction of renal vascular resistance [32, 33]. Differences may be observed in subjects with chronic renal insufficiency, whose renal blood flow and glomerular filtration rate are more tenuous. Subjects with renal artery stenosis, particularly of bilateral origin, may also be prone to severe hypotension and reduction of renal blood flow, as a result of hypoperfusion beyond the stenosis, and increased basal renin secretion. In addition to a reduction of renal resistance, converting enzyme inhibitors can produce a favorable effect in glomerular hemodynamics [34, 35].

Perspectives and future trends

There are at least eight converting enzyme inhibitors currently under evaluation in clinical trials. Based on the known hemodynamic effects of this drug class in hypertension, it is unlikely that major hemodynamic differences will exist amongst future converting enzyme inhibitors, except for differences of bioavailability and half-life. The more important conclusion drawn from these data, is that converting enzyme inhibitors have a desirable hemodynamic profile from the standpoint of safety and efficacy. It may also be important to consider the potential hemodynamic impact of alternate methods of renin systems blockade, such as the renin inhibitory peptides. These compounds are effective in vivo [36–38], and orally active chemical moieties are under development. Finally, it is also important to consider the maladaptive cardiovascular response in hypertension, as part of a cardiovascular continuum ultimately expressed as congestive heart failure of systolic and diastolic origin. Converting enzyme inhibitors have an excellent efficacy record in heart failure patients, including an improvement of patient survival. This is not simply manifest by a change in cardiac output or systemic vascular resistance, but rather as outlined in this chapter, an integrated cardiovascular response affecting systemic and regional hemodynamics and the morphologic changes in the myocardium and vascular smooth muscle, where tissue renin system activity resides [39–41]. It seems logical that early utilization of these agents in hypertension, with their favorable hemodynamic profile, may considerably reduce long-term cardiac morbidity and mortality, which heretofore has eluded other anti-hypertensive regimens.

References

1. Cody RJ (1984): Hemodynamic responses to specific renin-angiotensin inhibitors in hypertension and heart failure: A review. *Drugs* 28: 144–169.
2. Todd PA, Heel RC (1986): Enalapril: A review of its pharmacodynamic and pharmacokinetic properties, and therapeutic use in hypertension and congestive heart failure. *Drugs* 31: 198–248.
3. Weinberger MH (1987): Angiotensin-converting enzyme inhibitors. *Med Clin North Am* 71: 979–990.
4. Fitzpatrick MA, Julius S (1985): Hemodynamic effects of angiotensin converting enzyme inhibitors in essential hypertension: A Review. *J Cardiovasc Pharmacol* 7(suppl 1): 359–369.
5. Devereux RB, Savage DD, Sachs I, Laragh JH (1983): Relation of hemodynamic load to left ventricular hypertrophy and performance in hypertension. *Am J Cardiol* 51: 171–176.
6. Guazzi MD, DeCesare N, Fiorentini C, Galli C, Moruzzi P, Tamborini G (1987): The lesser circulation in patients with systemic hypertension. *Circulation* 75(suppl I): I 56–62.
7. Fagard R, Bulpitt C, Lijnen P, Amery A (1982): Response of the systemic and pulmonary circulation to converting-enzyme inhibition (captopril) at rest and during exercise in hypertensive patients. *Circulation* 65: 33–42.
8. Lund-Johansen P (1987): The role of drugs in countering adverse pathophysiological profiles: influence on hemodynamics. *Am Heart J* 114: 958–964.
9. Cody RJ, Kubo SH, Covit AB, Muller FB, Lopez-Ovejero J, Laragh JH (1986): Exercise

hemodynamics and oxygen delivery in human hypertension: response to verapamil. *Hypertension* 8: 3–10.

10. Cody RJ, Kubo SH, Ryman KS, Shaknovich A, Laragh JH (1987): Systemic and pulmonary hemodynamic responses to nicardipine during graded ergometric exercise in patients with moderate to severe essential hypertension. *J Am Coll Cardiol* 10: 647–654.

11. Cody RJ, Tarazi RC, Bravo EL, Fouad FM (1978): Haemodynamics of orally-active converting enzyme inhibitor (SQ 14225) in hypertensive patients. *Clin Sci Mol Med* 55: 453–459.

12. Lumbers ER, McCloskey DI, Potter ER (1979): Inhibition by angiotensin II of baroreceptor-evoked activity in cardiac vagal efferent nerves in the dog. *J Physiol* London 294: 69–80.

13. Reid JL, Millar JA, Campbell BC (1983): Enalapril and autonomic reflexes and exercise performance. *J Hypertension* 1(suppl 1): 129–134.

14. Curtiss C, Cohn JN, Vrobel T, Franciosa JA (1978): Role of the renin-angiotensin system in the systemic vasoconstriction of chronic congestive heart failure. *Circulation* 58: 763–770.

15. Fouad FM, Tarazi RC, Bravo EL, Textor SC (1984): Hemodynamic and antihypertensive effects of the new oral angiotensin-converting-enzyme inhibitor MK-421 (enalapril). *Hypertension* 6: 167–174.

16. van Schaik Ba, Geyskes GG, Boer P, Dorhout-Mees EJ (1986): Changes in haemodynamics and body fluid volume due to enalapril in patients with essential hypertension on chronic diuretic therapy. *Eur J Clin Pharmacol* 31: 381–385.

17. Dunn FG, Digman W, Ventura HO, Messerli FH, Kobrin I, Frohlich ED (1984): Enalapril improves systemic and renal hemodynamics and allows regression of left ventricular mass in essential hypertension. *Am J Cardiol* 53: 105–108.

18. Omvik P, Lund-Johansen P (1984): Combined captopril and hydrochlorothiazide therapy in severe hypertension: Long-term haemodynamic changes at rest and during exercise. *J Hypertension* 2: 73–80.

19. Fouad FM, Tarazi RC, Gallagher JH, MacIntyre WJ, Cook SA (1980): Abnormal left ventricular relaxation in hypertensive patients. *Clin Sci* 59(suppl 6): 411s–414s.

20. Smith V, White WB, Meeran MK, Karimeddini MK (1986): Improved left ventricular filling accompanies reduced left ventricular mass during therapy of essential hypertension. *J Am Coll Cardiol* 8: 1449–1454.

21. Hartford M, Wikstrand J, Wallentin I, Ljungman S, Wilhelmsen L, Berglund G (1984): Diastolic function of the heart in untreated primary hypertension. *Hypertension* 6: 329–338.

22. Savage DD, Garrison RJ, Kannel WB, Levy D, Anderson SJ, Stokes J, Feinleib M, Castelli WP (1987): The spectrum of left ventricular hypertrophy in a general population sample: The Framingham Study. *Circulation* 75(suppl I) I 26–33.

23. Casale PN, Devereux RB, Milner M, Zullo G, Harshfield GA, Pickering TG (1986): Value of echocardiographic measurement of left ventricular mass in predicting cardiovascular morbid events in hypertensive men. *Ann Intern Med* 105: 173–178.

24. Nakashima Y, Fouad FM, Tarazi RC (1984): Regression of left ventricular hypertrophy from systemic hypertension by enalapril. *Am J Cardiol* 53: 1044–1049.

25. Devereux RB, Pickering TG, Cody RJ, Laragh JH (1987): Relation of renin-angiotensin system activity to left ventricular hypertrophy and function in experimental and human hypertension. *J Clin Hypertens* 3: 87–103.

26. Pfeffer JM, Pfeffer MA, Mirsky I, Braunwald E (1983): Prevention of the development of heart failure and the regression of cardiac hypertrophy by captopril in the spontaneously hypertensive rat. *Eur Heart J* 4(suppl A): 143–148.

27. Daly P, Rouleau JL, Cousineau D, Burgess JH (1984): Acute effects of captopril on the coronary circulation of patients with hypertension and angina. *Am J Med* 76: 111–115.

28. Levenson JA, Peronneau PP, Simon AC, Safar ME (1981): Pulsed Doppler: Determination

of diameter, blood flow velocity and volumic flow of brachial artery in man. *Cardiovasc Res* 15: 164–172.

29. Folkow B (1983): Structural changes: the vascular wall. Consequences of treatment. *Hypertension* 5(suppl III): 58–62.

30. Simon AC, Levenson JA, Bouthier JL, Safar ME (1984): Captopril-induced changes in large arteries in essential hypertension. *Am J Med* 76: 71–75.

31. Safar ME, London GM, Safavian A, St Laurent, Pannier B (1987): Changes in arterial distensibility produced by converting enzyme inhibitors in hypertensive humans. *Clin Exp Hypertens* 9: 189–195.

32. Hollenberg NK (1984): Renal hemodynamics in essential and renovascular hypertension influence of captopril. *Am J Med* 76: 22–28.

33. Bauer JH, Reams GP (1986): Renal effects of angiotensin converting enzyme inhibitors in hypertension. *Am J Med* 81: 19–27.

34. Zatz R, Dunn BR, Meyer TW, Anderson S, Rennke HG, Brenner BM (1986): Prevention of diabetic glomerulopathy by pharmacological amelioration of glomerular capillary hypertension. *J Clin Invest* 77: 1925–1930.

35. Meyer TW, Anderson S, Rennke HG, Brenner BM (1987): Reversing glomerular hypertension stabilizes established glomerular injury. *Kidney Int* 31: 752–759.

36. Burton J, Cody RJ, Herd JA, Haber E (1980): Specific inhibition of renin by an angiotensin analog: studies in sodium depletion and renin-dependent hypertension. *Proceedings of the National Academy of Science* 77: 5476–5479.

37. Cody RJ, Burton J, Evin G, Poulsen K. Herd JA, Haber E (1980): A substrate analog inhibitor of renin that is effective in vivo. *Biochemical and Biophysical Research Communication* 97: 230–235.

38. Zusman RM, Burton J, Christensen D, Nussberger J, Dodds A, Haber E (1983): Hemodynamic effects of a competitive renin inhibitory peptide in humans: Evidence for multiple mechanisms of action. *Transactions of the Association of American Physicians* 96: 365–375.

39. Unger T, Scholkens BA, Ganten D, Lang RE (1987): Tissue converting enzyme inhibition and cardiovascular effects of converting enzyme inhibitors. *Clin Exp Hypertension* 9: 417–426.

40. Swales JD, Abramovici A, Beck F, Bing RF, Loudon M, Thurston H (1983): Arterial wall renin. *J Hypertension* 1(suppl 1): 17–22.

41. Re R, Fallon JT, Dzau V, Ouay SC, Haber E (1982): Renin synthesis by canine aortic smooth muscle cells in culture. *Life Sci* 30: 99–106.

31. Cardiovascular structure and function after treatment with calcium entry inhibitors in hypertension

ROBERTO PEDRINELLI

An intense research in the field of the structural cardiovascular alterations in experimental and clinical hypertension has carefully evaluated the heterogeneous nature and the clinical and physiopathological implications of either cardiac hypertrophy [1] or its vascular counterpart [2]. Thus, the importance of nonemodynamic factors in myocardial hypertrophy development, such as sympathetic stimuli [3, 4], has been elucidated even through the study of the effect of antihypertensive treatment [5, 6]. The lack of changes in myocardial mass during treatment with arteriolar vasodilators such as hydralazine or minoxidil was instrumental in developing that concept [6]. This chapter will focus on another group of vasodilators, the so called calcium entry blocker (CEB)s [7–23], rather recently brought to the front stage of antihypertensive treatment.

The deceiptevely simple term calcium entry inhibitor (calcium entry blocker, CEB) describes a highly heterogeneous group of compounds-mainly the dihydropiridine (nifedipine and congeners), benzothiazepine (diltiazem) and phenalkylamine (verapamil) derivatives [24]-whose common pharmacological trait is to antagonize the entry of extracellular calcium into the cell, thus decreasing the amount of available intracellular ion. For the interested reader, several recent reviews have dealt with their complex pharmacological characteristics and their vascular effect [e.g. 25, 26]. *In vitro*, CEBs relax potassium-depolarized preconstricted vessels, through interference with the socalled potential operated channels [27], but they are also active against a host of agonists including norepinephrine, possibly by altering the function of receptor operated channels [27]. Thus, to the extent of the dependence of alpha-adrenergic mediated vasoconstriction on calcium influx in hypertension, CEBs, and mainly the dihydropiridine derivatives, may also act through antagonism for alpha-mediated adrenergic vasoconstriction [28–30] even in

M.E. Safar & F. Fouad-Tarazi (eds.), The heart in hypertension.
© 1989 Kluwer Academic Publishers, Dordrecht –

man. The hemodynamic and reflexogenic consequences originating from the arteriolar vasodilating effect of those compounds has been overwied [e.g. 31, 32].

Although the antianginal effect of CEBs was exploited since the early seventies, the clear identification of their hypotensive potential was delayed until the midseventies [33]. Thereafter, however, the various aspects of the consequences of CEB administration in hypertension have been extensively explored [e.g. 34, 35, 36], including those on cardiovascular structural alterations [7–23]. In the animals studies addressing this point, CEBs caused consistent hemodynamic effects such as drops in blood pressure, no change or decreases in heart rate, and maintained [11] or increased cardiac output and ejection fraction [9, 10, 15]. This latter effect was attributed to a decreased wall stress, i.e. afterload), since neither preload, myocardial contractility or heart rate changed [37], a conclusion disputed by other authors [15] who found evidence for increased preload during calcium entry blockade, at least as obtained through felodipine administration. On the other hand, the effects on cardiac mass were more variable. Thus, Kazda et al reported the beneficial effects of nifedipine in preventing either hypertension or myocardial hypertrophy in a very specific model of hypertension such as the Dahl sensitive rat [7]. Comparable resullts were found by Kobayashi and Tarazi]10] in nitrendipine treated two-kidney, 1 clip (2k–1C) renal hypertensive rat (RHR)s, where, however, myocardial hypertrophy regressed less than predicted from the drop in blood pressure. Therefore, the data allowed speculations about a role for a subtle increase in reflex sympathetic activity in opposing full myocardial regression in this model where cardiac mass is strictly related to blood pressure levels. Further data are available regarding the effect of nifedipine [8, 9, 13], nitrendipine [11] and felodipine [12, 14, 15] in the spontaneously hypertensive rat (SHR), an animal model close, to an extent, to human essential hypertension. The absence of relationship between average percent differences in systemic blood pressure and cardiac mass indices of CEB-treated SHR vs their untreated controls (Figure 1, as recalculated from the available figures in the pertinent papers) further stresses the importance of nonhemodynamic factors in modulating cardiac mass, as commonly found in this animal model [3, 4]. More importantly in this context, however, CEBs not always prevented or reverted left ventricular hypertrophy in SHR [see data in 13, 14, 15], attenuating the strength of those statements claiming intrinsic differences between CEBs as a class and other non specific vasodilators [8]. Even more when considering that, under the appropriate experimental conditions, a classical non specific vasodilator such as hydralazine itself reverted myocardial hypertrophy [e.g. 38, 39, 40].

The issue of vascular hypertrophy in hypertension and its behavior during antihypertensive treatment as related to cardiac hypertrophy, has been raising

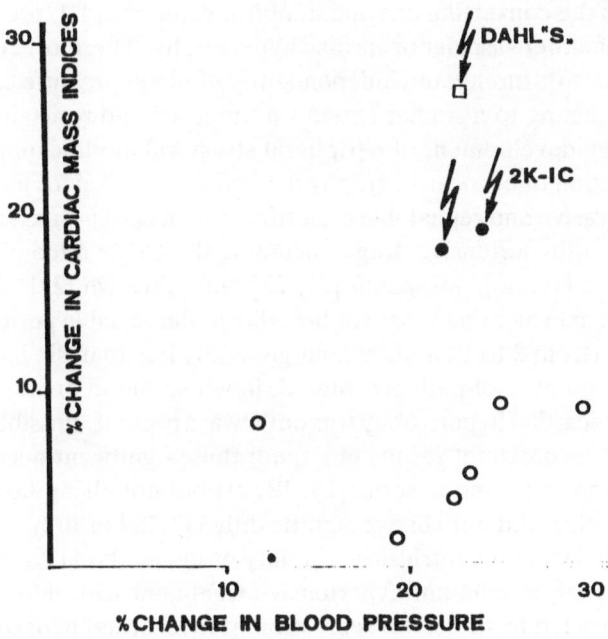

Figure 1. Relationship between average percent differences in blood pressure and cardiac mass indices (left ventricular weight / body weight ratio *or* heart weight / body weight ratio) in CEB-treated SHR vs. untreated controls (o). Data recalculated from figures reported in references 8, 9, 11–15.

Results obtained in studies performed in unrelated rat models of hypertension, such as the Dahl Sensitive (S) rat [7], or the two-kidney, one clip (2K–1C) renal hypertensive rat [8, 10] are also reported.

great interest in recent years. Some studies already evaluated the effect of CEBs in experimental animals, although the restriction to the use of dihydro-piridine derivatives precludes the extrapolation of the data to unrelated CEBs owing to the intrinsic heterogeneity of this class of compounds. Thus, felodi-pine-mediated hypotension was accompanied by decreased minimal vascular resistances during maximal vasodilation in in-vitro perfused hindlimbs of SHRs [12], a functional evidence for successful regression of vascular alter-ations [2]. However, in spite of a decrease in cardiac mass, no difference in minimal coronary resistances during maximal or near-to-maximal coronary vasodilation was found between nitrendipine-treated and untreated RHRs [10], thus suggesting the possibility of discrepancies in the hypertrophic re-sponse of vascular and cardiac tissue in experimental hypertension. On the same line, no changes in mesenteric arteriolar medial thickness occurred during felodipine treatment in SHR [14], at similarity with data obtained in SHR during hydralazine [39, 41], while a pharmacologically unrelated vasodilator, such as the converting enzyme inhibitor captopril [41], prevented the development of either vascular or cardiac hypertrophy. Therefore, even at the vascular level factors modulated independently of blood pressure control and not necessarily acting to a similar extent on the heart and resistance vessels, may mediate the development of peripheral structural modifications.

The introduction of echocardiography has offered the tool for a sufficiently precise, non invasive and repeatable quantification of cardiac mass in man per se and during antihypertensive drugs, including the CEBs nifedipine [16–18, 21], nitrendipine [19, 20], verapamil [21, 23] and diltiazem [22]. Difficulties arise, however, in evaluating those studies, due to the variable periods of drug administration (from 2 to 12 months, but generally less than six months) and the overall low number of patients studied, in whom blood pressure differed widely, and myocardial hypertrophy was not always present. Possibly for these reasons, rather inconsistent results emerged: thus, significant decrements in cardiac mass were reported in some [16, 18, 21] but not all studies, in which cardiac mass indices did not change significantly [17, 20] or only to an extent barely detectable from the intrinsic variability of the method [19]. Therefore, as in animals, even in man antihypertensive treatment with dihydropiridine CEBs not always led to successful regression of myocardial hypertrophy. On the other hand, either verapamil [21, 23] or diltiazem [22] treatment was associated with a reduced cardiac mass in the few clinical trials utilizing those drugs, but more data are needed before admitting differences among CEBs in this regard. Interestingly, during antihypertensive treatment, either through CEB treatment or else [1, 3], cardiac mass changes were independent of blood pressure levels, suggesting non hemodynamic determinants of myocardial hypertrophy even in man.

In conclusion, CEBs represent by now an established antihypertensive treatment but their effect on cardiovascular structure in hypertension needs further clarification in view of the importance of this issue. In fact, to the extent that myocardial hypertrophy represents a major independent risk for cardiac mortality [42], and as a function of the contribution of cardiovascullar hypertrophy in general to the evolution of hypertension itself [1, 2], the choice of drugs capable of normalizing either cardiac mass or an altered wall-lumen ratio in resistance vessels may become a must. Much more awaits to be learnt from future (especially human) studies on this topic.

References

1. Tarazi RC (1986): Cardiovascular hypertrophy in hypertension. *Hypertension* 8 (suppl II): II 187–190.
2. Folkow B (1982): Physiological aspects of primary hypertension. *Physiol Rev* 62: 347–504.

3. Frohlich ED, Tarazi RC (1979): Is arterial pressure the sole factor responsible for hypertensive cardiac hypertrophy? *Am J Cardiol* 44: 956–961.
4. Tarazi RC, Sen S, Saragoca M, Khairallah P (1982): The multifactorial role of catecholamines in hypertensive cardiac hypertrophy. *Eur Heart J* 3 (suppl A): 103–110.
5. Tarazi RC, Fouad FM (1984): Reversal of cardiac hypertrophy in humans. *Hypertension* 6 (suppl III): III 140–146.
6. Sen S (1983): Regression of cardiac hypertrophy: Experimental models. *Am J Med* 75 (suppl 3): 87a–93a.
7. Kazda S, Garthoff B, Dycka J, Iwai J (1982): Prevention of malignant hypertension in salt loaded 'S'Dahl rats with the calcium antagonist nifedipine. *Clin Exp Hyp* A4: 1231–1241.
8. Kazda S, Garthoff B, Thomas G (1982): Antihypertensive effect of calcium antagonists in rat differs from that of other vasodilators. *Clinical Science* 63: 363s–365s.
9. Motz W, Ploeger M, Ringsawandl G, Goeldel N, Garthoff B, Kazda S, Strauer BE (1983): Influence of nifedipine on ventricular function and myocardial hypertrophy in spontaneously hypertensive rats. *J Cardiovasc Pharmacol* 5: 55–61.
10. Kobayashi K, Tarazi RC (1983): Effect of nitrendipine on coronary flow and ventricular hypertrophy in hypertension. *Hypertension* 5 (suppl II): II 45–51.
11. Kobrin I, Sesoko S, Pegram BL, Frohlich ED (1984): Reduced cardiac mass by nitrendipine is dissociated from systemic or regional haemodynamic changes in rats. *Cardiovasc Res* 18: 158–162.
12. Lundin SA, Hallback-Nordlander M (1984): Regression of structural cardiovascular changes by antihypertensive therapy in spontaneously hypertensive rats. *J Hypertension* 2: 11–18.
13. Zaahringer J, Stangl E, Danninger B, Aschauer W, Motz W, Strauer B (1985): Regression of heart muscle hypertrophy after nifedipine therapy: Changes in cardiac gene expression. *J Hypertension* 3 (suppl 3): s493–s495.
14. Nyborg CB, Mulvany MJ (1985): Lack of effect of antihypertensive treatment with felodipine on cardiovascular structure of young spontaneously hypertensive rats. *Cardiovasc Res* 19: 528–536.
15. Friberg P, Folkow B, Nordlander M (1986): Cardiac dimensions in spontaneously hypertensive rats following different modes of blood pressure reduction by antihypertensive treatment. *J Hypertension* 4: 85–92.
16. McLeay RAB, Stallard TJ, Watson RDS, Littler WA (1983): The effect of nifedipine on arterial pressure and reflex cardiac control. *Circulation* 67: 1084–1090.
17. Ferrara LA, De Simone G, Mancini M, Fasano ML, Pasanisi F, Vallone G (1984): Changes in left ventricular mass during a double-blind study with chlortalidone and slow-release nifedipine. *Eur J Clin Pharmacol* 27: 525–528.
18. Strauer BE, Mahmoud MA, Mayer F, Bohn I, Motz U (1984): Reversal of left ventricular hypertrophy and improvement of cardiac function in man by nifedipine. *Eur Heart J* 5 (sF): 53–60.
19. Ferrara LA, Fasano ML, De Simone G, Goro S, Gagliardi R (1985): Antihypertensive and cardiovascular effect of nitrendipine: A controlled study vs. placebo. *Clin Pharmacol Ther* 38: 434–438.
20. Drayer JIM, Hall WD, Smith VE, Weber MA, Wollam L, White WB (1986): Effect of the calcium channel blocker nitrendipine on left ventricular mass in patients with hypertension. *Clin Pharmacol Ther* 40: 679–685.
21. Muiesan G, Agabiti-Rosei E, Romanelli G, Muiesan ML, Castellano M, Beschi M (1986): Adrenergic activity and left ventricular function during treatment of essential hypertension with calcium antagonists. *Am J Cardiol* 57: 44D–49D.
22. Amodeo C, Kobrin I, Ventura HO, Messerli FH, Frohlich ED (1986): Immediate and short term hemodynamic effects of diltiazem in patients with hypertension. *Circulation* 73: 108–113.

23. Schmieder RE, Messerli FH, Garavaglia GE, Nunez BD (1987): Cardiovascular effects of verapamil in patients with essential hypertension. *Circulation* 75: 1030–1036.
24. Fleckenstein A (1977): Specific pharmacology of calcium, cardiac pacemakers and vascular smooth muscle *Ann Rev Pharmacol Toxicol* 17: 149–166.
25. Schwartz A, Triggle DJ (1984): Cellular action of calcium channel blocking drugs. *Ann Rev Med* 35: 325–339.
26. Cauvin C, Loutzenhiser R, Van Breemen C (1983): Mechanisms of calcium antagonist-induced vasodilation. *Ann Rev Pharmacol Toxicol* 23: 373–396.
27. Bolton TB (1979): Mechanisms of action of transmitters and other substances on smooth muscle. *Physiol Rev* 59: 606–718.
28. Pedrinelli R, Tarazi RC (1984): Interference of calcium entry blockade in vivo with pressor responses to alpha-adrenergic stimulation: Effects of two unrelated blockers on responses to both exogenous and endogenously released norepinephrine. *Circulation* 69: 1171–1176.
29. Pedrinelli R, Tarazi RC (1985): Calcium entry blockade by nitrendipine and alpha-adrenergic responsiveness in vivo: comparison of systemic vs local effects. *J Pharmacol Exp Ther* 233: 643–649.
30. Pedrinelli R, Taddei S, Salvetti A: Interference by calcium entry blockade with vaso-constrictor responses to alpha adrenergic stimulation in human beings: Effects of two unrelated blockers on forearm vascular responses to exogenous norepinephrine. *Clin Pharmacol Ther* 45: 285–290.
31. Guazzi MD, Polese A, Fiorentini C, Bartorelli A, Moruzzi P (1983): Treatment of hypertension with calcium antagonists: A review. *Hypertension* 5 (suppl II): II 85–90.
32. Zsoter TT, Church JG (1983): Calcium antagonists: Pharmacodynamic effects and mechanisms of action. *Drugs* 25: 93–112.
33. Guazzi M, Olivari MT, Polese A, Fiorentini C, Magrini F, Moruzzi P (1977): Treatment of hypertension with nifedipine, a calcium antagonist agent. *Clin Pharmacol Ther* 22: 528–53.
34. Stornello M, Di Rao G, Iachello M, Pisani R, Scapellato L, Pedrinelli R, Salvetti A (1983): Hemodynamic and humoral interactions between captopril and nifedipine. *Hypertension* 5 (suppl III): III 154–156.
35. Fouad FM, Pedrinelli R, Bravo EL, Abi-Samra F, Textor SC, Tarazi RC (1984): Clinical and systemic hemodynamic effects of nitrendipine. *Clin Pharmacol Ther* 35: 768–775.
36. Pedrinelli R, Fouad FM, Tarazi RC, Bravo EL, Textor SC (1986): Nitrendipine, a calcium entry blocker: Renal and humoral effects in human arterial hypertension. *Arch Intern Med* 146: 62–65.
37. Motz W, Strauer BE (1983): Nifedipine in the long term management of hypertensive heart disease. *Hypertension* 5(suppl II): II 39–44.
38. Pfeffer JM, Pfeffer MA, Flethcher P, Fishbein MC, Braunwald E (1982): Favorable effects of therapy on cardiac performance in spontaneously hypertensive rats. *Am J Physiol* 242: H 776–784.
39. Sano T, Tarazi RC (1987): Differential structural responses of small resistance vessels to antihypertensive therapy. *Circulation* 75: 618–626.
40. Motz W, Strauer BE (1984): Regression of structural cardiovascular changes by antihypertensive therapy. *Hypertension* 6 (suppl III): III 133–139.
41. Freslon JL, Giudicelli JF (1983): Compared myocardial and vascular effects of captopril and dihydralazine during hypertension development in spontaneously hypertensive rats. *Br J Pharmac* 80: 533–543.
42. Frohlich ED (1987): Cardiac hypertrophy in hypertension. *New Eng J Med* 317: 831–833.

PART FIVE

The heart and reversion of arterial and arteriolar structural changes

32. Baroreceptor mechanisms and the control of vascular resistance

ALBERTO U. FERRARI, GIUSEPPE MANCIA and
ALBERTO ZANCHETTI

Introduction

Animal studies have documented that arterial baroreflexes subserve crucial functions in cardiovascular control. First of all, arterial baroreflexes minimize moment-to-moment blood pressure oscillations [1], thereby reducing the extent of spontaneous blood pressure variability and its possible impact on cardiovascular disease [2]. Secondly, they participate in the cardiovascular modulation of a number of behaviours (sleep, exercise,, emotion, etc.), ultimately determining the size of their heart rate and blood pressure effects [3, 4]. Thirdly, arterial baroreflexes may be important in the long-term determination of mean blood pressure levels, as shown by the sustained rise in blood pressure that has been reported to follow chronic section of the carotid sinus and aortic nerves [5].

All these findings raise the possibility that abnormalities in baroreceptor reflexes are involved in the pathogenesis of arterial hypertension in man. This was investigated in the late 60's following the introduction of a technique by which baroreceptor activity could be altered through an i.v. injection of a vasopressor or a vasodepressor drug and the reflex response assessed as the attendant change in heart interval [6]. This approach, however, did not allow to gather information on the most important target organ of the baroreflex, i.e. the control of blood pressure and peripheral circulation.

Such limitation was overcome by adopting a variable pressure neck chamber technique which allows to alter in a controlled fashion transmural pressure across the carotid sinuses [7]. This can increase or reduce carotid baroreceptor activity in a way that permits simultaneous assessment of the reflex effects not only on heart rate but also on blood pressure and vascular resistance.

In the last 10 years we have remodeled this technique and applied it to baroreflex studies in normotensive and hypertensive subjects. The basic prin-

M.E. Safar & F. Fouad-Tarazi (eds.), The heart in hypertension.
© *1989 Kluwer Academic Publishers, Dordrecht –*

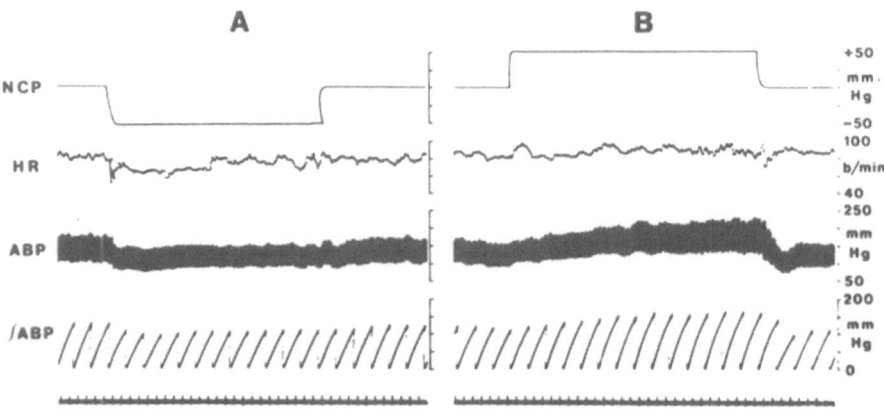

Figure 1. Original record from a normotensive subject illustrating the effects on arterial blood pressure (ABP) of carotid baroreceptor stimulation (A) and deactivation (B) obtained by respectively lowering and raising the pneumatic neck chamber pressure (NCP). Also represented are heart rate (HR) and mean arterial pressure (10 sec-period integration, ABP). Bottom trace represents 5 sec time divisions.

ciple is to enclose the neck into a plastic collar equipped with rubber seals and adapted inferiorly to the shoulders and superiorly to the occiput, the ear lobes and the chin. This allows the air pressure in the compartment between the collar and the neck skin to be altered in a positive or a negative direction within a range of ± 50 mmHg. By percutaneously advancing a small cannula into the vicinity of the carotid bifurcation we demonstrated that these pneumatic changes are accompanied by linear changes in the pressure around the carotid sinuses, thereby modifying carotid baroreceptor activity. We also showed that pneumatic pressure is incompletely and asymmetrically transmitted, insofar only 86% of the positive and 64% of the negative applied pressures reach the carotid sinus region. This allowed to adopt correction factors to properly estimate the stimulus affecting the baroreceptors [8].

Baroreceptor reflex in normotension

In 11 normotensive subjects with arterial blood pressure continuously recorded (femoral catheter), carotid baroreceptors were stimulated and deactivated by respectively applying negative and positive neck chamber pressures. At least 4 positive and 4 negative pressures of different intensity were applied in a random sequence. Each application was maintained for 120 sec, the reflex effects being evaluated in the initial 10 sec and in the final 30 sec of each episode, and referred to as the 'transient' (or 'early') and the 'steady state'

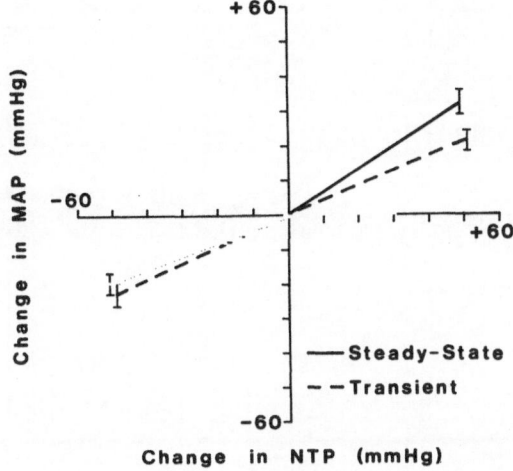

Figure 2. Means ± SE of individual regression coefficients relating transient and steady-state changes in mean arterial pressure (MAP) to changes in neck tissue pressure (NTP) in the whole group of normotensive subjects (n = 11).

responses respectively. Because in all subjects a linear stimulus-response relationship was present, the baroreflex sensitivity was expressed as regression coefficient separately for the condition of increased and reduced baroreceptor activity [9]. As shown in the example of Figure 1 and in the average data of Figure 2, (1) baroreceptor stimulation was accompanied by a blood pressure fall and baroreceptor deactivation by a blood pressure rise, (2) the depressor response reached a maximum in the early phase of the stimulus and then partially regressed to a sustained plateau while the pressor response developed more slowly and reached its maximum in the steady-state phase, and (3) in the steady-state phase the responses were asymmetric, i.e. the blood pressure rise accompanying carotid baroreceptor deactivation was larger than the blood pressure fall accompanying carotid baroreceptor stimulation. This asymmetry could not be accounted for by the intervention of the aortic baroreceptors because in both animals and man these reflexes probably have little tonic influence on blood pressure and thus little ability to counteract more a blood pressure fall than a blood pressure rise [10]. Therefore the most likely explanation is that normally the set-point of the carotid baroreceptor-blood pressure reflex is shifted towards the upper inflection of its stimulus-response curve. This means that this reflex mechanism is more effective for a deactivation than for a further stimulation of the receptors, i.e. that it has a better antihypotensive than an antihypertensive function.

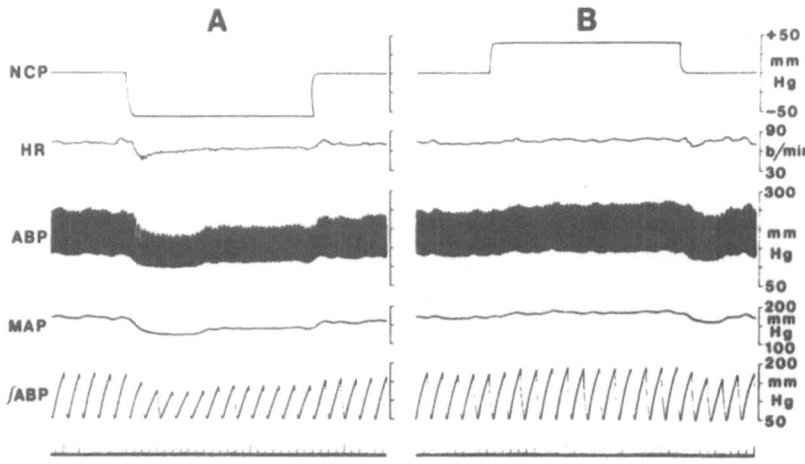

Figure 3. Original record from a hypertensive subject illustrating the effects on arterial blood pressure (ABP) of carotid baroreceptor stimulation (A) and deactivation (B) obtained by respectively lowering and raising the pneumatic neck chamber pressure. MAP, mean arterial pressure (NCP). Other abbreviations as in Figure 1.

Baroreceptor reflex in essential hypertension

In 35 patients with essential hypertension of various severity the carotid baroreflex was manipulated in a fashion identical to that described for the normotensive subjects [11]. This allowed to show that the direction and time course of the blood pressure changes attending baroreceptor stimulation and deactivation were unaltered by a chronic blood pressure elevation. However in hypertensive subjects the asymmetry of the reflex function observed in normotensive individuals was replaced by an asymmetry in the opposite direction, i.e. the blood pressure effects of carotid baroreceptor stimulation were larger than those of carotid baroreceptor deactivation and more pronouncedly so as the severity of hypertension increased. A further important observation was that this was not accompanied by a reduction in the overall ability of this reflex system to modulate blood pressure as (1) the total blood pressure excursions induced by the alterations in baroreceptor activity employed in our study were not different in subjects with normal and high blood pressure, and (2) the maximal sensitivity of the baroreflex (i.e. the slope of the curve showing maximal changes in arterial blood pressure for a given change in carotid transmural pressure) was also similar in the two groups (Figures 3 and 4, upper panels).

These data shed light on the longstanding controversy concerning baroreflex sensitivity in hypertension. Data obtained by the vasoactive drug technique [6, 11, 12] clearly show that in the high blood pressure state barorecep-

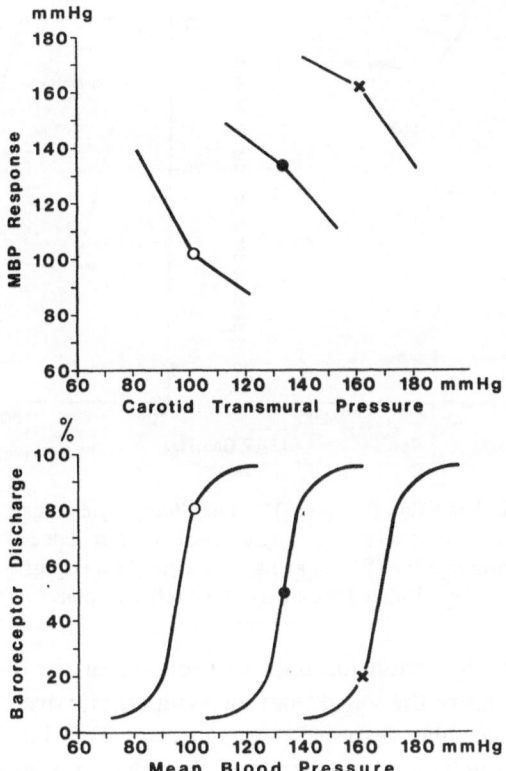

Figure 4. In each panel the open circle, filled circle and cross represent the average resting mean blood pressure (MBP) of normotensive, moderate hypertensive and severe hypertensive subjects respectively. In the upper panel, each line represent the mean regression coefficient relating steady-state MBP responses to carotid transmural pressure, calculated as systemic MBP minus neck tissue pressure during carotid baroreceptor manipulation by the neck chamber technique. In the lower panel a possible explanation of the marked resetting of the baroreflex in hypertension is illustrated by schematically drawing the stimulus-response curve relating MBP to carotid barore-ceptor discharge in each group. At resting MBP the discharge may be near saturation in normoten-sives and be progressively shifted towards threshold in moderate and severe hypertensives.

tors have a limited ability to modulate heart rate. However, this is not the case for the ability of baroreceptors to modulate blood pressure which is rearranged but not blunted in even severely hypertensive patients. The reason for this differential effect of hypertension on the cardiac and blood pressure influences of the baroreflex is not known but data obtained by other investigators suggest two possible (and not mutually exclusive) explanations. One, at the vascular level any hypertension-induced reduction in the baroreceptor influence may be counteracted by a hypertrophy of the vessel wall increasing the changes in vascular resistance and blood pressure resulting from changes in sympathetic

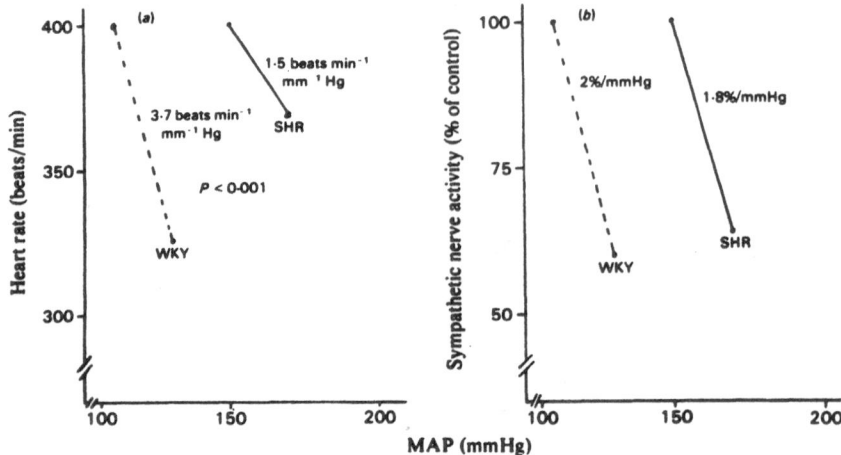

Figure 5. Responses in heart rate (left panel) and in efferent sympathetic nerve activity (right panel) to baroreceptor stimulation obtained by a vasoactive drug-induced rise in mean arterial pressure (MAP) in normotensive (WKY) and spontaneously hypertensive (SHR) rats. Figures siding each line refer to the calculated sensitivity of the reflex response.

drive [13]. Two, the hypertension-induced reduction in the baroreceptor influence may involve more the vagal than the sympathetic drive which modulate the cardiac and vascular responses respectively. This latter explanation is supported by the unchanged baroreceptor modulation of muscle sympathetic activity which has been shown in essential hypertension [14]. It is also elegantly documented by the fact that in experimental hypertensive models a clearcut reduction in the sensitivity of the baroreceptor-heart rate reflex coexists with an unchanged sensitivity of the baroreceptor effects on efferent sympathetic nerve activity (Figure 5) [15]. Although circumstantial evidence favours the hypothalamus [16], the site(s) at which this differential effect of hypertension on these two components of the baroreceptor reflex is established remains to be investigated.

The reversed asymmetry of the baroreceptor-blood pressure reflex observed in hypertension deserves a further comment. In descriptive terms this means that during chronic blood pressure elevations there are small reflex effects when baroreceptors are unloaded and large reflex effects when baroreceptors are stimulated above their tonic level of activity. Thus in hypertension the baroreceptor-blood pressure reflex does not move towards further saturation but paradoxically shifts towards threshold (Figure 4, lower panels) [17]. This reflects a resetting phenomenon much more pronounced than that described in experimental hypertension. This phenomenon may protect hypertensive patients against influences tending to further raise the already elevated blood pressure. It may also, however, reduce the efficiency of a homeostatic mechanism preventing blood pressure falls, facilitating the occurrence of postural hypotension [18].

Hemodynamic changes associated with carotid baroreceptor manipulation

In 27 hypertensive patients we characterized the hemodynamic changes accompanying baroreceptor manipulation by adding to the experimental set-up described above a thermodilution catheter which measured cardiac output changes occurring during the steady-state phase of a marked degree of positive or negative neck pressure application. It was shown that the blood pressure fall accompanying the negative neck pressure application, i.e. carotid baroreceptor stimulation, was due to a reduction both in cardiac output and in total peripheral resistance. In contrast, the blood pressure rise accompanying the positive neck pressure application, i.e. carotid baroreceptor deactivation, was exclusively due to a vasoconstrictor response with no change in cardiac output (Figure 6) [17]. This pattern is different from that described in normotensive subjects, in whom the reflex depressor response is due to a reduction in cardiac output and total peripheral resistance but the reflex pressor response is almost solely mediated via a cardiac output rise [19]. This may reflect a greater responsiveness of the peripheral vasculature to sympathetic stimulation in hypertensive subjects. It may also depend, however, on the fact that these subjects had a somewhat reduced inotropic reserve which makes an already burdened left ventricle less capable of raising its output in response to a further elevation of the afterload.

In normotensive subjects carotid baroreceptor manipulation modulates splanchnic vasomotor tone but only transiently affects sympathetic activity and vasomotor tone of skeletal muscle circulation [20]. A similar pattern has been described in hypertensive patients [21] but no systematic comparison between the two conditions has been reported.

Baroreceptor reflex in renovascular hypertension

Does the alteration of the baroreceptor-blood pressure reflex observed in essential hypertension precede the increase in blood pressure, or is it merely secondary to the blood pressure elevation? Our approach to this question was to examine the carotid baroreceptor reflex in a type of hypertension which is not initiated by baroreceptor-dependent mechanisms, namely renovascular hypertension. In 18 patients affected by this condition the blood pressure responses to applications of graded degrees of positive and negative neck pressure were similar to those observed in age- and blood-pressure-matched

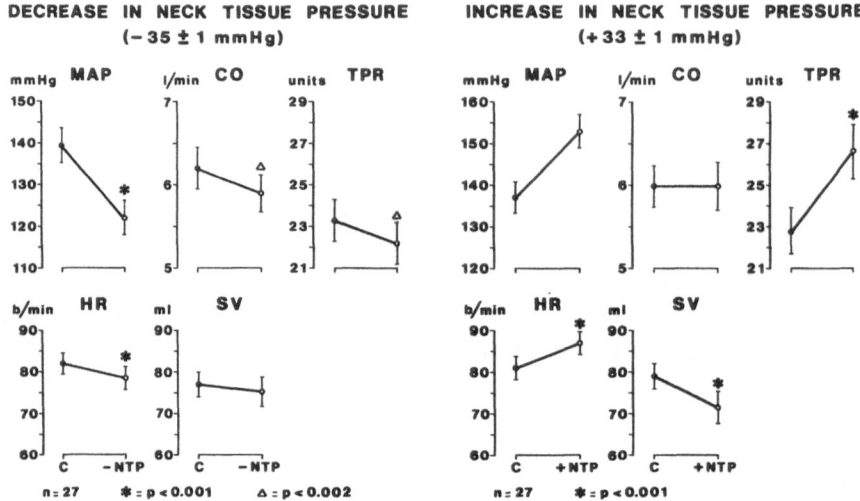

Figure 6. Changes in mean arterial pressure (MAP), cardiac output (CO), total peripheral resistance (TPR), heart rate (HR) and stroke volume (SV) induced by stimulating (*left*) and deactivating (*right*) carotid baroreceptors by the neck chamber technique (stimulus intensity in parenthesis) in 27 essential hypertensive subjects.
Closed circles indicate control values (C) and open circles the values observed during the final 30 sec of the neck tissue pressure change (± NTP).

individuals with essential hypertension. In particular the reversed asymmetry of the pressor and depressor responses indicating an exaggerated resetting phenomenon was evident in the renovascular hypertensive patients as well and the sensitivity of the baroreflex was not significantly different in the two groups (Figure 7) [22]. This finding is against a peculiar baroreflex alteration in essential hypertension and rather points towards a common secondary mechanism affecting the reflex in chronically elevated blood pressure states irrespective of their origin.

Modulation of baroreceptor reflex in man

The studies described above were designed to examine the baroreceptor control of blood pressure in untreated, quietly resting, supine subjects. In daily life, however, this control operates under environmental conditions which can be markedly different from those existing in the laboratory. As shown below these conditions may modify the baroreflex in a complex fashion.

Carotid baroreflexes and exercise. In normotensive subjects [23] and in patients with essential hypertension of variable severity [24] the hypotensive and

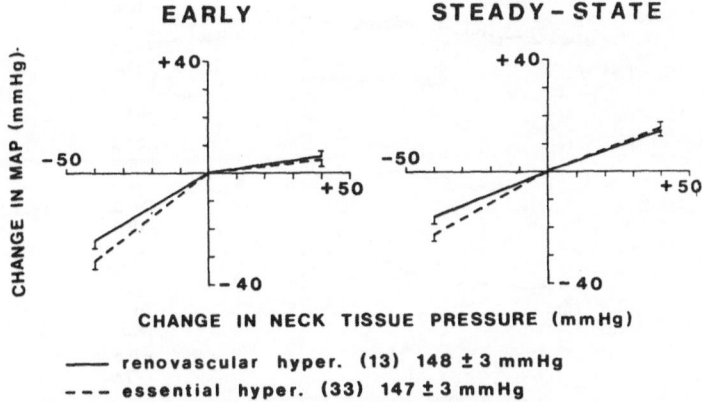

Figure 7. Mean regression coefficients relating early and steady-state changes in mean arterial pressure (MAP) to changes in neck tissue pressure observed by the neck chamber technique in renovascular hypertensive subjects (continuous lines). The responses provided by essential hypertensive subjects are shown for comparison (dashed lines). No significant differences between the two groups were ever observed.

bradycardic responses to carotid baroreceptor stimulation (negative neck chamber pressure) were compared at rest and during an isometric handgrip exercise of moderate intensity. The bradycardia induced by the baroreceptor stimulation at rest (see Figure 1) was almost completely abolished when the stimulation was performed during handgrip; in contrast, the concomitant hypotensive response was largely preserved (Figure 8). Thus during exercise baroreceptors loose their cardiac modulating ability but retain their ability to control blood pressure. This selective rearrangement of the baroreflex functions is physiologically appropriate because it allows heart rate (and presumably cardiac output) to increase while preventing an eccessive blood pressure rise. It is likely that this occurs as a result of central volitional factors selectively suppressing reflex parasympathetic influences with no impairment of the sympathetically mediated ones. This is confirmed by the demonstration that suppression of the baroreceptor effects on heart rate can be seen since the very beginning of isometric exercise, prior to any exercise-induced hemodynamic changes [25].

Baroreflexes, emotional behaviors and sleep. Suppression of the baroreceptor-heart rate reflex has also been observed during emotional behaviors deprived of any exercise component [26]. In contrast, this reflex function has been shown to increase its sensitivity during sleep [27, 28]. In neither instance, however, the observations could be extended to the baroreceptor-blood pres-

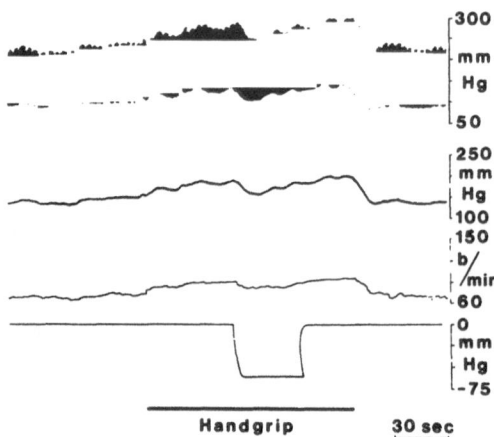

Figure 8. Original record showing the effects of isometric exercise (handgrip) on the responses to carotid baroreceptor stimulation. Traces from top to bottom are: pulsatile arterial pressure, mean arterial pressure, heart rate and neck chamber pressure. Note the marked blood pressure fall but the modest bradycardia accompanying the negative neck chamber pressure application.

sure control, which makes any correlation with the effects of exercise on the baroreflex difficult.

Baroreflexes and salt intake. In the past decade animal experiments have shown that a reduction in sodium intake impairs neural cardiovascular control and that this involves to an important extent baroreceptor control of circulation [29]. Human data on this topic are still preliminary. However, in elderly subjects in whom a negative sodium balance was produced by dietary salt restriction or diuretic administration, an increased rate of orthostatic or post-prandial hypotension was observed [30]. Although other explanations are possible, this is interpretable as to represent a reduction in the efficiency of the reflex mechanisms devoted to blood pressure homeostasis. Interestingly, salt loading has been reported to be accompanied by the opposite effect, i.e. an increased effectiveness of baroreceptor mechanisms [31], and late studies suggest that this may also be the case in man [32].

Baroreflexes and cardiovascular drugs. Most hypertensive patients receive chronic drug treatment, which makes theoretically and practically important to determine whether the baroreceptor reflex is modified by antihypertensive drugs. We investigated this point by measuring the blood pressure responses to carotid baroreceptor stimulation and deactivation (neck chamber technique) before and after administration of many of these drugs. In brief, these responses were not affected by the acute or chronic administration of clonidine

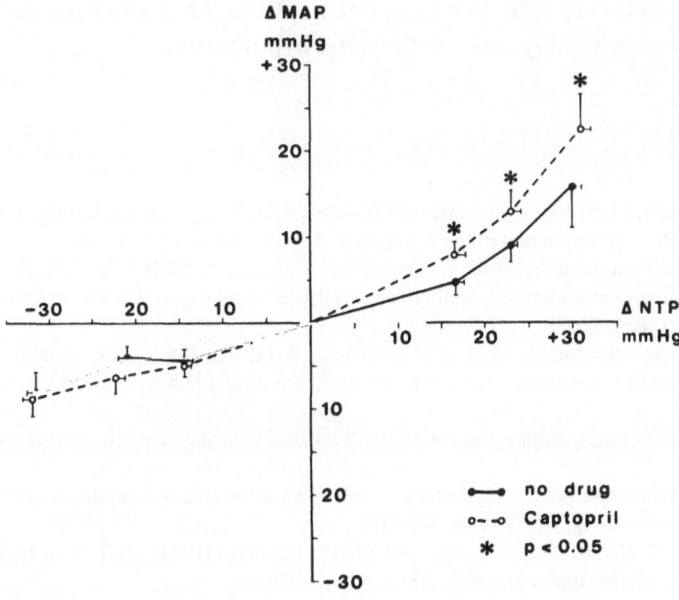

Figure 9. Effects of captopril administration on the steady-state responses in mean arterial pressure (Δ MAP) accompanying changes in neck tissue pressure (Δ NTP) obtained by the neck chamber technique to alter carotid baroreceptor activity. Note the significant captopril-induced augmentation of the MAP responses to baroreceptor deactivation.

[33], methyldopa [34], prazosin [35], nitrendipine [36], and beta-blockers [37], demonstrating that their interference with sympathetic vasoconstrictor influences, although capable of reducing blood pressure, is not so pronounced as to impair neural mechanisms responsible for cardiovascular homeostasis. In all instances, however, the curve relating baroreceptor stimuli to reflex blood pressure responses was shifted towards lower blood pressure values. This means that the upward resetting of the baroreflex observed in hypertension is a rapidly reversible phenomenon, the clinical implication being that it does not oppose the blood pressure lowering effect of several antihypertensive drug regimens.

A regression of the upward resetting of the baroreflex was also observed following captopril administration (Figure 9) [38]. In this instance, however, the magnitude of the blood pressure responses to carotid baroreceptor deactivation was enhanced as compared to the untreated condition. This was the case also for the heart rate responses either to carotid and to overall baroreceptor deactivation induced by injection of a vasodepressor drug. Thus ACE-inhibition seems to offer an advantage over other antihypertensive drugs in that following its induction, the antihypotensive effect of the baroreflex is improved. This may explain why in uncomplicated hypertension ACE-inhibition only exceptionally cause orthostatic hypotension.

References

1. Cowley AW, Liard JF, Guyton AC (1973): Role of the baroreceptor reflex in daily control of arterial blood pressure and other variables in dogs. *Circ Res* 32: 564–576.
2. Parati G,, Pomidossi G, Albini F, Malaspina D, Mancia G (1987): Relationship of 24-hour blood pressure mean and variability to severity of target organ damage in hypertension. *J Hypertension* 5: 93–98.
3. Baccelli G, Albertini R, Mancia G, Zanchetti A (1976): Interactions between sinoaortic reflexes and cardiovascular effects of sleep and emotional behavior in the cat. *Circ Res* 38: 1130–1134.
4. Ludbrook J (1983): Reflex control of blood prerssure during exercise. *Ann Rev Physiol* 45: 155–168.
5. Ito CS, Scher AM (1981): Hypertension following arterial baroreceptor denervation in the unanesthetized dog. *Circ Res* 48: 576–586.
6. Bristow JD, Honour AJ, Pickering GW, Sleight P, Smyth HS (1969): Diminished baroreflex sensitivity in high blood pressure. *Circulation* 39: 48–54.
7. Ernsting J, Parry DJ (1957): Some observations on the effects of stimulating the stretch receptors in the carotid artery of man (abstract). *J Physiol* (London) 137: 45P–46P.
8. Ludbrook J, Mancia G, Ferrari A, Zanchetti A (1977): The variable-pressure neck chamber method for studying the carotid baroreflex in man. *Clin Sci Mol Med* 53: 165–171.
9. Mancia G, Ferrari A, Gregorini L, Valentini R, Ludbrook J, Zanchetti A (1977): Circulatory reflexes from carotid and extracarotid baroreceptor areas in man. *Circ Res* 41: 309–315.
10. Thoren P, Saum W, Brown AM (1977): Characteristics of rat aortic baroreceptors with nonmedullated afferent nerve fibers. *Circ Res* 40: 231–237.
11. Mancia G, Ludbrook J, Ferrari A, Gregorini L, Zanchetti A (1978): Baroreceptor reflexes in human hypertension. *Circ Res* 43: 170–177.
12. Korner PI, West J, Shaw J, Uther JB (1974): Steady-state properties of the baroreceptor-heart rate reflex in essential hypertension in man. *Clin Exp Pharmacol Physiol* 1: 65–76.
13. Folkow B (1982): Physiological aspects of primary hypertension. *Physiol Rev* 62: 347–404.
14. Wallin BG, Delius W, Hagbarth KE (1973): Comparison of sympathetic nerve activity in normotensive and hypertensive subjects. *Circ Res* 33: 9–21.
15. Ricksten SE, Thoren P (1981): Reflex control of sympathetic nerve activity and heart rate from arterial baroreceptors in conscious spontaneously hypertensive rats. *Clin Sci* 61: 169s–172s.
16. Djojosugito AM, Folkow B, Kylstra PH, Lisander B, Tuttle RS (1971): Differentiated interaction between the hypothalamic defence reaction and baroreceptor reflexes, I: Effects on heart rate and regional flow resistance. *Acta Physiol Scand* 78: 376–385.
17. Mancia G, Ferrari A, Gregorini L, Parati G, Pomidossi G, Zanchetti A (1979): Control of blood pressure by carotid sinus baroreceptors in human beings. *Am J Cardiol* 44: 895–902.
18. Cuche JL, Kuchel O, Barbean A, Langlois Y, Boucher R, Genest J (1974): Autonomic nervous system and benign essential hypertension in man. *Circ Res* 35: 290–297.
19. Bjurstedt H, Rosenhamer G, Tyden G (1975): Cardiovascular responses to changes in carotid sinus transmural pressure in man. *Acta Physiol Scand* 94: 497–505.
20. Mancia G, Mark AL (1983): Arterial baroreflexes in humans, in: Shepherd JT, Abboud FM

(eds), *Handbook of Physiology*, section 2, The Cardiovascular System, Vol 3. Peripheral circulation and organ blood flow, Part 2, pp 755–793. Washington D.C.: American Physiological Society.

21. Wallin GB (1979): A quantitative study of muscle nerve sympathetic activity in resting normotensive and hypertensive subjects. *Hypertension* 1: 67.

22. Mancia G, Ferrari A, Leonetti G, Pomidossi G, Zanchetti A (1982): Carotid sinus baroreceptor control of arterial pressure in renovascular hypertensive subjects. *Hypertension* 4: 47–50.

23. Ludbrook J, Faris IB, Iannos J, Jamieson GG, Russel WS (1978): Lack of effect of isometric handgrip exercise in the responses of the carotid sinus baroreceptor reflex in man. *Clin Sci Mol Med* 55: 189–194.

24. Mancia G, Ferrari A, Gregorini L, Parati G, Pomidossi G (1982): Effects of isometric exercise on the carotid baroreflex in hypertensive subjects. *Hypertension* 4: 245–250.

25. Mancia G, Iannos J, Jamieson GG, Lawrence HH, Sherman PR, Ludbrook J (1978): The effect of isometric handgrip exercise on the carotid sinus baroreceptor reflex in man. *Clin Sci Mol Med* 54: 33–37.

26. Sleight P, Fox P, Lopez R, Brooks DE (1978): The effect of mental arithmetic on blood pressure variability and baroreflex sensitivity in man. *Clin Sci Mol Med* 55: 381s–382s.

27. Smyth HS, Sleight P, Oickering GW (1969): Reflex regulation of arterial pressure during sleep in man: A quantitative method for measuring baroreflex sensitivity. *Circ Res*: 109–121.

28. Bertinieri G, Di Rienzo M, Parati G, Pomidossi G, Pedotti A, Zanchetti A, Mancia G (1987): Baroreceptor-heart rate reflex studied in normotensives and essential hypertensives by beat-to-beat analysis of 24-hour blood pressure and heart rate. *J Hypertension* 5 (suppl 5): S 333–335.

29. Rocchini AP, Cant JR, Barger AC (1977): Carotid sinus reflex in dogs with low- to high-sodium intake. *Am J Physiol* 233: H 196–202.

30. Shannon RP, Wei SY, Rosa RM, Epstein FH, Rowe JW (1986): The effect of age and sodium depletion on cardiovascular response to orthostasis. *Hyppertension* 8: 438–443.

31. Ferrari AU, Mark AL (1987): Sensitization of aortic baroreceptors by high salt diet in Dahl salt-resistant rats. *Hypertension* 10: 55–60.

32. Mark AL, Lawton WJ, Abboud FM, Fitz AE, Connor WE, Heistad DD (1975): Effects of high and low sodium intake on arterial pressure and forearm vascular resistance in borderline hypertension. *Circ Res* 36/37 (suppl 2): 94–98.

33. Mancia G, Ferari A, Gregorini L, Zanchetti A (1979): Clonidine and carotid baroreflex in essential hypertension. *Hypertension* 1: 362–370.

34. Mancia G, Ferrari A, Gregorini L, Bianchini C, Terzoli L, Leonetti G, Zanchetti A (1980): Methyldopa and neural control of circulation in essential hypertension. *Am J Cardiol* 45: 1237–1243.

35. Mancia G, Ferrari A, Gregorini L, Ferrari MC, Bianchini C, Terzoli L, Leonetti G, Zanchetti A (1980): Effects of prazosin on autonomic control of circulation in essential hypertension. *Hypertension* 2: 700–707.

36. Gregorini L, Perondi R, Grassi G, Sino A, Giannattasio C, Mancia G, Zanchetti A (1987): Hemodynamic effects of acute and prolonged administration of nitrendipine in essential hypertension. *J Cardiovasc Pharmacol* 10 (suppl 10): s126–s128.

37. Grassi G, Parati G, Pomidossi G, Ramirez A, Ferrari A, Bertinieri G, Gavazzi C, Mancia G (1983): Baroreceptor control of the cardiovascular system during administration of beta-adrenergic blocking drugs in man. *J Hypertension* 1 (suppl 2): 332–334.

38. Mancia G, Parati G, Pomidossi G, Grassi G, Bertinieri G, Buccino N, Ferrari A, Gregorini L, Rupoli L, Zanchetti A (1982): Modification of arterial baroreflexes by captopril in essential hypertension. *Am J Cardiol* 49: 1415–1419.

33. Structural changes of small resistance vessels in essential hypertension

ENRICO AGABITI-ROSEI and GIULIO MUIESAN

Introduction

The main hemodynamic characteristic of established essential hypertension is a raised peripheral resistance, while cardiac output is usually within normal limits [1]. Precapillary resistance vessels give the major contribution to the total peripheral resistance in the systemic circulation. Although the high peripheral resistance in essential hypertension can be related to an elevated vasoconstrictor tone, it has been demonstrated that an increased wall thickness in relation to the lumen in the precapillary vessels is of great importance for the maintenance and probably also for the progressive worsening of the hypertensive disease [2, 3]. In fact, many years ago Folkow and coworkers showed that as a consequence of the increased wall-to-lumen ratio, there must always be a greater change in resistance for any given degree of smooth muscle shortening in blood vessels [4].

Structural vascular changes are related to the prevailing level of arterial pressure, and it has been shown that raised blood pressure per se, irrespective of the cause, may induce smooth muscle cell hypertrophy and also synthesis of collagen in the vascular wall [5]. However, there is also evidence that genetic and neurohumoral factors – particularly the sympathetic tone and possibly the renin-angiotensin system – may have a marked influence in the development of vascular structural changes [2]. For the assessment of vascular structural changes in man several methodological and technical problems must be taken into consideration. In addition, from the clinical point of view it seems particularly important to determine whether a regression of vascular structural changes in essential hypertension could be induced by an antihypertensive treatment, to establish whether such a possible regression may be different with different drugs and to correlate the response to treatment of cardiac hypertrophy with that of small resistance vessels.

M.E. Safar & F. Fouad-Tarazi (eds.), The heart in hypertension.
© *1989 Kluwer Academic Publishers, Dordrecht –*

Methodological aspects in the evaluation of structural changes of small resistance vessels

The assessment of vascular structural changes can be performed either by histologic or hemodynamic methods. Some difficulties intrinsic to an hystologic evaluation of arteriolar structural changes are related to muscle tone; in fact an increase in smooth muscle tone will decrease the inner radius and increase the wall thickness, and viceversa; in addition, the variables will be also affected in opposite directions by changes in intravascular pressure. Therefore, morphometric evaluation of vessels wall can be performed only at known smooth muscle tone. Recently, however, a micromyographic technique has been developed for the examination of functional and morphologic characteristics of isolated resistance vessels taken from human subcutaneous biopsies during local anesthesia [6].

Repeated histologic estimations are obviously difficult to perform in vivo, particularly in man. Therefore, an evaluation of vascular structural changes in humans has mainly rested on hemodynamic measurements [7]. In fact, Folkow and coworkers have demonstrated a close correlation between minimal perfusion pressure and the ratio of wall thickness to internal radius in small resistance vessels [5]. For this approach it is very important that the vascular bed under study is at maximal dilatation. In man it is possible to bring vascular beds to maximal dilatation with a combination of ischemia, muscle work and possibly also heat, mainly in skin and muscle vascular beds. It is not possible to obtain the same high flow levels by pharmacological means such as intraarterial administration of acetylcholine, isoproterenol, histamine and adenosine triphosphate [8, 9]. From maximal blood flow, minimal vascular resistance, an index of structural vascular changes, may be calculated. This method has the advantage that it evaluates exactly the vessels responsible for the flow resistance in vivo.

Structural changes of resistance vessels in essential hypertension

Several studies have demonstrated significantly higher resistance at maximal vasodilatation in various vascular beds of patients with established essential hypertension compared with normotensive control subjects, thus indicating the presence of a structural vascular abnormality in the resistance vessels. In particular, high minimal vascular resistance has been demonstrated in the hand, calf and forearm vascular beds of hypertensive patients [10, 11, 12]. Conway [13] observed that this abnormality in the forearm vascular bed was related to the level of blood pressure but not to the duration of hypertension. Takeshita and coworkers [14, 15] have also demonstrated the presence of vascular structural changes, as inferred from high forearm vascular resistance at maximal vasodilatation, in patients with borderline hypertension, and in normotensive young men with a family history of hypertension. However, in their as well as in other studies, only a small portion of the variability in minimal vascular resistance could be explained by the variability in mean blood pressure at the time of the study. In addition, structural changes have been observed not only in resistance, but also in capacitance vessels. Taken together, these observations suggest that in addition to the magnitude of blood pressure elevation, structural vascular changes may be induced and influenced by other factors, such as the sympathetic nervous system tone, humoral mechanisms, local factors or primary vascular abnormalities.

Vascular structural changes have been demonstrated in man also by histologic measurements usually performed on autopsy material or on biopsy material obtained in connection with surgery on patients for various reasons [16, 17, 18]. Recently, Aalkjaer and coworkers examined the functional and morphologic characteristics of isolated artery segments (about 170 μm internal diameter) dissected from biopsies of skin and subcutaneous tissue taken under local anesthesia from the gluteal region. They found that vessels from hypertensives had a 29% increase in the media-thickness-to-lumen-diameter ratio in respect to those taken from matched controls. They observed an increased pressor response in hypertensive patients and concluded that this abnormal response can, to a large extent, be explained by altered vascular structure. This technique is very promising as it seems to allow a pathophysiological and clinical evaluation of vascular structural changes in essential hypertension.

Regression of vascular structural changes by antihypertensive treatment

Studies in animal models have demonstrated that arteriolar structural changes are reversible with long term reduction in arterial pressure. In fact, blood vessels can be completely normalized provided an adequate antihypertensive treatment is started early [19]. However, the longer the duration of hypertension, the less complete the reversal. In addition, antihypertensive therapy prevents development of vascular changes in young SHR, but does not result in complete regression in adult SHR [20].

Studies in man on the possible regression of vascular structural changes by antihypertensive treatment have been performed mainly by haemodynamic investigations in skin and muscle vascular beds. In the hand vascular bed of 12 hypertensive patients a significant regression of structural vascular changes after 5 years of antihypertensive therapy was demonstrated, but a complete normalization could not be achieved [10]. The effect of antihypertensive treatment in the calf muscle vascular bed was evaluated in a large group of patients by Sivertsson and coworkers [10, 11] and by Svensson and coworkers [12]. A total of 90 patients with essential hypertension underwent repeated plethysmographic investigations after 6 weeks, 6 months and 18 months of therapy with either a diuretic or a beta-blocker. In these patients, despite a significant reduction of blood pressure, no evidence of decrease of minimal vascular resistance, and hence of regression of vascular structural changes, was observed. It has been proposed that these negative results could be due to men's erect posture which increases the transmural pressure in the calf vessels as the effect of gravity is added to intravascular pressure.

As far as the forearm vascular bed is concerned, some conflicting results have been reported using different beta-blockers [12]. In fact, minimal vascular resistance in the forearm was significantly reduced by long term treatment for 6 months with pindolol, which possesses marked intrinsic sympathomimetic activity (ISA), but not by metoprolol, a β_1-selective blocker devoided of ISA. It is possible that antihypertensive drugs that induce vasodilatation without stimulation of the sympathetic nervous system activity, may induce more easily a regression of vascular structural changes. In fact, pindolol, owing to its ISA, may cause a β_2-mediated vasodilatation of the vessels when general sympathetic tone is low. In addition, we have recently reported [21, 22] for the first time that long-term treatment for 6 months with the calcium antagonist nitrendipine and the ACE inhibitor captopril, in some cases combined respectively with atenolol or hydrochlorothiazide, may significantly decrease forearm minimal vascular resistance in hypertensive patients. Thus, it is possible that different antihypertensive drugs have different effects on structural vascular changes. This hypothesis is supported by the results obtained in animal studies. In fact, Sano and Tarazi [23] have observed that thickening of small resistance vessels in the hindlimbs of pithed SHR was reduced significantly more in captopril+hydrochlorothiazide treated than in hydralazine treated groups of animal.

These results confirmed those obtained by Freslon and coworkers [24] in the mesenteric artery of SHR, and indicate that regression of vascular structural changes by antihypertensive treatment is not dependent on blood pressure control alone. It must be pointed out that even in the studies showing a relationship between blood pressure control and regression of structural changes, the correlation was not close. Although studies in experimental animals have shown that the blood vessels can be completely normalized through early blood pressure lowering treatment, studies in man have indicated that complete normalization of vascular changes occurs very rarely. The difficulty of inducing a decrease of minimal vascular resistance within normal limits in hypertensive patients may be related to the fact that long standing hypertension may induce fibrosis of the arteriolar media whose regression by antihypertensive therapy is probably more incomplete than regression of mere smooth muscle cell hypertrophy. A recent study of Aalk-jaer and coworkers in isolated subcutaneous resistance vessels of patients with essential hypertension has shown that, despite long term normalization of blood pressure with various drugs, the structural abnormalities were only partially reversed [25].

Interrelationship of cardiac and vascular wall hypertrophy in essential hypertension

Tarazi emphasized the particular importance of the relationship between the structural responses of the heart and of the vessels to hypertension or to antihypertensive treatment [26]. He pointed out that hypertrophy of both the large and smaller arterial vessels was shown to follow the same general pattern of development and regression as in the heart, although the studies reported were scanty and, particularly in man, the evidence still fragmentary.

In a recently published study we observed that in a total group of 80 patients with essential hypertension the degree of vascular alterations in the limbs, as evaluated by resistance at maximal vasodilatation, and that of left ventricular hypertrophy were reciprocally correlated, and that the cardiovascular structural changes were proportional to the severity of hypertension. All these correlations were statistically significant, but not very close; in fact, the indices of determination were never greater than 25%. The low correlation coefficient observed between minimal vascular resistance and left ventricular mass suggested that structural changes in the systemic arteries and in the heart did not develop simultaneously. Thus, patients were categorized according to whether they had left ventricular hypertrophy or impaired blood flow: although the majority of patients had at the same time presence or absence of hypertrophy in the heart and in the vessels, in a small number of cases cardiac hypertrophy was observed in combination with normal minimal vascular resistance in the limbs. Thus, the results suggested that the development of left ventricular hypertrophy may be more frequently and easily detectable at an earlier phase than the development of arterial structural changes in the limbs.

To the extent that cardiovascular hypertrophy contributes to the evolution and complications of hypertension, its reversal should be a primary goal of antihypertensive therapy. However few, if any of the studies on the regression of cardiovascular hypertrophy have specifically addressed the effects of anti-hypertensive treatment on the heart and vascular structural changes in the same patients. We have recently undertaken a study with the purpose of assessing whether long term antihypertensive treatment may induce a parallel chronological and quantitative regression of left ventricular hypertrophy and arterial structural changes [27]. We studied 14 essential hypertensive patients,

8 were given Captopril (plus diuretics, when necessary) and 6 were given Nitrendipine (plus Atenolol, when necessary). After 6 months of treatment both Captopril and Nitrendipine significantly reduced blood pressure, left ventricular mass and forearm minimal vascular resistance; left ventricular mass was normalized in 7 patients and minimal vascular resistance in 1 patient only. After 12 months of treatment blood pressure, left ventricular mass and minimal vascular resistance were further reduced; left ventricular mass was normalized in 9 patients and minimal vascular resistance in 2 patients only. Our results indicate therefore that long-term antihypertensive treatment may normalize left ventricular mass before minimal vascular resistance returns to normal. The different behaviour in the response to treatment of cardiac and vascular hypertrophy may have, in our opinion, relevant clinical implications, since before normalization of vascular structural changes, the load on the heart could be significantly increased, particularly during stress. Consequently we have evaluated the cardiac systolic performance, both at rest and during stress, after regression of cardiovascular hypertrophy. In all the patients left ventricular systolic performance was evaluated considering shortening fraction in relation to end-systolic stress. All data points obtained at rest and at the peak of handgrip and cold pressor tests, before and after 6 and 12 months of treatment, fell within 95% confidence limits of the correlation previously established in normal subjects. Therefore, after normalisation of left ventricular mass, systolic function was well maintained both at rest and during stress. This observation deserves further investigation, as its importance from the point of view of the achievement of a more complete therapeutic goal in antihypertensive therapy is indeed relevant.

Conclusion

The present review emphasizes the pathophysiological and clinical importance of the development, detection and regression of structural changes of small resistance vessels in essential hypertension. Since the hypertrophy of these vessels can maintain elevated vascular resistance and amplify the response to hypertensive stimuli, it is conceivable that return toward normal of the wall-to-lumen ratio will make control of arterial pressure easier and possibly result in long lasting period of remission. However, the studies so far performed indicate that a large number of patients with essential hypertension may have structural changes that are only partially reversible. This could be due, in the first place, to the fact that only rarely blood pressure is completely and persistently normalised by antihypertensive therapy. Furthermore the hypertensive disease in human subjects is often treated relatively late in its course, when structural changes are already, at least in part, irreversible. Regression of vascular changes in the calf muscle bed has never been demonstrated. Further studies are needed to determine whether regional differences in the regression of vascular structural changes do actually occur or whether different antihypertensive drugs have different effects on structural vascular changes. The new micromyographic techniques on isolated human resistance vessels might in the future add important contributions to the understanding and control of vascular structural changes in hypertension.

References

1. Frohlich ED, Tarazi RC, Dustan HP (1969): Re-examination of the hemodynamics of hypertension. *Am J Med Sci* 257: 9–23.
2. Folkow B, Hansson L, Sivertsson R (1983): Structural vascular factors in the pathogenesis of hypertension, in: Robertson JIS (ed), *Handbook of Hypertension,* Vol I, pp 133–150. Amsterdam-New York-Oxford: Elsevier.
3. Hansson L, Sivertsson R (1984): Regression of structural vascular changes by antihypertensive therapy. *Hypertension* 6 (suppl III): III 147–149.
4. Folkow B, Grimby G, Thulesius O (1958): Adaptive structural changes of the vascular walls in hypertension and their relation to control of peripheral resistance. *Acta Physiol Scand* 44: 255–272.
5. Folkow B (1983): Structural factors: The vascular wall. *Hypertension* 5 (suppl III): III 58–62.
6. Aalkjaer C, Heagerty AM, Petersen K, Swales J, Mulvany M (1987): Evidence for increased media thickness, increased neuronal amine uptake, and depressed excitation-contraction coupling in isolated resistance vessels from essential hypertensives. *Circ Res* 61: 181–186.
7. Sivertsson R (1970): The hemodynamic importance of structural vascular changes in essential hypertension. *Acta Physiol Scand* (Suppl 343): 1–56.
8. Duff F, Greenfield ADM, Sheperd JT, Thompson ID (1953): A quantitative study of the response to acetylcholine and hystamine of the blood vessels of the human hand and forearm. *J Physiol* (London) 120: 160–170.
9. Duff F, Patterson GC, Shepherd JT (1954): A quantitative study of the response to adenosine triphosfate of the blood vessels of the human hand and forearm. *J Physiol* (London) 125: 581–589.
10. Sivertsson R, Hansson L (1976): Effects of blood pressure reduction on structural vascular abnormality in skin and muscle vascular beds in human essential hypertension. *Clin Sci Mol Med* 51 (suppl 3): 77s–79s.
11. Sivertsson R, Andersson O, Hansson L (1979): Blood pressure reduction and vascular adaptation: A study on long-term effects of treatment with mefruside or atenolol. *Acta Med Scand* 205: 477–482.
12. Svensson A, Gudbrandsson T, Sivertsson R, Hansson L (1982): Haemodinamic effects of metoprolol and pindolol: A comparison in hypertensives patients. *Br J Clin Pharmacol* 13 (suppl 2): 259s–267s.
13. Conway J (1963): A vascular abnormality in hypertension: A study of blood flow in the forearm. *Circulation* 27: 520–529.
14. Takeshita A, Mark AL (1980): Decreased vasodilator capacity of forearm resistance vessels in borderline hypertension. *Hypertension* 2: 610–616.
15. Takeshita A, Imaizumi T, Ashihara T, Yamamoto K, Hoka S, Nakamura M (1982): Limited

maximal vasodilator capacity of forearm resistance vessels in normotensive young men with a familial predisposition to hypertension. *Circ Res* 50: 671–677.

16. Short D (1966): Morphology of the intestinal arterioles in chronic human hypertension. *Br Heart J* 28: 184–192.

17. Horwitz D, Clineschmidt BV, Vanburen JM, Ommaia AK (1974): Temporal arteries from hypertensive and normotensive man. *Circ Res* 34/35 (suppl 1): 109–115.

18. Thulesius O, Gjores JE, Berlin E (1983): Vascular reactivity of normotensive and hypertensive human arteries. *Gen Pharmacol* 14: 153–154.

19. Weiss L (1974): Aspects of the relation between functional and structural cardiovascular factors in primary hypertension. *Acta Physiol Scand* (suppl 401): 1–58.

20. Lundgren Y (1974): Adaptive changes of cardiovascular design in spontaneous and renal hypertension. *Acta Physiol Scand* (suppl 408): 1–62.

21. Agabiti-Rosei E, Muiesan ML, Geri A, Muiesan G (1987): Interrelationship of cardiac and vascular wall hypertrophy in essential hypertension: Effects of treatment. *J Cardiovasc Pharmacol* 10 (suppl 5): S 116–119.

22. Agabiti-Rosei E, Muiesan ML, Geri A, Romanelli G, Montani G, Muiesan G (1988): Relation between cardiac hypertrophy and forearm vascular structural changes before and during long term antihypertensive treatment. *Am J Med* 84 (suppl 3A): 124–128.

23. Sano T, Tarazi RC (1987): Differential structural responses of small resistance vessel to antihypertensive therapy. *Circulation* 3: 618–626.

24. Freslon J, Giudicelli JF (1983): Compared myocardial and vascular effects of captopril and dihydralazine during hypertension development in spontaneously hypertensive rats. *Br J Pharmacol* 80: 533–543.

25. Aalkjaer C, Mulvany MJ, Biskjær H, Jespersen B, Kjær T, Sørensen SS, Pedersen BB (1988): Morphological and functional abnormalities of resistance vessels from patients with essential hypertension are not normalized by antihypertensive therapy. *12th Scientific Meeting of the International Society of Hypertension*, Abst. Book 720, Kyoto.

26. Tarazi RC (1983): Regression of left ventricular hypertrophy by medical treatment: Present status and possible implications. *Am J Med* 26: 80–86.

27. Agabiti-Rosei E, Muiesan ML, Geri A, Romanelli G, Beschi M, Castellano M, Muiesan G (1988): Long term antihypertensive treatment may induce normalization of left ventricular mass before complete regression of vascular structural changes. Consequences for cardiac function at rest and during stress. *J Hypertension*, 6 (suppl 4): 94s–96s.

34. Hemodynamic response to exercise in hypertension and its modulation by anti-hypertensive therapy

PER OMVIK and PER LUND-JOHANSEN

Introduction

The rise in blood pressure (BP) during exercise is the result of hemodynamic adjustments initiated by metabolic and neurohumoral reflex changes. These hemodynamic responses varies considerably in hypertensive as well as in normotensive subjects and is dependent on several factors such as training and body configuration and also on the type of exercise (i.e. static *vs* dynamic) [1]. Since a rise in BP increases the myocardial oxygen demand [2] exercise testing may be of importance in evaluation of hypertensives wanting to take part in vigorous physical activity or patients with target organ manifestations like left ventricular hypertrophy or coronary artery disease but it is generally not used on a routine basis [3]. It is possible, however that exercise testing could be of importance in determining the prognosis of hypertension, but long-term data are limited [4]. It should also be stressed that standard noninvasive measurements of diastolic BP during exercise are unreliable and that accurate measurements can only be obtained by intraarterial recordings [5, 6].

During antihypertensive therapy the BP is lowered either by reduction in cardiac index (CI), total peripheral resistance index (TPRI) or both [7]. Since the primary goal of therapy is reduction of BP and of hypertensive morbidity it could be argued that the underlying mechanism behind the fall in BP is merely hemodynamic cosmetics. However, it should be pointed out that the work burden on the heart is not determined by BP alone [2] and also that restoration of tissue perfusion requires a normal cardiac performance. It has been shown that changes in cardiac pump function in essential hypertension (EH) are most readily demonstrated during exercise [8]. In our laboratory invasive studies on the hemodynamic response to exercise have been performed in more than 500 men with EH in different stages. Furthermore, the hemodynamic modulation

M.E. Safar & F. Fouad-Tarazi (eds.), The heart in hypertension.
© *1989 Kluwer Academic Publishers, Dordrecht –*

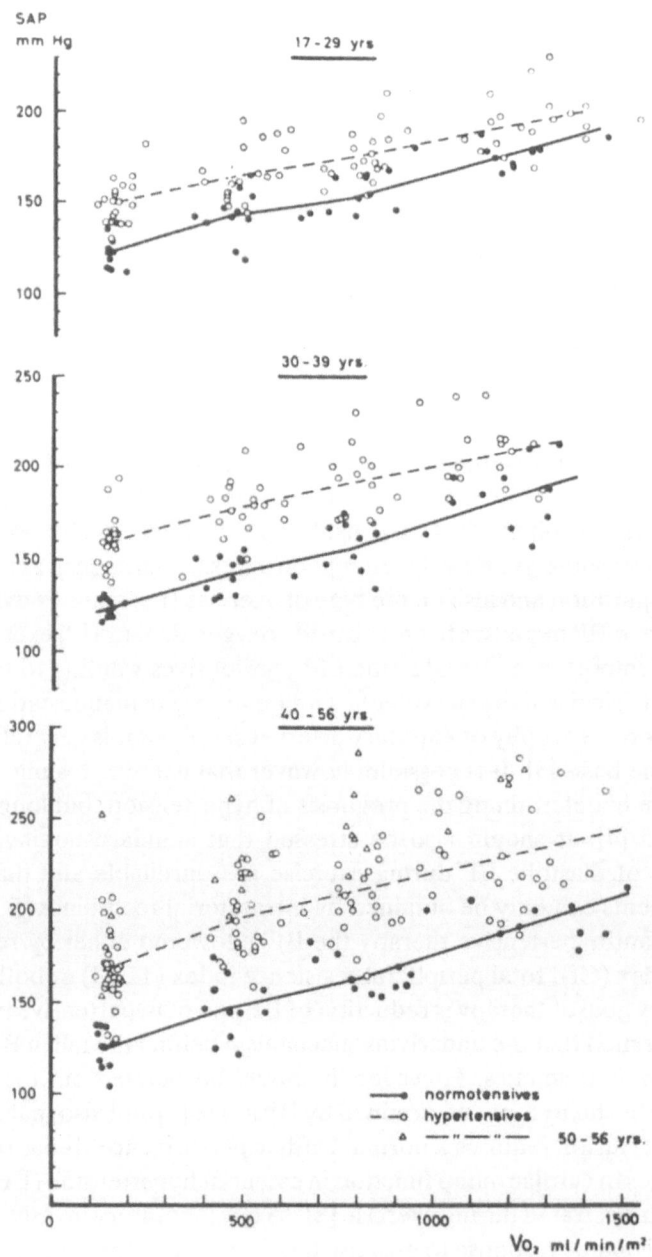

A

Figure 1.

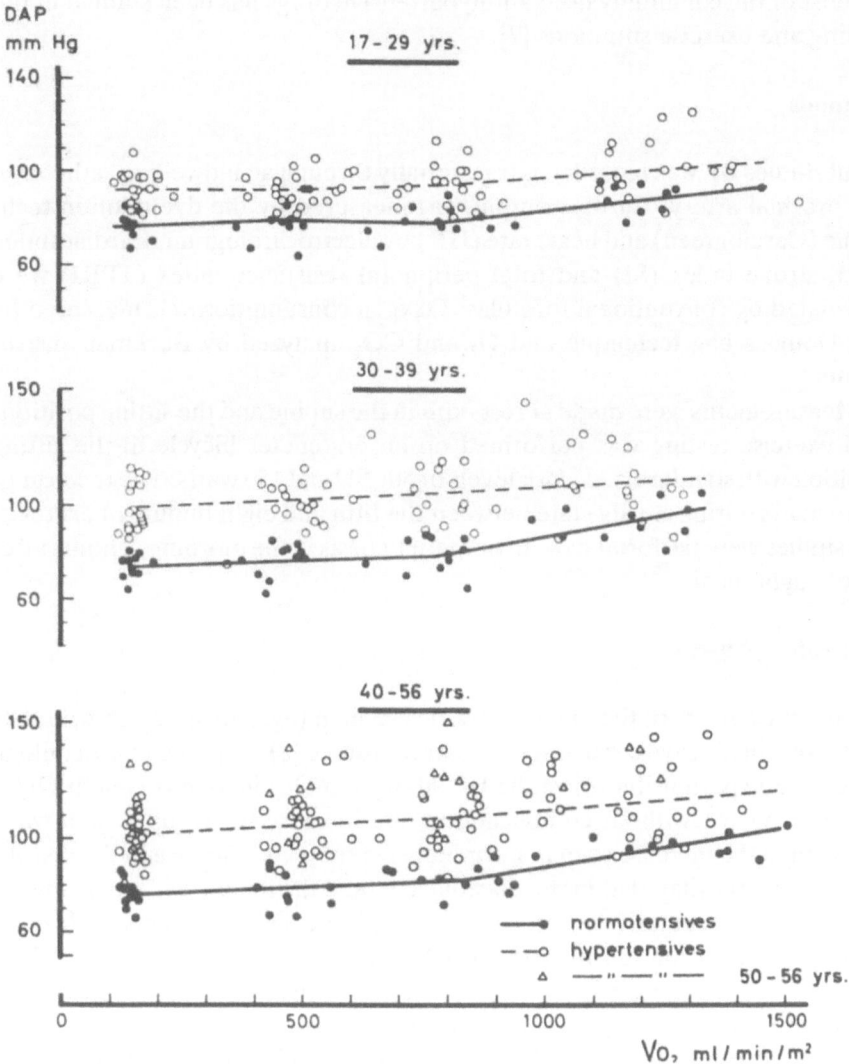

B

Figure 1. Intraarterial systolic (A) and diastolic (B) blood pressure at rest, sitting and during dynamic exercise in normotensive (●) and hypertensive (○) men. The lines represent mean values. VO$_2$ = oxygen uptake.

to most of the commonly used antihypertensive drugs has been studied in the resting and exercise situations [7].

Methods

In all studies BP was recorded intraarterially through an indwelling catheter in the brachial artery. Cardiac output was measured by the dye dilution technique (Cardiogreen) and heart rate (HR) by electrocardiogram. Cardiac index (CI), stroke index (SI) and total peripheral resistance index (TPRI) were calculated by conventional formulas. Oxygen consumption was measured by the Douglas bag technique and O_2 and CO_2 analyzed by Beckman Instruments [8].

Measurements were made at rest both in the supine and the sitting positions and exercise testing was performed on an ergometer bicycle in the sitting position with standardized work levels of 50, 100 and 150 watts. The recordings were made during steady state between the fifth and eight minute of exercise. All studies were performed on an outpatient basis in the morning, 2 hours after a very light meal.

Untreated patients

Dynamic exercise. In the untreated series 93 men (ages 18–65 years) with EH and 33 normotensive control subjects were studied [8]. In patients with mild to moderate hypertension (diastolic BP 90–105 mmHg) in World Health Organization stage I without complications, the increase in BP up to 150 watts parallelled the increase seen in normotensive subjects. The rise in the systolic BP was greater than that in the diastolic BP, and the increase in mean arterial pressure was generally between the two (Figure 1). In patients with more severe hypertension the increase in BP during exercise was steeper. When related to CI the rise in BP also became steeper with increasing age, particularly during severe exercise. Several large invasive studies from the 1960s to the 1980s have confirmed these findings [10–14], and similar results were also reported in a recent noninvasive study [15].

A rise in TPRI is usually considered the hemodynamic hallmark of EH [8] but at rest this was only apparent in the patients with moderate or more severe hypertension. Physical exercise is associated with a fall in TPRI due to increased tissue perfusion. However, for any given level of CI during exercise the TPRI was higher in the hypertensive patients-including those with very mild hypertension – than in the normotensive control subjects. Thus, exercise testing may be useful to disclose early changes in total peripheral vascular resistance.

During exercise the HR increased in proportion with the work load. The

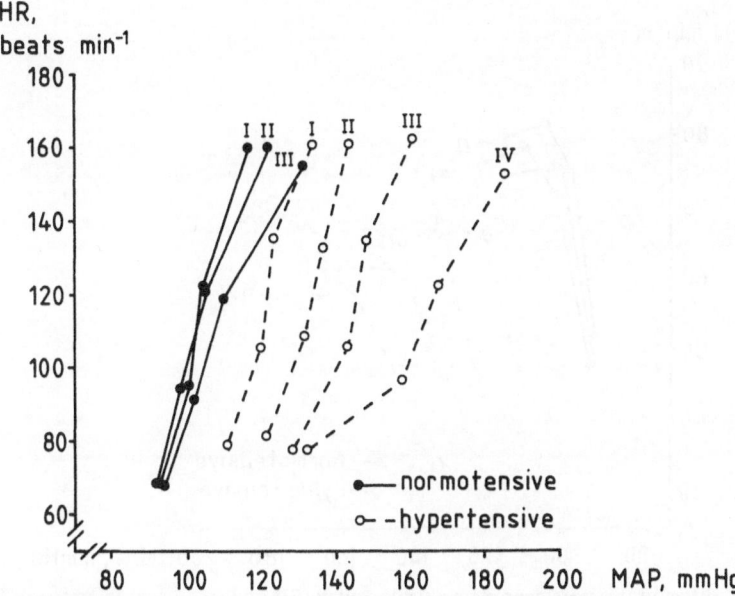

Figure 2. Relationship between heart rate (HR) and mean arterial pressure (MAP) during exercise in normotensive (●) and hypertensive (○) males. (Lund-Johansen, 1967 [8])

ratio between the rise in HR and BP was the same in mild and moderate hypertensives as in the control subjects (range 2.9–5.7 *vs* 2.9–4.6 beats min − $1 \, mmHg^{-1}$) but the curves were shifted to the right (Figure 2).

The SI rapidly increases during exercise – usually by 50% from the SI at rest sitting – reaching a plateau at a workload of about 50 watts. In the young hypertensive patients no change in SI was observed at rest, but during exercise the SI was reduced 15–20% (Figure 3). Thus, in hypertensives early changes in heart pump function may be more readily disclosed during exercise testing than at rest. The patients with more severe hypertension also had lower SI at rest; during exercise the SI was reduced 28% compared with normotensive controls.

It is not known what causes the reduction in SI during exercise in hypertension but one factor might be an increased afterload. However, when comparing the SI during exercise at a fixed level of BP and HR in the hypertensive and normotensive groups the SI is still reduced in the hypertensive patients. Initially it was suggested that the subnormal stroke volume response to exercise was due to incipient coronary artery disease [8]. However, as first pointed out by Tarazi it is well possible that early structural changes may reduce the filling rate of the left ventricle [16, 17]. This has also been supported in recent years by echocardiographic studies and by isotope methods [18].

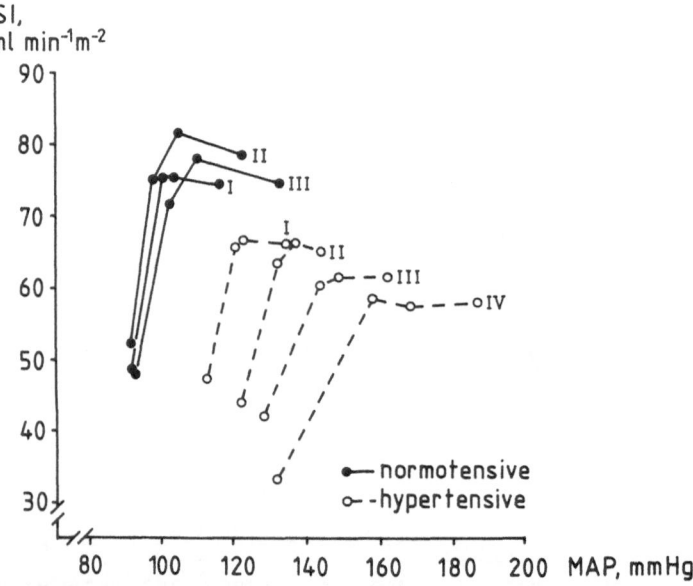

Figure 3. Effect of dynamic exercise on stroke index (SI) and mean arterial pressure (MAP) in normotensive (●) and hypertensive (○) males at different age groups. I = 17–29 years; II = 30–39 years; III = 40–49 years; IV = 50–59 years. (Lund-Johansen, 1967 [8])

Static exercise. Static exercise such as weight lifting and handgrip testing induce marked increases in the systolic as well as the diastolic BP. Figure 4 illustrates the difference between the BP response to dynamic exercise (bicycling) and static exercise (weight lifting). The mechanism of BP rise during static exercise is an increase in CI which is mainly due to an increase in HR [19–21]. The SI is generally not increased, but due to the rise in pressure load the stroke work index and myocardial oxygen demand increase significantly [2, 20]. It has been shown that abnormalities of the filling rate of the left ventricle, suggesting diminished left ventricular compliance may be disclosed in early stages of hypertension during static exercise [22]. This was supported by the demonstration of a greater increase in pulmonary wedge pressure in early essential hypertension. In hypertensive patients the TPRI may increase during isometric exercise while it does not increase significantly in normotensive subjects [23].

The hemodynamic response to isometric work is due to a reflex originating in the contracting muscle and may be elicited by activation of small muscle groups. Correspondingly, the total body oxygen consumption is less than during dynamic exercise and the increase in CI disproportionately large [20]. The difference between the dynamic and isometric exercise seem to be, at least partly, related to active muscle mass since a gradual transition from a 'static' to

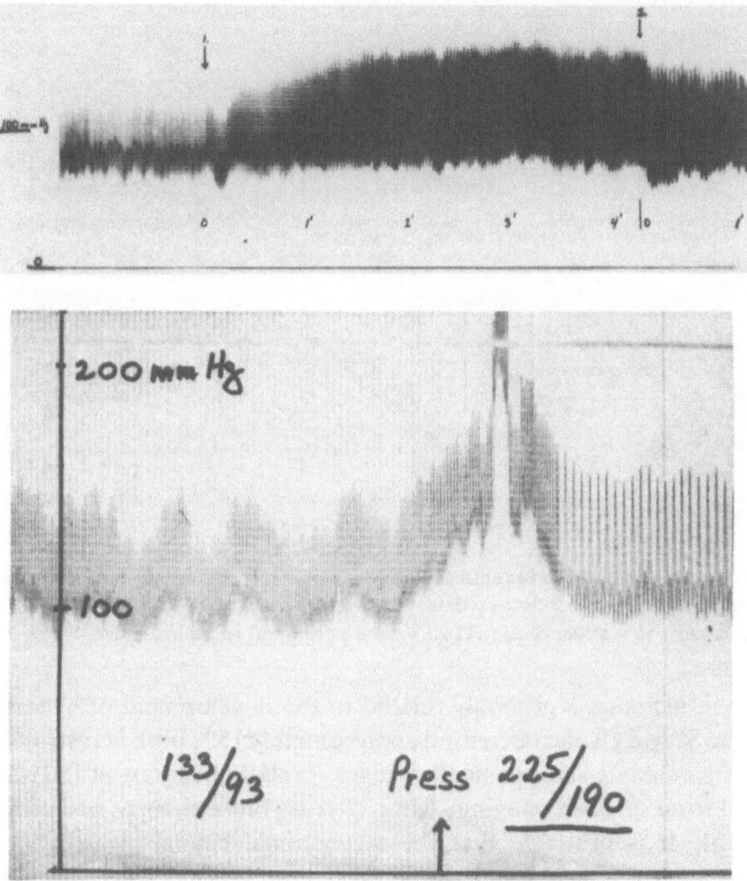

Figure 4. Intraarterial blood pressure in a 65-year-old hypertensive man at rest sitting and during 150 watts bicycle exercise (upper panel), and during maximal static (biceps contraction) exercise (lower panel). Arrows show start of exercise and the numbers the blood pressure.

a 'dynamic' hemodynamic pattern is seen when smaller muscle groups are engaged in dynamic work [24].

Long-term hemodynamic changes in untreated essential hypertension. The patients younger than 40 years left untreated (n = 28) were restudied after 10 years by exactly the same methods as in the first study [25]. Whereas the BP at rest sitting and supine had changed remarkably little over the 10 year period, the BP during severe exercise (150 watts) was slightly but significantly increased. In spite of the small changes in pressure there was an increase of about 25% in TPRI at rest as well as during exercise. Part of this must be due to aging, since a similar increase in TPRI is seen in normotensive subjects, while

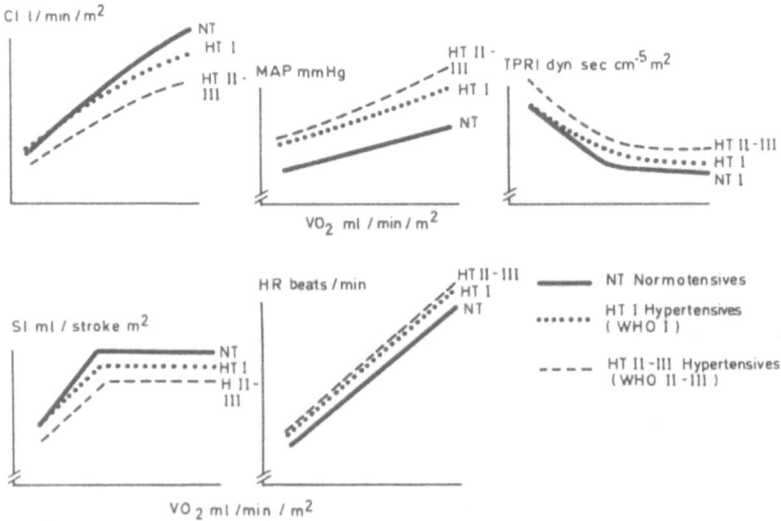

Figure 5. Spontaneous changes in central hemodynamics at rest, sitting and during 50, 100 and 150 watts exercise from 17-year follow-up data. CI = cardiac index; HR = heart rate; MAP = mean arterial pressure; SI = stroke index; TPRI = total peripheral resistance index.

part of the increase is probably related to the development of hypertension itself. The SI and CI had decreased approximately 15% both at rest and during exercise. Heart rate showed small changes – a slight decrease at 150 watts – as expected from 10 years of aging. After 17 years these changes had progressed (Figure 5). It is probable that these functional changes reflect increased stiffness and reduced compliance of the left ventricle and also reduced elasticity – possibly due to structural changes – in the arterioles [26]. In addition to lowering of BP it would be a primary goal to counteract such changes with antihypertensive therapy.

Modulation of exercise hemodynamics by antihypertensive treatment

Diuretics. Few studies have been done on the acute effects of diuretics in hypertensive patients during exercise. At rest the TPRI is unchanged and the decrease in BP is due to reduction in plasma volume and CI [27]. During chronic therapy the decrease in exercise BP is usually similar to that seen at rest, and is maintained through a long-term reduction in TPRI.

In our study of hydrochlorothiazide [28] there was no significant decrease in cardiac pump function either at rest or during exercise, but the SI tended to be slightly decreased during exercise at 150 watts. A similar effect was also seen in a group of severely hypertensive patients during submaximal exercise after

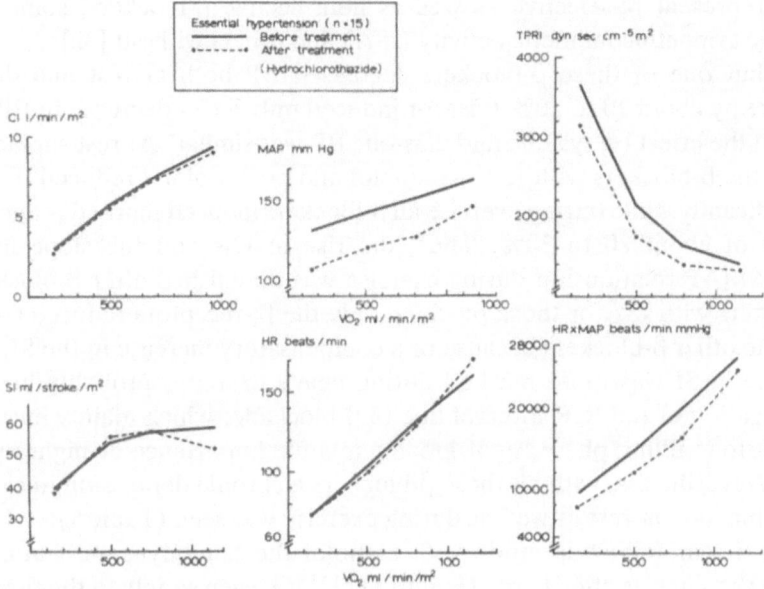

Figure 6. Hemodynamic effects of chronic thiazide therapy (100 mg hydrochlorothiazide daily for 1 year; n = 15). Mean values. Abbreviations as in Figure 5. VO_2 = oxygen uptake.

long-term treatment with the combination of hydrochlorothiazide and captopril [29]. During maximal exercise any factor reducing ventricular filling rate would tend to reduce the SI. Since plasma volume is slightly diminished (7%) during chronic diuretic therapy it is suggested that the fall in SI at the highest level of exercise is due to a reduction in preload.

At the high dosage of hydrochlorothiazide (100 mg) used in our study the fall in TPRI was similar at rest and during exercise – about 15% – but as the subnormal CI was not increased (Figure 6) only partial normalization of central hemodynamics was achieved.

Beta blockers. From an exercise performance point of view, treatment of hypertension with β-blockers seem to be an even greater paradox than it is when using these compounds for treating hypertension during rest. It is well established that short-term effect of the classic β-blocker propranolol is an immediate decrease in HR, SI and CI, a compensatory increase in TPRI and practically no change in BP. Over time, TPRI and BP decrease slowly with propranolol [30] and more rapidly with other β-blockers [31] (Figure 7).
In our laboratory the long-term effects of eight β-blockers (atenolol, metoprolol, timolol, alprenolol, bunitrol, penbutolol, pindolol and visacor) was studied at rest and during exercise in 101 men with mild and moderate EH. The

drugs represent β_1-selective as well as nonselective β-blockers, some with intrinsic sympathicomimetic activity (ISA) and others without [32].

All but one of these β-blockers decreased BP both at rest and during exercise by about 10 to 20% (visacor induced only a 6% decrease in BP). In general the effect on systolic and diastolic BP was similar. At rest supine and sitting the β-blockers with ISA – pindolol and penbutolol – reduced the HR insignificantly while during exercise all β-blockers induced marked reductions in HR of about 20 to 30%. Thus, the rise in HR and the slope of the ΔHR/ΔMAP relationship during exercise was diminished after β-blockade. β-blockers with ISA or those blocking only the β_1-receptors reduced CI less than the other β-blockers because of a compensatory increase in the SI. This increase in SI was more marked during heavy exercise, probably because prolongation of the R-R interval due to β-blockade, which mainly increases the diastolic filling phase, is of greater relative importance at higher pulse rates. Nevertheless, with all these β-blockers a chronic depression in cardiac pump function at rest as well as during exercise was seen (Table 1).

In a 5-year follow-up study with atenolol the hemodynamic status was largely the same as after 1 year (Figure 8) [33]. Oxygen supply to the tissues is maintained by increase in the arteriovenous oxygen difference while muscle blood flow is reduced. The first weeks of treatment with a β-blocker many patients accustomed to vigorous physical activity complain of reduced exercise capacity and a feeling of tiredness and heavy legs (Table 2) [32]. These complaints seem to disappear and most patients are able to continue their level of habitual physical exercise in spite of the long-term depression in CI.

In an extensive study on physical performance and muscle metabolism during β-blockade, Kaiser reported that muscle strength – measured as maximal isokinetic torque- and maximal dynamic muscle power – measured as highest power output during a 30 second maximal cycle-exercise test – were unaltered by β-blockade [34]: However, when maximal exercise was prolonged to 30 to 60 seconds, anaerobic endurance time was decreased and aerobic power – measured as maximal oxygen uptake (VO_2 max) – during cycle exercise was also reduced. When comparing the effects of β_1-selective and nonselective β-blockers on work capacity, no differences were demonstrated with regard to muscle strength, muscle power and VO_2 max. However, anaerobic endurance was decreased more by nonselective than by a β_1-selective β-blocker when similar decreases in HR and VO_2 were attained. This is probably due to different effects of metabolic factors.

Other studies have also failed to show differences between the β_1-selective and the nonselective blockers on short-term isometric and dynamic exercise [35, 36]. However, during long-term exercise it has been shown that propranolol caused a greater reduction in total exercise time than metoprolol [37].

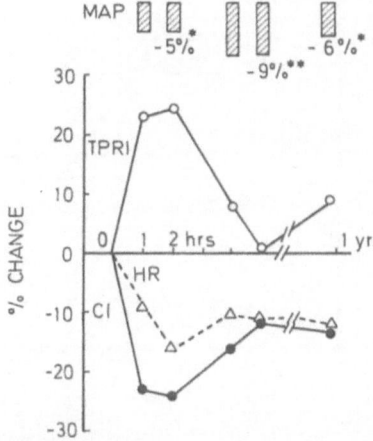

Figure 7. Immediate and chronic hemodynamic effects of the cardioselective β-blocker visacor. Mean values n = 12. Note the decrease in TPRI starting already after 2 hours. Abbreviations as in Figure 5.

Table 1. Relative changes in heart rate, mean arterial pressure and cardiac index of 7 different β-blockers.

Group	n	HR (%)			MAP (%)			CI (%)		
		Rest		Work 100 W	Rest		Work 100 W	Rest		Work 100 W
		Supine	Sitting		Supine	Sitting		Supine	Sitting	
Atenolol	13	− 24	− 28	− 29	− 17	− 17	− 19	− 16	− 27	− 20
Metoprolol	12	− 21	− 24	− 20	− 13	− 11	− 9	− 20	− 24	− 17
Timolol	16	− 26	− 28	− 27	− 18	− 17	− 14	− 28	− 32	− 25
Penbutolol	13	− 23	− 24	− 25	− 17	− 19	− 17	− 20	− 24	− 15
Alprenolol	10	− 20	− 20	− 18	− 11	− 7	− 6	− 13	− 23	− 10
Bunitrolol	11	− 13	− 15	− 17	− 15	− 13	− 12	− 18	− 23	− 24
Pindolol	14	− 11	− 11	− 19	− 15	− 15	− 15	− 13	− 17	− 14

Table 2. Side-effects during start of beta-blocker therapy.

Group	n	Side-effects
Atenolol	13	Muscular fatigue 3
Metoprolol	12	0
Timolol	16	Muscular fatigue 3, Dizzy 1, Cold feet 1
Penbutolol	13	Muscular fatigue 3, Dizzy 2
Alprenolol	10	0
Bunitrolol	11	Muscular fatigue 3
Pindolol	14	Sleeping problems 2, Muscular fatigue 1, Dizzy 1

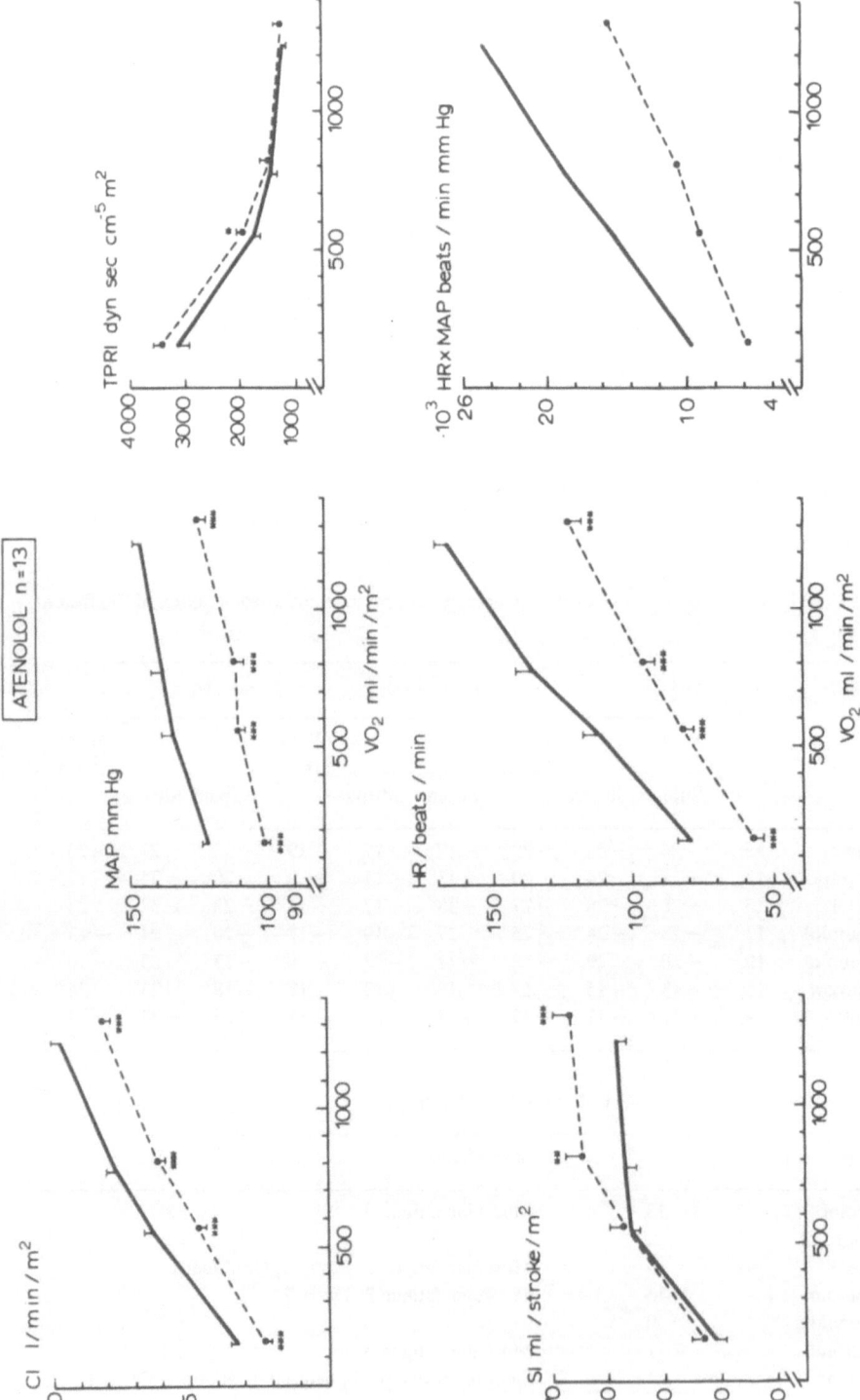

Figure 8. Mean hemodynamic changes at rest sitting and during three exercise levels before (——) and after 1 year (–––) treatment with atenolol. N = 10. Abbreviations as in Figure 5.

Reduced exercise capacity has also been demonstrated after long-term treatment with other β-blockers [38, 39].

For this reason there has been an increasing interest in treating hypertension by drugs that do not cause a decrease in CI or exercise performance, particularly when dealing with very physically active subjects.

Alpha-receptor blockers. Both acutely and chronically the alpha-receptor blockers reduce BP through entirely different hemodynamic mechanisms than the β-blockers. Only a few minutes after doxazosin injection (0.7 to 1.0 mg intravenously) a dramatic decrease in TPRI and in BP (about 9%) is seen without any decrease in CI or any reflex tachycardia [40]. During exercise there is a slight increase in CI (4%) due to a rise in HR while SI is unchanged. After long-term use doxazosin induced an even more marked increase in CI due to a rise in SI while the HR changes were remarkably small. Thus, both at rest and during exercise the fall in BP, which was greater than after the first dose (15 *vs* 9%), was entirely due to a decrease in TPRI (Figure 9). Comparable results with a rise in CI and SI rather than a fall were also observed with prazosin [41]. The results with trimazosin were similar but due to slightly less reduction in TPRI the fall in BP was less pronounced than for the other two quinazoline derivatives [42]. However, all of these compounds with vasodilating properties induce greater normalization in central hemodynamics at rest as well as during dynamic exercise than do diuretics and β-blockers.

Combined alpha and beta receptor blockers. Combination of the effects of β-blockade and vasodilatation has been achieved by compounds like prizidilol [43] and labetalol [44–46]. Short- and long-term hemodynamic studies have shown that the combined alpha and beta blocker labetalol induces a marked decrease in BP at rest as well as during exercise of about 15 to 25%, partly through a decrease in TPRI (by alpha blockade) and partly by a decrease in HR and CI (by beta blockade). In patients with severe EH the immediate fall in BP was correlated with the reduction in CI, mainly due to a fall in HR [47]. However, during long-term treatment the SI increases both at rest and during exercise, thereby compensating for the decrease in HR. Thus, the fall in CI during long-term treatment with labetalol is much less than that achieved by pure β-blockade. In a 6-year follow-up the CI had returned to pretreatment (but slightly subnormal) level, and the decrease in BP was entirely due to reduction in TPRI [46]. Combined alpha and beta receptor blockade might therefore also serve to partly normalize central hemodynamics in EH.

Calcium blockers. Although all the calcium antagonists used in hypertension basically have the same mode of action-reduction in TPRI by arteriolar smooth muscle relaxation due to blockade of slow channel calcium transport

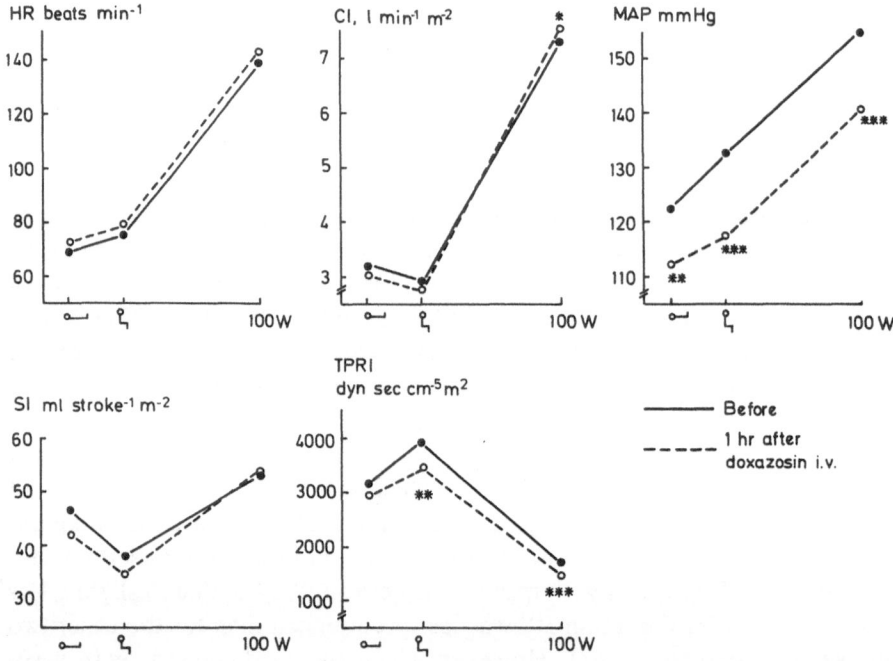

Figure 9. Acute hemodynamic profile of doxazosin. Mean values ± 1 SEM. N = 12. Abbreviations as in Figure 5. ⌐ = at rest supine; ↳ = at rest sitting; 100 W = during 100 watts bicycle exercise.

[48] – it should be emphasized that the effect on HR varies. The negative inotropic effect demonstrated experimentally does not seem to be of clinical significance.

Verapamil decreases TPRI and BP at reast and during exercise. The HR at rest is hardly affected, but during exercise it is reduced by approximately 10% (hence, much less than by conventional beta blockade). There is a compensatory increase in SI, probably due to prolonged diastolic filling phase. Thus, no impairment in heart pump function, measured as CI, is seen either at rest or during dynamic exercise [49].

Diltiazem induces similar hemodynamic effects both at rest and during exercise as verapamil [50]. In a comparison with propranolol in hypertensive patients Yakamodo et al. reported that both propranolol and diltiazem reduced BP and HR at rest and during exercise, but the decrease in HR was greatest with propranolol [51]. In that study maximal exercise duration was not different while in another placebo controlled study Pool et al. found that diltiazem increased the maximum duration of exercise [52]. In a study on the short-term effects of diltiazem (0.2 mg per kg intravenously) on central and peripheral hemodynamics a decrease in TPRI was found and also dilatation of large arteries [53]. Cardiac index and HR increased initially, but returned to pretreatment values while TPRI and BP remained reduced. Comparable hemodynamic changes as with diltiazem and verapamil – fall in TPRI at rest as well as during exercise and a moderate reduction in HR with compensatory increase in SI during exercise – were also found with tiapamil [54]. Shortly after the first dose a small increase in HR (reflex tachycardia) is observed but the effect disappears during long-term treatment.

When treatment with calcium channel blockers of the dihydropyridine derivatives is begun, central hemodynamics change very quickly. In an acute study on nisoldipine, we found that 1 hour after a 10 mg oral dose TPRI had decreased 20%. The decrease in BP was partly counteracted by reflex tachycardia (12% increase in HR) leading to an increase in CI, but still the immediate decrease in BP was 10% [55]. With continued treatment reflex tachycardia disappeared and 1 year after treatment was started HR was unchanged and the fall in BP (about 15%) was related to a decrease in TPRI (about 18%) at rest as well as during exercise (Figure 10).

Also with nifedipine the long-term hemodynamic effect is a reduction in BP and TPRI of about 17% both at rest and during exercise without any changes in HR, SI or CI [56]. Neither with nisoldipine nor with nifedipine there were any complaints of reduced physical capacity. Because SI was subnormal before therapy and because a fall in TPRI implies afterload reduction, an increase in SI after 1 year was expected but was not found. It is possible that the lack of increase in exercise SI could be related to a slight degree of negative ionotropic effect of both nifedipine and nisoldipine that is not seen in the resting situation but unveiled during exercise. Since development of peripheral edema is seen in some patients treated with dihydropyridine calcium blockers, it is suggested that reduced preload due to smaller intravascular volume could contribute to the small reduction in SI. However, plasma volume and extracellular fluid volume measurements did not reveal any significant changes in body fluid distribution [54, 55].

Also other dihydropyridine derivatives, nitrendipine, felodipine and amlodipine have been reported to induce good BP control during exercise [57, 58].

In summary, the calcium blockers have been shown to induce satisfactory control of BP at rest and during exercise. The decrease in BP is clearly related to reduction in TPRI without any decrease in cardiac pump function measured as CI at rest and with a modest reduction during exercise. However, the subnormal CI seen in untreated hypertensive patients is not corrected. Complaints of reduced physical capacity have not been reported and a few studies have indicated a slight increase in endurance time-in contrast to β-blocker treatment, which tends to diminish physical capacity.

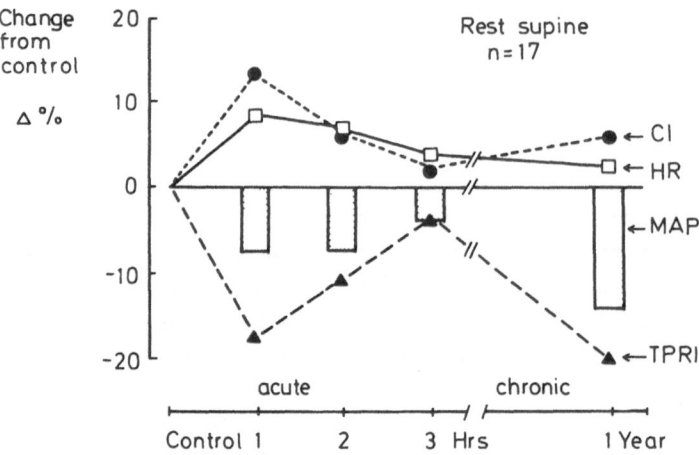

Figure 10. Acute and chronic hemodynamic effects of nisoldipine at rest and during exercise in essential hypertension. N = 19. Abbreviations as in Figure 5.

Angiotensin converting enzyme inhibitors. The angiotensin converting enzyme (ACE) inhibitors is a new and important class of antihypertensive agents that induce satisfactory BP control at rest as well as during exercise. In our study on enalapril BP was reduced 28/17 mmHg (13%) during 150 watts bicycle exercise and 34/19 mmHg (20%) at rest sitting after 1 year treatment (Figure 11). Both at rest and during exercise the reduction in BP was entirely due to reduction in TPRI while the SI and CI remained unchanged [59]. In spite of the marked vasodilatation there was no reflex tachycardia.

All of these patients were actively working and many were engaged in vigorous physical activity (jogging, skiing) but no one had any complaints about reduced physical capacity.

The group of patients treated with captopril also demonstrated significant reduction in TPRI at rest, but during exercise the reduction in BP was due to fall in CI and SI while the HR was unaltered [29]. It is possible that the reduction in SI during work in these patients was related to the more advanced hypertensive disease (WHO class II and III) with an average intraarterial BP at rest sitting of 205/119 mmHg (as opposed to 184/108 mmHg in the enalapril study). Nevertheless, ACE inhibitors seem to induce adequat BP reduction both at rest and during physical exercise even in patients with severe EH. However, as with the calcium blockers the ACE inhibitors only partially normalize the central hemodynamics of EH since the subnormal CI is not increased.

Other antihypertensive drugs. The hemodynamic modulations induced by other antihypertensive agents will be discussed very briefly (see reference 7 for

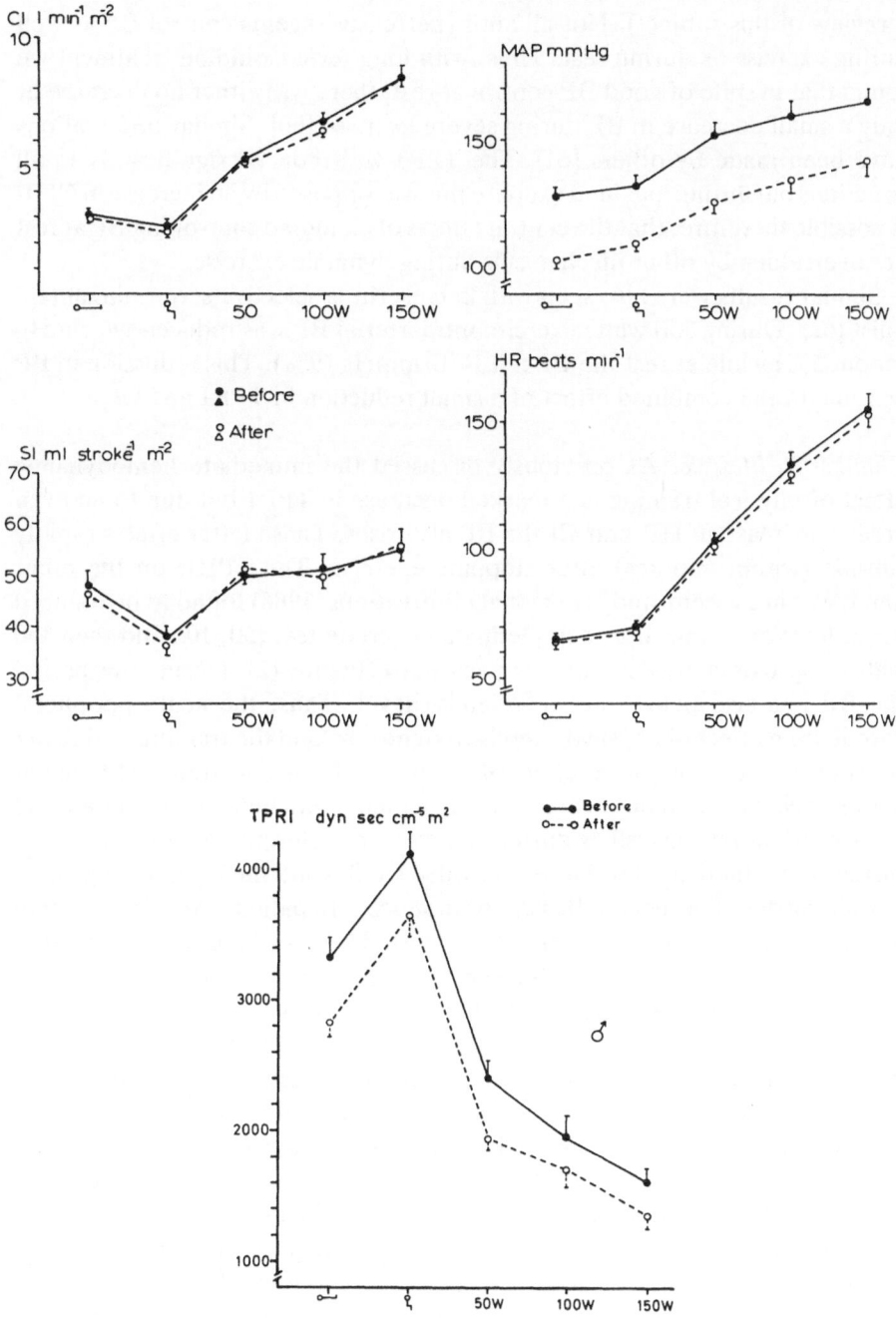

Figure 11. Hemodynamic long-term effects of enalapril at rest and during exercise in 12 essential hypertensive males. Mean values ± 1 SEM. Cardiac index (CI), stroke index (SI), heart rate (HR) and mean arterial pressure (MAP), total peripheral resistance index (TPRI).

a review of this subject). Not all antihypertensive agents control BP as well during exercise as during rest. Thus, with long-term clonidine treatment we found that in spite of good BP control at rest, there was either no decrease or only a small decrease in BP during severe exercise [60]. Similar observations have been made by others [61]. The TPRI was reduced significantly in all situations but during maximal exercise this was opposed by an increase in CI. It is possible therefore, that the central effects of clonidine controlling BP at rest are overridden by other mechanisms during dynamic exercise.

Similar results were also seen with ketanserin, a selective serotonin$_2$ antagonist [62]. During 150 watts exercise intraarterial BP was reduced 9/6 mmHg (about 5%) while at rest the BP fell 14/10 mmHg (9%). This reduction in BP was due to the combined effect of a small reduction in TPRI and CI.

Changes in lifestyle. As previously discussed the immediate hemodynamic effect of physical training is a marked decrease in TPRI but due to an even greater increase in HR and CI the BP also rises. These latter effects rapidly subside (within minutes) after stopping exercise. The TPRI, on the other hand, was in a recent study (personal observations, 1986) found to be reduced for at least one hour after completing an exercise test (50, 100 and then 150 watts; approximately 8 minutes at each step) (Figure 12). During this period the BP was also below the pre-exercise level. Thus, the acute peripheral vasodilating effect of physical exercise extends beyond the training period *per se*. However, the long-term effect of training of BP is uncertain. Although it has been claimed that physical training in patients with mild and moderate EH reduces BP at rest as well as during exercise (see reference 63 for a review of this subject), there are few large controlled studies and the BP lowering effect of training does not seem to be very pronounced. In patients with more severe hypertension, drug treatment should be started first, and it is unclear whether physical training will lower BP further. However, because endurance training has other beneficial effects on the heart; e.g. an increase in end diastolic volume, myocardial contraction and in SI- and on systemic circulation in general, it should be encouraged in hypertensive patients. Furthermore, regular physical training often leads to other beneficial lifestyle changes like stopping smoking, less caloric intake and weight reduction.

Low salt diet was advokated in the 1940'ies by Kempner and others for treatment of hypertension [64]. In the 1970'ies sodium restriction was revived as antihypertensive therapy, first by Parijs [65] and later by Morgan [66] and many other investigators. However, the efficacy of low salt diet in the treatment of mild EH has been disputed [67, 68]. In a group of 19 men with borderline or mild hypertension we studied the effect of a 35% cut in salt intake (from 210 mmols per day). After about 1 year the changes in BP at rest as well as during exercise were disappointingly small – only about a 4%

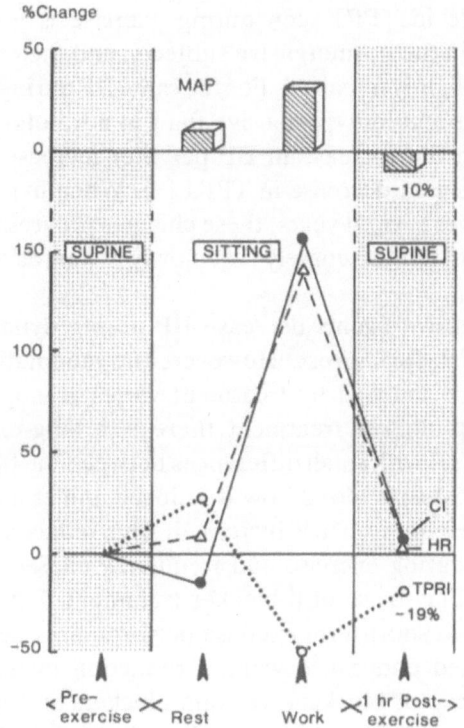

Figure 12. Hemodynamic changes induced by 150 watt bicycle exercise and then followed by one hour supine rest in 11 essential hypertensive patients. Mean values. Shaded areas indicate supine position and open area sitting position. Abbreviations as in Figure 5.

decrease in intraarterial BP [69]. The modest BP reduction was associated with a decrease in CI, partly due to a slight decrease in HR and partly due to a slight decrease in SI. There was no reduction in TPRI, either at rest or during exercise.

Conclusions

Exercise testing challenges left ventricular pump function and is useful in evaluation of the functional capacity of the heart and the circulatory control mechanisms. However, exercise testing is time-consuming and the difficulty in obtaining accurate diastolic BP measurements during exercise makes it unlikely that such testing will be used to any great extent in the diagnostic work-up of hypertensive patients. In untreated patients with mild to moderate hypertension, the BP response to dynamic exercise is similar to what is seen in normotensive age-matched control subjects, but the hemodynamic changes differ. The decrease in TPRI seen during exercise is less marked in the hypertensives than in the normotensive subjects, and the cardiac pump function during work is slightly impaired. For the same BP during dynamic exercise the stroke volume is less in hypertensive than in normotensives. With more severe hypertension the increase in BP per liter increase in CI is steeper, reflecting the insufficient decrease in TPRI [9]. When hypertensive subjects are left untreated over several years, these changes progress. The heart pump function deteriorates, but fortunately very slowly as long as coronary disease is not developed [25].

Most antihypertensive agents decrease BP during dynamic exercise to a similar extent as that during rest. However, the modulation of the central hemodynamic profile induced by treatment varies greatly for the different compounds. With β-blocker treatment there is a long-term depression in cardiac output and HR with small differences between the β_1-selective and the nonselective drugs. Muscle blood flow is reduced and as a compensation the arteriovenous oxygen difference is increased. This reduced heart pump function is maintained during exercise and frequently causes impaired physical capacity in the starting phase of β-blocker treatment. During chronic treatment the reduction in short-term exercise performance seems to be modest, but during prolonged endurance work a reduction in the performance is common. Alpha receptor blockers, calcium blockers and ACE inhibitors all reduce BP at rest as well as during exercise by a decrease in TPRI, but through very different mechanisms. The calcium antagonists of dihydropyridine-type cause initial reflex tachycardia; in contrast, verapamil and diltiazem tend to decrease the HR, especially during work. During long-term use the reflex tachycardia tends to disappear also for the dihydropyridine derivatives. The calcium antagonists do not decrease CI or muscle blood flow, and complaints of reduced physical capacity are rare. Some studies indicate an increased endurance time. Although all of these compounds – alpha blockers, calcium blockers and ACE inhibitors – induce afterload reduction through peripheral vasodilatation, only alpha blockers have been shown to increase the slightly subnormal CI at rest as well as during exercise. An additional beneficial effect of the ACE inhibitors is regression of left ventricular hypertrophy [70] but in spite of this there is no increase in cardiac output either at rest or during exercise.

Today a large variety of antihypertensive agents are available. It is still not known which type of antihypertensive treatment will lead to the best prognosis with respect to morbidity and mortality. Large-scale trials have been designed to define the cardiovascular protective effect of the newer classes of antihypertensive drugs [71], but as long as this is unsettled, it would seem logical to treat – in particular physically active patients – with drugs that will not reduce heart pump function or physical endurance. All the vasodilating antihypertensive drugs would suit these requirements.

References

1. Mitchell JH, Blomquist G, Haskell WL, James FW, Miller Jr HS, Miller WW, Strong WB (1985): Classification of sports. *JACC* 6: 1198–1199.
2. Sarnoff SJ, Braunwald E, Welch Jr GH, Case RB, Stainsby WN, Macruz R (1958): Hemodynamic determinants of oxygen consumption of the heart with special reference to the tension-time index. *Am J Physiol* 192: 148.
3. Frohlich ED, Lowenthal DT, Miller Jr HS, Pickering TH, Strong WB (1985): Task force IV: Systemic arterial hypertension. *JACC* 6: 1218–1221.
4. Dlin RA, Hanne N, Silverberg DS, Bar-Or O (1983): Follow-up of normal men with exaggerated blood pressure response to exercise. *Am Heart J* 106: 316–320.
5. Rasmussen PH, Staats BA, Driscoll DJ, Beck KC, Bonekat W, Wilcox WD (1985): Direct and indirect blood pressure during exercise. *Chest* 87: 743–748.
6. Karlfors T, Nielsen R, Westling H (1966): On the accuracy of indirect auscultatory blood pressure measurement during exercise. *Acta Med Scand* 180 (suppl 449): 91–102.
7. Lund-Johansen P (1988): Haemodynamic effects of antihypertensive agents, in: Doyle AE (ed), *Handbook of Hypertension*. Vol. 5: *Clinical Pharmacology of Antihypertensive Drugs*, pp 41–72. Amsterdam: Elsevier Science Publishers.
8. Lund-Johansen P (1967): Haemodynamic changes in early essential hypertension. *Acta Med Scand* suppl 482: 1–102.
9. Lund-Johansen P (1983): The hemodynamics of essential hypertension. in: Robertson JIS (ed), *Handbook of Hypertension*, Vol. 1: *Clinical Aspects of Essential Hypertension*, pp 151–173. Amsterdam: Elsevier Science Publishers.
10. Sannerstedt R (1966): Hemodynamic response to exercise in patients with arterial hypertension. *Acta Med Scand* 180 (suppl 458): 1–83.
11. Amery A, Julius S, Whitlock LS, Conway J (1967): Influence of hypertension on the hemodynamic response to exercise. *Circulation* 36: 231–237.
12. Julius S, Amery A, Whitlock LS, Conway J (1967): Influence of age on the hemodynamic response to exercise. *Circulation* 36: 222–230.
13. Levy AM, Tabakin BS, Hanson JS (1967): Hemodynamic responses to graded treadmill exercise in young untreated labile hypertensive patients. *Circulation* 35: 1063–1072.
14. Widimsky J, Jandova R, Ressl J (1981): Haemodynamic studies in juvenile hypertension at rest and during supine exercise. *Eur Heart J* 2: 307–315.
15. Schulte W, Fehring C, Neus H (1983): Cardiovascular reactivity to ergometric exercise in mild hypertension. *Cardiology* 70: 50–56.
16. Tarazi RC, Ferrario CM, Dustan HP (1977): The heart in hypertension. in: Genest J, Koiw E, Kuchel O (eds), *Hypertension*, pp 738–754. New York: McGraw-Hill Book.
17. Averill DB, Ferrario CM, Tarazi RC, Sen S, Bajbus R (1976): Cardiac performance in rats with renal hypertension. *Circ Res* 38: 280–288.
18. Fouad FM, Tarazi RC, Gallagher JM, McIntyre WJ, Cook SA (1980): Abnormal left ventricular relaxation in hypertensive patients. *Clin Sci* 59: 411S–415S.
19. Perez-Gonzales JF, Schiller NB, Parmley WW (1981): Direct and non-invasive evaluation of the cardiovascular response to isometric exercise. *Circ Res* 48 (suppl 1): I 138–148.

20. Shepherd JT, Blomquist CG, Lind AR, Mitchell JH, Saltin B (1981): Static (isometric) exercise. Retrospection and introspection. *Circ Res* 48 (suppl 1): I 179–188.

21. Keul J, Dickhuth H-H, Simon G, Lehman M (1981): Effect of static and dynamic exercise on heart volume, contractility, and left ventricular dimensions. *Circ Res* 48 (suppl 1): I 161–170.

22. Alicandri C, Fouad FM, Tarazi RC, Bravo EL, Greenstreet RL (1983): Sympathetic contribution to the cardiac response to stress in hypertension. *Hypertension* 5: 147–154.

23. Dustan HP, Tarazi RC, Bravo EL (1973): Physiologic characteristics of hypertension, in: Laragh JH (ed), *Hypertension manual,* pp 227–256. New York: Dun-Donnelly Publishing Corporation.

24. Blomquist CG, Lewis SF, Taylor WF, Graham RM (1981): Similarity of the hemodynamic responses to static and dynamic exercise of small muscle groups. *Circ Res* 48 (suppl 1): I 87–92.

25. Lund-Johansen P (1979): Spontaneous changes in central hemodynamics in essential hypertension – a 10-year follow-up study, in: Onesti G, Klimt CR (eds), *Hypertension.* Determinants, complications, and intervention, pp 201–209. New York: Grune & Stratton.

26. Folkow B (1985): Vascular changes in hypertension. Therapeutic considerations. *Drugs* 29 (suppl 2): 1–8.

27. Dustan HP, Bravo EL, Tarazi RC (1973): Volume-dependent essential and steroid hypertensions. *Am J Cardiol* 31: 606–615.

28. Lund-Johansen P (1970): Hemodynamic changes in long-term diuretic therapy of essential hypertension. *Acta Med Scand* 187: 509–518.

29. Omvik P, Lund-Johansen P (1984): Combined captopril and hydrochlorothiazide therapy in severe hypertension: long-term haemodynamic changes at rest and during exercise. *J Hypertension* 2: 73–80.

30. Tarazi RC, Dustan HP (1972): Beta-adrenergic blockade in hypertension. *Am J Cardiol* 29: 633–640.

31. Lund-Johansen P, Omvik P, Haugland H (1984): The first dose hemodynamic responses to visacor. (ICI 141 292) in essential hypertension. *Acta Med Scand* suppl 693: 121–125.

32. Lund-Johansen P (1983): Central haemodynamic effects of beta-blockers in hypertension. A comparison between atenolol, metoprolol, timolol, penbutolol, alprenolol, pindolol and bunitrolol. *Eur Heart J* 4 (suppl D): 1–12.

33. Lund-Johansen P (1979): Hemodynamic consequences of long-term beta-blocker therapy – a 5-year follow-up study of atenolol. *J Cardiovasc Pharmacol* 1: 487–495.

34. Kaiser P (1984): Physical performance and muscle metabolism during beta-adrenergic blockade in man. *Acta Physiol Scand* suppl 536: 1–44.

35. Houben H, Thien T, de Boo T, Lemmens W, Binkhorst R, van 't Larr A (1983): Hemodynamic effects of isometric exercise and mental arithmetic in hypertension treated with selective and nonselective beta-blockade. *Clin Pharmacol Ther* 34: 164–169.

36. Leenen FHH, Coenen CHM, Zonderland M, Maas AHJ (1980): Effects of cardioselective and nonselective beta-blockade on dynamic exercise performance in mildly hypertensive men. *Clin Pharmacol Ther* 28: 12–21.

37. Lundborg P, Astrom H, Bengtsson C, Fellenius E, von Schenck H, Svensson L, Smith U (1981): Effect of beta-adrenoceptor blockade on exercise performance and metabolism. *Clin Sci* 61: 299–305.

38. von Lehmann M, Keuhl J, Wybitul K, Fischer H. Auswirkung einer selektiven und nicht-selektiven Adrenozeptorblockade während Korparbeit auf den Energiestoffwechsel und das sympatho-adrenerge System. *Drug Res* 32: 261–266.

39. Kindermann W, Scheerer W, Salas-Fraire O, Biro G, Wolfing A (1984): Verhalten der korperlichen Leistungsfähigkeit und des Metabolismus unter akuter Beta$_1$- und Beta$_2$-Blockade. *Z Kardiol* 73: 380–387.

40. Lund-Johansen P, Omvik P, Haugland H (1986): Acute and chronic haemodynamic effects of

doxazosin in hypertension at rest and during exercise. *Br J Clin Pharmacol* 2i (suppl): 45s–54s.

41. Lund-Johansen P (1975): Hemodynamic changes at rest and during exercise in long-term prazosin therapy for essential hypertension. *Postgrad Med J* 58 (suppl 1): 45–52.

42. Omvik P, Lund-Johansen P (1987): Review of central haemodynamic effects of alpha-blockers and their future use in essential hypertension. *Br J Clin Practice* 41 (syppl 54): 15–21.

43. Lund-Johansen P, Omvik P (1982): Prizidilol in essential hypertension: long-term effects on plasma volume, extracellular fluid volume, and central hemodynamics at rest and during exercise. *J Cardiovasc Pharmacol* 4: 1012–1017.

44. Fagard R, Lijnen P, Amery A (1982): Response of the systemic and pulmonary circulation to labetalol at rest and during exercise. *Br J Clin Pharmacol* 13 (suppl 1) 13S–17S.

45. Koch G (1979): Haemodynamic adaptation at rest and during exercise to long-term anti-hypertensive treatment with combined alpha- and beta-adrenoceptor blockade by labetalol. *Br Heart J* 41: 192–198.

46. Lund-Johansen P (1983): Short- and long-term (six year) hemodynamic effects of labetalol in essential hypertension. *Am J Med* 74: 24–31.

47. Omvik P, Lund-Johansen P (1982): Acute hemodynamic effects of labetalol in severe hypertension. *J Cardiovasc Pharmacol* 4: 915–920.

48. Fleckenstein A (1977): Specific pharmacology of calcium in myocardium, cardiac pacemakers, and vascular smooth muscle. *Annu Rev Pharmacol Toxicol* 17: 149–166.

49. Lund-Johansen P (1984): Hemodynamic long-term effects of verapamil in essential hypertension at rest and during exercise. *Acta Med Scand* Suppl 681: 109–115.

50. Aoki K, Sato K, Kondo S, Yamamoto M (1983): Hypotensive effects of diltiazem to normals and essential hypertension. *Eur J Clin Pharmacol* 25: 475–480.

51. Yakamodo T, Oonishi N, Kondo S, Noziri A, Nakano T, Takezawa H (1983): Effects of diltiazem on cardiovascular responses during exercise in systemic hypertension and comparison with propranolol. *Am J Cardiol* 52: 1023–1027.

52. Pool PE, Seagren SC, Salel AF, Skalland ML (1985): Effects of diltiazem on serum lipids, exercise performance and blood pressure: randomized, double blind, placebo-controlled evaluation for systemic hypertension. *Am J Cardiol* 56: 86H–91H.

53. Safar ME, Simon AC, Levenson JA, Cazor JL (1983): Hemodynamic effects of diltiazem in hypertension. *Circ Res* 52 (suppl 1): 174–181.

54. Omvik P, Lund-Johansen P (1989): Acute and long-term hemodynamic effects of tiapamil at rest and during exercise in essential hypertension. *Cardiovasc Drugs Ther* (in press).

55. Omvik P, Lund-Johansen P, Haugland H (1987): Nisoldipine: central hemodynamic effects at rest and during exercise in essential hypertension. Acute and chronic studies. *J Hypertension* 6: 95–103.

56. Lund-Johansen P, Omvik P (1983): Haemodynamic effects of nifedipine in essential hypertension at rest and during exercise. *J Hypertension* 1: 159–163.

57. Franz I-W, Wiewel D (1984): Antihypertensive effects on blood pressure at rest and during exercise of calcium antagonists, beta-receptor blockers, and their combination in hypertensive patients. *J Cardiovasc Pharmacol* 6: S1037–S1042.

58. Lorimer AR, McAlpine HM, Rae AP, Simpson IA, Barbour MP, Forret EA, Kent Hill TW, Veitch Lawrie TD (1985): Effects of felodipine on rest and exercise heart rate and blood pressure in hypertensive patients. *Drugs* 29 (suppl 2): 154–164.

59. Lund-Johansen P, Omvik P (1984): Long-term haemodynamic effects of enalapril (alone and in combination with hydrochlorothiazide) at rest and during exercise in essential hypertension. *J Hypertension* 2 (suppl 2): 49–56.

60. Lund-Johansen P (1976): Hemodynamic effects of clonidine in man, in: Onesti G, Fernandes

M, Kim KE (eds), *Regulation of blood pressure by the central nervous sytem,* pp 355–365. New York: Grune & Stratton.

61. Virtanen K, Janne J, Frick MH (1982): Response of blood pressure and plasma norepine-phrine to propranolol, metoprolol and clonidine during isometric and dynamic exercise in hypertensive patients. *Eur J Clin Pharmacol* 21: 275–279.

62. Omvik P, Lund-Johansen P (1983): Long-term effects on central hemodynamics and body-fluid volumes of ketanserin in essential hypertension. Studies at rest and during exercise. *J Hypertension* 1: 405–412.

63. Martin JE, Dubbert PM (1987): The role of exercise in preventing and moderating blood pressure elevation, in: Blaufox MD, Langford HG (eds), *Non-pharmacologic therapy of hypertension,* pp 120–142. Basel: Karger.

64. Kempner W (1948): Treatment of hypertensive vascular disease with rice diet. *Am J Med* 4: 545–577.

65. Parijs J, Joosens JV, Van der Linden L, Verstreken G, Amery AKPC (1973): Moderate sodium restriction and diuretics in the treatment of hypertension. *Am Heart J* 25: 22–34.

66. Morgan T, Gillies A, Morgan G, Adam W, Wilson M, Carney S (1978): Hypertension treated by salt restriction. *Lancet* 1978/1: 227–230.

67. Simpson FO (1979): Salt and hypertension: a sceptical review of the evidence. *Clin Sci* 57: 463S–469S.

68. Swales JD (1980): Dietary salt and hypertension. *Lancet* 1980/1: 1177–1179.

69. Omvik P, Lund-Johansen P (1986): Is sodium restriction effective treatment of borderline and mild essential hypertension? A long-term hemodynamic study at rest and during exercise. *J Hypertension* 4: 535–541.

70. Fouad FM, Tarazi RC, Bravo EL (1983): Cardiac and hemodynamic effects of enalapril. *J Hypertension* 1 (suppl 1): 135–142.

71. Stamler J, Prineas RJ, Neaton JD, Grimm RH, McDonald RH, Schnapper HW, Schoenber-ger JA, Elmer PJ, Cutler JA (1987): Background and design of the new U.S. trial on diet and drug treatment of 'mild' hypertension. *Am J Cardiol* 59: 51G–60G.

35. Reversion of cardiac, arteriolar and arterial changes following antihypertensive treatment

PIERRE G. CARLIER, NICOLE S. SMELTEN and
GEORGES L. RORIVE

The goal of an antihypertensive treatment is to reduce and ultimately suppress the excess of mortality and morbidity caused by hypertension. The current therapeutic strategies have, at least partly, failed to fulfil this criterium: the coronary events, the most frequent complications in mild and moderate hypertensive patients, do not unambiguously diminish following antihypertensive therapy [1]. The cardiovascular structural changes might play a crucial role in this situation and it is now widely accepted that the normalisation of the cardiovascular structures should be the second objective of hypertension treatment [2]. Unfortunately, the conditions to meet for an optimal prevention or regression of the structural changes are still largely unknown. This might be attributed for one part to the multiplicity of the possible remodeling patterns during the natural course of hypertension (another illustration of Page's mosaic theory) and for another to the diversity of the responses to the antihypertensive agents. Because of these difficulties in collecting, interpreting and integrating the scientific data, the therapeutic guidelines available at the present time are often confined to quasi-dogmatic considerations, inappropriate for an optimal reversion of the structural changes.

In this brief review, we shall not consider the possibilities and the conditions of regression of cardiac hypertrophy, a topic discussed in detail in the previous chapters, and we shall primarily analyze the response of cardiac hypertrophy in relation to the arterial remodeling during therapy. We shall address a number of questions pertinent for a definition of therapeutic strategies aiming both at the correction of hypertension and the reversion of the associated structural changes. They are:
1) is the course of arteriolar hypertrophy reversible and dependent on blood pressure level?
2) is the course of large arteries hypertrophy reversible and dependent on blood pressure level?

M.E. Safar & F. Fouad-Tarazi (eds.), The heart in hypertension.
© *1989 Kluwer Academic Publishers, Dordrecht –*

3) do the cardiac, arterial and arteriolar structural changes respond similarly to an antihypertensive treatment or do they possibly show divergent evolutions?
4) do the major cellular processes (i.e. cell proliferation, cell hypertrophy, extracellular matrix accumulation) that result in a tissue macroscopic hypertrophy respond in block to an antihypertensive treatment or do they evolve independently?
5) does the duration of hypertension condition the reversibility of the structural changes?
6) are monotherapy and drugs associations equipotent?
7) are all classes of antihypertensive agents equivalent or is one or several types of drugs specially effective in controlling hypertrophy?
8) are there non-antihypertensive drugs that can heal the hypertensive structural changes?
9) can the course of atherosclerosis be modified by some antihypertensive agents?

Regression of arteriolar hypertrophy:
Can it be achieved? Is the return to normotension the sole requirement?

Even if they are often based on indirect evidence derived from hemodynamic studies, convincing arguments have been published showing that a reversal of the hypertensive microangiopathy can be obtained in animal models as well as in humans.

The Goteborg school first demonstrated that the structural resetting of the hindlimb vascular bed of renovascular hypertensive rats was reversed after unclipping the animals at an early stage [3]. Recent studies have shown that similar results could be obtained with antihypertensive agents both in secondary and genetic hypertension [4, 5]. Morphometric analysis of resistance vessels, i.e. branches of the mesenteric artery, provided direct evidence of regression of arteriolar hypertrophy and strongly supported the conclusions derived from the hemodynamic studies [6, 7].

Clinical investigators, also from Sweden, established that correction of the vascular abnormalities was possible in patients with essential hypertension as it was in animal models [8, 9].

In most of these studies, return to the blood pressure genetically determined for the species seemed to be a requisite for the correction of the structural abnormalities. Unloading the stressed arterial wall is apparently a most critical factor in vascular trophicity control.

Some authors have found a very significant, if not close correlation, between the degree of normotension and the subsequent correction of the structural changes [4, 6]. They concluded that the physical factors were the most important and possibly, the only factors controlling hypertrophy.

On the other hand, many studies have failed to demonstrate a significant regression of the arterial hypertrophic changes despite an effective and/or prolonged antihypertensive treatment [10, 11]. Similarly, with the same level of blood pressure reduction, different and possibly divergent responses of the structural abnormalities were observed on many occasions [5, 12]. Factors other than blood pressure, but not clearly identified and usually named 'neurohormonal trophic influences' modulate, the extent and gravity of the structural changes following antihypertensive therapy, as they do in untreated hypertension [13].

Regression of large conduits hypertrophy:
Can it be achieved? Is the return to normotension the sole requirement?

The contribution of the large arteries to the pathogenesis of hypertension was long ignored but the functional consequences of the hypertensive macroangiopathy are now largely demonstrated and increasingly acknowledged [14]. Still, not many researchers have directed their investigations to the response of the large arteries to an antihypertensive therapy, compared with the many studies devoted to the reversal of the cardiac and arteriolar changes.

Wolinsky [15] did not observe a significant regression of the aortic hypertrophy in unclipped renovascular hypertensive after 3 or even 9 months of normotension. In our laboratory, a number of antihypertensive agents were tested in Goldblatt one-kidney, one-clip rats (Figure 1). No correlation was found between blood pressure and the degree of hyperplasia of the aorta, even when treatment was begun at the early stage of hypertension [16, 17]. By contrast, in treated SHRs, we and others observed a significant relationship between the blood pressure evolution and the aortic, mesenteric or tail artery hypertrophy [18, 19]. This is the exact opposite image of what was observed on the dependence of cardiac hypertrophy on the blood pressure control. In renovascular hypertension Goldblatt two-kidneys as well as one kidney models, left ventricular mass and blood pressure generally evolved in parallel during therapy [16, 20], whereas a great number of discrepancies were noted by most investigators between the evolution of heart hypertrophy and hypertension in SHRs [21, 22].

In human hypertension, few data are available on the long-term effects of hypertensive macroangiopathy treatment. Chronic administration of nicardipine improved the buffering function of the brachial artery [23]. For a similar decrease in diastolic blood pressure, chronic enalapril therapy increased large vessels compliance, but propranolol did not [24]. Achimastos et al. [25]

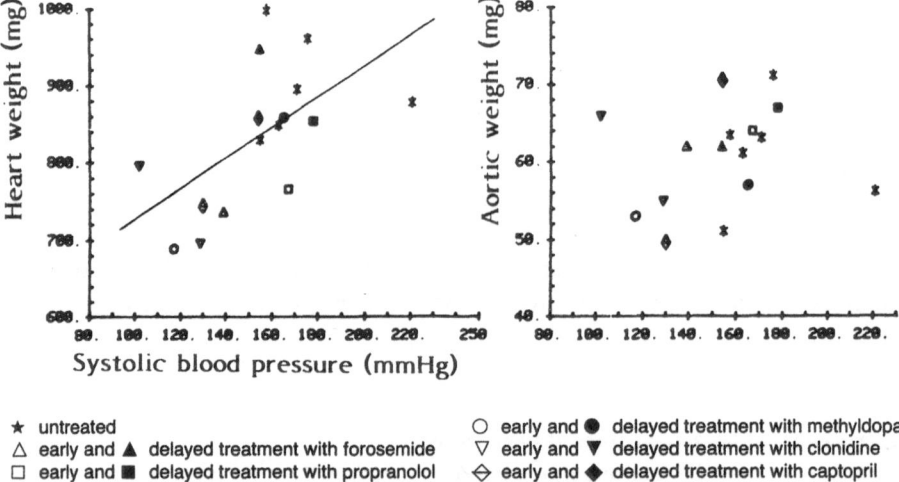

★ untreated
△ early and ▲ delayed treatment with forosemide
□ early and ■ delayed treatment with propranolol
○ early and ● delayed treatment with methyldopa
▽ early and ▼ delayed treatment with clonidine
◇ early and ◆ delayed treatment with captopril

Figure 1. Dissociated responses of heart and aorta to antihypertensive therapy in Goldblatt one-kidney, one-clip rats. Renovascular hypertensive rats were treated with furosemide, propranolol, methyldopa, clonidine or captopril for 2 weeks. Treatment was started after one week (early) or three weeks (delayed) hypertension. The degree of prevention or reversion of cardiac hypertrophy was significantly correlated with the effect of treatment on blood pressure (Heart weight = 1.84 blood pressure + 548; r = 0.57; p = 0.02). A similar relationship was not observed between aortic wet weight changes and blood pressure changes (r = 0.18; p > 0.10).

studied the effects of a 12-week treatment period by clonidine in mild and moderate hypertensive patients and did not detect any improvement in humeral artery distensibility.

Regression of the large arteries structural changes appears to be uncertain following antihypertensive therapy and, in many circumstances, poorly related to the blood pressure changes.

Smooth muscle cell hypertrophy, smooth muscle cell proliferation, fibrous proteins in arteries following an antihypertensive therapy

The global hypertrophy of the arterial wall in hypertension is the result of multiple cellular events: smooth muscle proliferation (hyperplasia and polyploidy) [26–29], cell hypertrophy [30], fibrous proteins synthesis and deposit in the extracellular matrix [30–32]. With the exception of malignant forms leading rapidly to the disruption of the arteriolar architecture, the early phases of hypertension usually respect the normal appearance of the arterial wall [31]. All the cellular components participate in the process of hypertrophy, which appears relatively homogenous. In chronic hypertension, collagen and glycosaminoglycans synthesis predominate and lead to a progressive arterial fibrosis [33]. One of the goals in hypertension treatment is a return to normal of the smooth muscle cell activity. Assuming that this objective is achieved, the return to a normal arterial trophicity will then depend on the turnover rate of the major structural proteins.

The first evidence of dissociated responses of the arterial components following an antihypertensive treatment were produced by Wolinsky [15]. Unclipping renovascular hypertensive rats made it possible to lower the aortic alcali-soluble proteins to normal values, indicating the reversal of the cellular hypertrophy. However, the collagen content remained unchanged or even increased in males after several months of normotension.

Other studies confirmed that smooth muscle cell hypertrophy is most rapidly and completely reversed among the arterial structural changes [34–37]. Extracellular deposition of fibrous proteins, mainly of collagen seems considerably more difficult to heal. A number of studies did not detect any change in arterial collagen content induced by treatment [15, 38–40]. It was however reported that collagen turnover remained high in arteries during antihypertensive treatment, allowing a progressive decrease in collagen content [41]. Moreover, we and others were able to induce long-lasting inhibition of collagen deposition in SHR arteries by an early and prolonged antihypertensive therapy [18, 42]. The intensity o this effect was directly related to blood pressure control during the treatment period and was apparently not facilitated by any of the six different antihypertensive drugs that we tested (Figure 2).

Smooth muscle cell hyperplasia seems to be the most difficult parameter to control. In the arteries of adult rats, muscle cell DNA metabolism is quiescent, as indicated by the very low labelling index after tritiated thymidine injections [26]. Arterial mitotic activity is high in two cases: during the first hours and day of acute blood pressure rise in secondary hypertension [26, 28] and at the prehypertensive phase of genetic hypertension (particularly the SHR) [33, 37]. In both cases, the intense DNA synthesis activity is a transient phenomenon. The nucleic acids metabolism returns to normal or quasi normal values in chronic hypertension and appears to be only slightly affected by an antihypertensive treatment [17, 36]. In our hands, arterial smooth muscle hyperplasia was virtually impossible to reverse. An experiment that we conducted in renovascular hypertensive rats illustrated the complete dissociation of cell hypertrophy and cell hyperplasia following a 12-week unclipping period (Figure 3). The aortic wet weight and the aortic alcali-soluble proteins content of the unclipped resumed normotensive values. By contrast, the aortic DNA content as well as the residual tritiated thymidine radioactivity injected after 4 days of hypertension, an estimate for the early DNA synthesis, was not different in the treated animals compared to the hypertensive controls [37].

Moreover, preventive administration of antihypertensive agents in prehy-

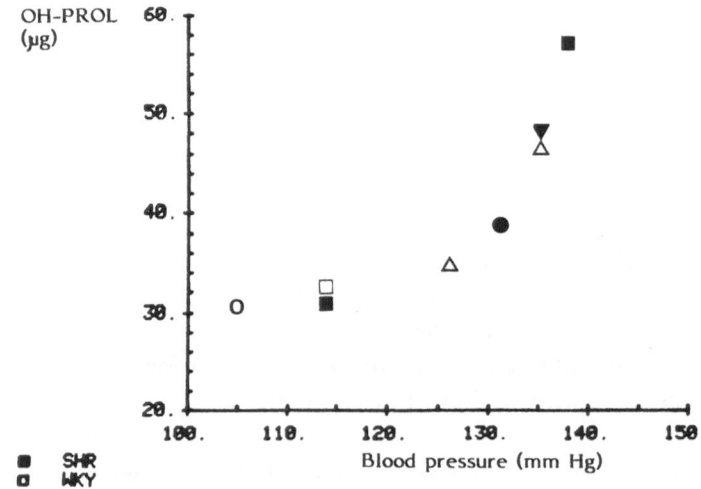

Figure 2. Long-term prevention of collagen deposition in the tail artery of spontaneously hypertensive rats. Young (3-week old) SHRs received one of the following antihypertensives for 12 weeks: methyldopa (▲), atenolol (●), hydrochlorothiazide (▼), nifedipine (△), captopril (○), and dihydralazine (▽). They were subsequently maintained without any treatment for another 12-week period. At the end of which, we noted a strong relationship between the arterial collagen content and the blood pressure during the treatment period, suggesting a long-term inhibition of collagen deposition by early and prolonged antihypertensive therapy.

pertensive SHR often had no effect on the smooth muscle cell hyperplasia that develops very early in the middle-size arteries of these animals [18]. Only methyldopa was able to prevent the early increase in DNA content, but nifedipine, captopril and hydralazine failed to despite significant inhibition of hypertension development.

Compared responses to treatment: The heart, the large arteries and the arterioles

In the natural course of hypertension, all segments of the cardiovascular system show signs of moderate to profound remodeling at one stage or another. However, there are large variations in the development of the structural changes [33]. The heterogenous installation of hypertrophy is most easily detected at the early phase of hypertension and is related to parameters such as the species, the age of the animals, the type of hypertension and the organs studied. This important characteristic is often not taken into account. This frequent underestimation of the 'polychromatism' of the structural changes helps understand why so few authors have so far studied the regression of cardiac and arterial hypertrophy in parallel.

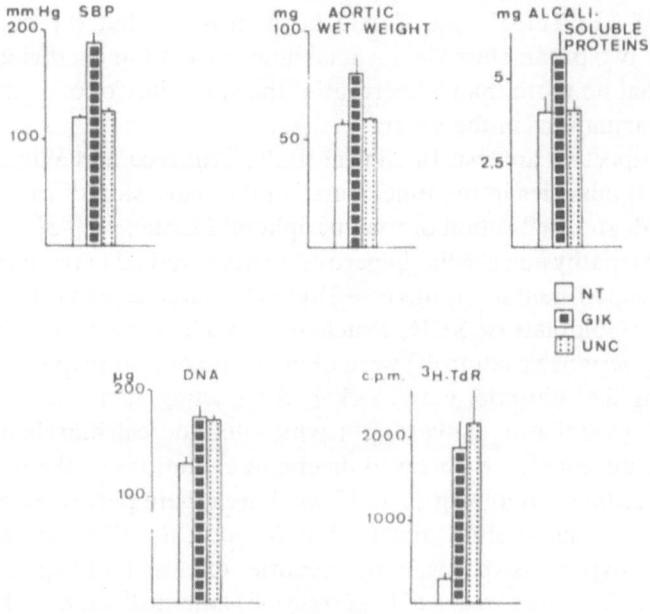

Figure 3. Persistence of the early proliferation changes in the aorta of Goldblatt one-kidney, one-clip rats following long-term unclipping. Renovascular hypertensive rats were unclipped after 3 weeks hypertension (UNC) and compared to normotensive (NT) and untreated hypertensive controls (G1K). After 12 weeks, removal of the renal clip resulted in a subtotal correction of hypertension (G1K-UNC; $p < 0.001$; UNC-NT: NS). At the same time, aortic hypertrophy, as estimated macroscopically by wet weight changes was reversed (G1K-UNC; $p < 0.01$; UNC-NT: NS). Similarly, cell hypertrophy, as determined by alcali-soluble proteins, was normalised in the UNC group (G1K-UNC: $p = 0.05$; UNC-NT: NS). However, the aortic proliferation changes were still present in the UNC group with the same intensity as in the G1K rats (DNA content: G1K-UNC: NS; UNC-NT: $p < 0.001$). The rats also had received intraperitoneal injections of tritiated thymidine (^{3}H-TdR) immediately after the onset of hypertension (day 4). The ^{3}H-TdR aortic residual activity was high and identical in the UNC and G1K rats (G1K-UNC: NS; UNC-NT: $p = 0.002$), suggesting the persistence of the early proliferation changes despite prolonged and efficient antihypertensive therapy.

Lundin et Hallback-Nordlander reported a significant correlation between the regression of cardiac hypertrophy and the normalisation of the niminum arteriolar resistance in SHR treated with several drug regimens [4]. In another study on SHRs, Sano and Tarazi found a significant correlation between the heart weight to body weight ratio and the minimum perfusion pressure in the hindlimb of the treated rats [5]. They confirmed previous histological results from Freslon and Giudicelli showing a parallelism between the morphometric changes of the heart and those of branches of the mesenteric artery [7]. The data presently available support the concept of a similar heart and microangiopathy behavior following an antihypertensive treatment. As already pointed out by Sano and Tarazi, one should keep in mind that the comparisons between the two parameters yield a maximum correlation coefficient of 0.70, indicating that no more than 50 percent of the variability of one parameter is related to fluctuations in the other.

In a retrospective analysis of clinical trials, Trimarco and Wikstrand also noted large similarities in the time-course of the regression of cardiac hypertrophy and the normalisation of total peripheral resistances [43].

Macroangiopathy and cardiac hypertrophy were studied in our laboratory in a variety of experimental settings (see Table 1). Thirty seven groups of hypertensive rats (Goldblatt or SHR, matched with adequate normotensive and untreated hypertensive controls) were treated with one antihypertensive from the following list: diuretic, beta-blocker, drug acting at the central nervous system level, vasodilator, converting enzyme inhibitor, calcium channel blocker. In many instances, we observed divergent evolutions of the aorta or tail artery and the heart following a 2 to 12-week treatment period. Left ventricle hypertrophy was successfully amended in 17 out of the 37 groups treated. In renovascular hypertensive rats, early (i.e. after one week of hypertension) or delayed (i.e. after three weeks of hypertension) administration of clonidine or propranolol, as well as early – but not delayed – treatment with methyldopa, furosemide and ticlopidine, successfully reduced cardiac hypertrophy. In spontaneously hypertensive rats, early and prolonged (i.e. begun at the age of 3 weeks for a 12-week period) administration of methyldopa, captopril, nifedipine, or hydralazine – but not of atenolol and hydrochlorothiazide – was able to prevent the development of cardiac hypertrophy. Despite a significant effect on the cardiac structural changes, the course of the hypertensive macroangiopathy was affected in only a minority (seven) of these groups. Only methyldopa and clonidine treatments had a simultaneous effect on the aortic hyperplasia in Goldblatt hypertensive rats. In SHRs, the hypertrophy of the caudal artery was prevented in the methyldopa and dihydralazine groups. In our hands, propranolol, furosemide, captopril, ticlopidine and nifedipine, which in a number of protocols efficiently reduced the ventricular mass of the treated animals, did not significantly affect the development of the large arteries lesions.

Dissociated responses of macroangiopathy and heart to antihypertensive treatments seem to be far more frequent than divergent evolutions of cardiac and arteriolar hypertrophy. There is no satisfactory explanation of this situation so far available but one must stress that the chances to heal the large arteries hypertensive lesions by a decrease in blood pressure are considerably lower than in other segments of the cardiovascular system. This might bear considerable pathological implications. The cardiovascular events whose incidence is poorly reduced by antihypertensive therapy, result from the aggravation of atherosclerosis by hypertension. As atheromas develop mainly in

Table 1. *Effect of different antihypertensive agents on blood pressure, cardiac and arterial hypertrophy in experimental hypertension.* All the experiments referred to were conducted in our laboratory on spontaneously and renovascular hypertensive rats. For each parameter, the figures represent the ratio of the successful studies (i.e. with a significant effect observed) to the total number of studies performed with each drug. -1 stands for a significant aggravation of the parameter by the treatment.

	Blood pressure	Heart hypertrophy	Arterial hypertrophy
1. Drugs altering the sympathetic system			
a) *Centrally acting*			
Methyldopa	6/7	5/7	4/7
Clonidine	3/4	3/4	1/4
b) *Postganglionic neuron blocking*			
Reserpine	1/1	—	1/1
Guanethidine	2/2	0/2	0/2
c) *β-adrenoceptor antagonist*			
Propranolol	0/2	2/2	0/2
Atenolol	1/3	0/3	1/3
d) *α-adrenoceptor antagonist*			
Prazosine	1/1	$-1/1$	0/1
2. Diuretic			
Thiazide	0/2	0/2	0/2
Furosemide	1/3	1/3	0/3
3. Vasodilator			
Hydralazine	1/1	1/1	1/1
4. Calcium antagonist			
Nifedipine	1/1	1/1	0/1
Cinnarizine	1/2	0/2	0/2
5. Converting-enzyme inhibitor			
Captopril	4/5	2/5	0/5
6. Platelet aggregation inhibitor			
Ticlopidine	3/3	2/3	0/3

large arterial conduits, the role of persistent hypertensive structural damages deserves further investigation with respect to their significance in atherogenesis. This is particularly true as far as the hypertensive smooth muscle cell hyperplasia is concerned, since smooth muscle multiplication is also a major event in atheroma formation.

Early versus late antihypertensive treatment

However controversial the definition of optimal conditions for the reversal of the arterial structural changes can be, there is general agreement on the prime importance of an early treatment. Among the first and yet most demonstrative evidence were the unclipping experiments in renovascular hypertensive rats. In this model, the removal of the renal clip after a few weeks of hypertension induced a rapid and complete normalisation of the cardiovascular design [3]. When the duration of hypertension exceeded 3months, the unclipping failed to correct the hemodynamic abnormalities and high blood pressure progressively reinstalled [44]. Similarly, drug treatments have proven to be more efficient in controlling the structural changes when administered at an early stage [34, 45].

Our own data demonstrate, at the large arteries level, the validity of the theory of the time-dependent efficacy of an antihypertensive therapy. After one week of hypertension, the unclipping of Goldblatt one-kidney, one-clip rats led to a subtotal normalisation of the aortic wall structure within the next two weeks. After three weeks of hypertension, the same procedure was then completely inefficient [16]. Still, in the same model, none of the delayed treatment protocols with methyldopa, clonidine, propranolol, furosemide, captopril or prazosin succeeded in modifying the course of the aortic wall changes. By contrast, preventive administration of methyldopa, clonidine and atenolol were able to inhibit the aortic hyperplasia [17, 37].

Monotherapy versus multiple therapy

A great number of factors have been shown to promote cardiac and arterial hyperplasia and/or hypertrophy. A non limitative list would include: physical stress, catecholamines, angiotensine, vasopressine, serotonine, platelet-derived growth factor, uremic factors, cholesterol, LDL, thrombine, STH, lymphokines, substance P, VIP, tobacco extracts.

One can easily conceive that, by giving different drugs with different modes of action, one could increase the chances of interfering with the numerous potential stimuli for hypertrophy. In accordance with this hypothesis, the most convincing evidence of an effective prevention or even correction of the arterial hypertrophy are from experimental studies where the animals were submitted to multiple therapy: clopamide, dihydroergocristine and reserpine in Grollman hypertensive rats [46], reserpine, hydrochlorothiazide and hydralazine [6, 47] or metroprolol and felodipine in SHRs [45], hydrochlorothiazide, propranolol and prazosin in dogs with aortic coarctation [48]. A better correction of hypertension in these studies cannot explain the reversal of the arterial structural changes since similar blood pressure levels can be obtained with vasodilators without benefit on arterial hypertrophy. This observation might lead to a reevaluation of the current therapeutic trend towards treatment simplification on the only basis of a better patient compliance. This attitude might have to be reconsidered with regard to the potential superiority of multiple therapy in controlling the cardiovascular structural changes.

Importance of the type of antihypertensive used for the reversal of the arterial structural changes

As mentioned above, the return to normotension cannot always guarantee a normalisation of the cardiovascular design. Other factors are likely to be involved and are, directly or indirectly, related to the mechanisms of action of the antihypertensive agents: changes in global and regional hemodynamics, drug-induced metabolic effects, interferences with trophic agents or direct pharmacological effect on the arterial wall composition.

It has long been suspected that sympathetic inhibitors are more likely to induce a regression of cardiovascular hypertrophy than other classes of anti-hypertensives.

First, the trophic role of the sympathetic system is supported by several lines of arguments: (1) catecholamines at non-pressive doses induce cardiac and arterial hypertrophy [49], (2) catecholamines stimulate cell proliferation in culture [50], (3) selective arterial denervation, without alteration in global hemodynamics, results in arterial wall atrophy [51], (4) the maturation of the sympathetic system precedes the normal blood pressure rise in weaning rats and the onset of hypertension in genetic animal models [52]. Whether the catecholamines directly stimulate protein synthesis or act indirectly through hemodynamic changes, which would be the real stimulus for hypertrophy, remains debated [13]. Recent data from our laboratory support the former hypothesis. We perfused terbutaline to paced isolated heart preparations. At a dose with no inotropic effect, the beta-2 adrenergic agonist was able to stimulate ornithine decarboxylase, an enzyme involved at the early stage of cardiac hypertrophy (Carlier et al., submitted for publication).

Secondly, an impressive number of experimental [21, 22, 37, 53–56] and clinical [57, 58] studies about the prevention or regression of the structural changes concluded to a better efficacy with the drugs that interfere with the sympathetic function.

Thirdly, in our study of the hypertensive macroangiopathy, we observed a higher incidence of large arteries responses to treatment with the agents acting at the central nervous system level (Figure 4). These results could not be accounted for by differences in antihypertensive potency of the various drug regimens.

So far, very few studies have raised the question of the mechanisms respons-ible for the superiority of the sympathetic inhibitors. Data, although not

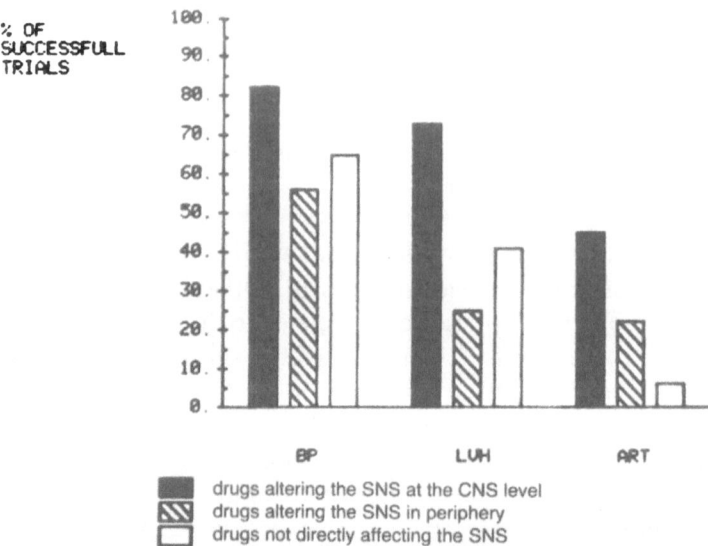

Figure 4. Comparisons of the effect of different types of antihypertensives on blood pressure (BP), cardiac (LVH) and large arteries (ART) hypertrophy. The results of the experiments performed in our laboratory are summarized according to the nature of the antihypertensive agent. As far as the aorta or tail artery hypertrophy is concerned, the drugs that act at the central nervous system level appears to be more efficient (5/11 successful trials, 45%), compared to the agents that do not interfere directly with the sympathetic function (vasodilators, diuretics, angiotensin converting enzyme inhibitor, calcium-channel blocker) (1/17; 6%).

absolutely conclusive, suggested that left ventricular mass in SHRs treated with clonidine and methyldopa did not better correlate with changes in cardiac work than with blood pressure [56], indicating that the beneficial action of these drugs was, at least partly, independent of their hemodynamical consequences. The antitrophic effect of the sympathetic inhibitors was also observed in vascular territories apparently inaffected by abnormal wall stress [59, 60]. The effect of clonidine and methyldopa was not suppressed despite simultaneous administration of phentolamine. In several instances (i.e. Table 1), drugs acting at the central nervous system yielded better results than peripheral antagonists. All these observations might reflect either a direct action of these drugs on the cardiovascular trophicity or regulatory influences exerted on mediators of the sympathetic system, other than catecholamines. There are indeed other substances cosecreted by the sympathetic neuronal endings [61]; some of them might be of prime importance in modulating the trophic action of the catecholamines. For instance, endogenous opiates are known to decrease protein synthesis in most tissues. Some antihypertensive agents might potentiate or inhibit the influences of one or several of these neurotransmitters. At the present time, this hypothesis remains pure speculation.

More recently, evidence have been accumulated showing that converting enzyme inhibitors and calcium channel blockers could also successfully treat hypertensive structural changes [62–65]. It is thought that the control of hypertrophy by captopril or enalapril is, at least partly, obtained by a diminished responsiveness to sympathetic stimuli during converting enzyme inhibition [66].

Conversely, two classes of antihypertensive agents (i.e. diuretics and vasodilators) were repetitively associated with the persistence of cardiovascular structural changes. This statement must immediately be amended: there are unquestionable reports that these agents actually did prevent or reverse cardiac and arterial hypertrophy, both in experimental and clinical settings. For example, Motz and Strauer [67] as well as our group [18] were able to prevent the development of cardiac hypertrophy by long-term dihydralazine administration to SHRs. Nevertheless, failures to maintain or obtain a normal cardiovascular design are undoubtedly more frequent with diuretics and vasodilators [10, 21, 22, 64, 68–72]. Treatment with these substances are generally accompanied by reflex activation of the renin-angiotensin-aldosterone system and increase in sympathetic activity. The two mechanisms are assumed to be responsible for the deleterious effect of these agents. Sen and Tarazi have raised the question of the relationship between blood pressure, sympathetic activity and cardiac hypertrophy during combined therapy with propranolol and hydralazine [72]. With the same blood pressure level achieved with different dosages of propranolol and hydralazine, they observed a range of left ventricular mass in the SHRs treated. There was a strong correlation between the degree of heart hypertrophy and the cardiac catecholamines content, suggesting that the cardiac response to vasodilation treatment might indeed be modulated by the level of reflex sympathetic activity.

'Anti-trophic' substances as specific treatment of the hypertensive structural changes

The relative inefficacy of the current therapeutic approaches to reverse or even prevent the hypertensive structural changes has encouraged the formulation of new strategies, aiming at more specific actions on arterial hypertrophy. There are scarce reports in the literature of a successful prevention of arterial remodeling by non-antihypertensive drugs. Schmitt et al. [73] observed a decrease in tritiated thymidine uptake, an index of cell proliferation, in arteries of renal hypertensive rats treated with cinnarizine, an antiplatelet agent. Attempts to reproduce these results using the same or similar drugs, including in our laboratory with ticlopidine and cinnarizine, generally failed [14]. Anti-tumoral agents have also been tested. Arabinoside-C, an inhibitor of DNA

transcription, given to Goldblatt one-kidney, one clip hypertensive rats immediately after surgery, inhibited the early DNA synthesis by the aorta of these
animals, and, interestingly, also delayed the blood pressure rise [75]. The
toxicity of arabinoside-C precluded any long-term study.

A more appealing approach is to interfere with the first intracellular signals
leading to hypertrophy and/or hypertrophy. The experiments aiming at the
inhibition of the polyamines synthesis illustrate this concept. The activity of
ornithine decarboxylase, the first and rate-limiting enzyme in the polyamines
synthesis (putrescine, spermidine, spermine) was found to be increased in
every modality of cardiac hypertrophy investigated so far, including the hypertensive ones [76, 77]. The blockade of the polyamines synthesis by an irreversible inhibitor of ornithine decarboxylase, difluoromethyl-ornithine, seemed of
potential interest for the control of hypertensive structural changes, as it had
proven to be for the catecholamine-induced cardiac hypertrophy. Such experiments are being conducted at Merrel Dow on SHRs (Mac Cann, personal
communication) and in our laboratory on renovascular hypertensive rats.
They have so far produced only one positive result: the prevention of the right
ventricular hypertrophy in Goldblatt one-kidney, one clip hypertension. The
association of DFMO and an antihypertensive, the vasodilator minoxidil, was
not more successful [78]. These frustrating data are puzzling because difluoromethyl-ornithine is able to block in vitro the arterial proliferations induced by
PDGF [79], a most powerful mitogen for the smooth muscle cells suspected to
promote arterial hyperplasia in renovascular hypertension.

Further investigation is needed to identify and validate other 'antitrophic'
substances as being specific therapeutic agents of cardiac and arterial hypertrophy.

Dietetic manipulations might also modulate the intensity of the structural
changes. A high-sodium diet induces or aggravates cardiac hypertrophy in
normotensive [80] as well as in hypertensive rats [81], without apparent
hemodynamic changes. Smooth muscle cells in culture proliferate more rapidly in sodium-enriched medium [82]. By contrast, potassium-enriched diet
prevented the development of aortic, renal and mesenteric arteriolar hypertrophy in SHR-SP and Dahl hypertensive rats, with minimum effect on hypertension but a strong reduction in mortality rate [83]. This most interesting
observation needs to be confirmed. Similarly, further investigation is required
into the mechanisms through which potassium inhibits the development of
hypertrophy.

Antihypertensive treatment and atherosclerosis

It was known that substances interfering with calcium metabolism, such as

EDTA, diphosphonates and lanthane, exert an antiatherosclerotic action. Recently, the possibility that clinically used calcium channel blockers might share the same property has raised enthusiasm in the scientific community. A number of experiments showed that several calcium channel blockers are able to prevent atheroma development in the aorta of cholesterol-fed rabbits [84–88]. Unfortunately, the demonstration was much less convincing in lesions developing in the coronary arteries [89] or in WHHL rabbits, with hereditary hypercholesterolemia [90, 91]. Calcium antagonists decrease cholesterol and cholesterol ester accumulation in smooth muscle cells probably by increasing arterial cholesterol esterase activity, as it was demonstrated in vitro in culltures of lipid-laden smooth muscle cells treated with nifedipine [92]. Interestingly, this enzyme activity is decreased in hypertensive animals. Other mechanisms have to be considered regarding the antiatherogenic property of the calcium channel blockers. They might prevent (1) platelet activation, (2) endothelial cell contraction and the subsequent increase in permeability, (3) LDL-glycosa-minoglycans interactions, (4) smooth muscle cell proliferation and intimal migration, (5) synthesis and secretion of connective tissue proteins by smooth muscle cells, (6) necrosis of damaged cells in fatty streaks. These events are calcium-dependent and involved in atherogenesis [93].

The beta-blockers are the other class of antihypertensive agents to which an antiatherogenic action was attributed. Hypertensive rabbits fed an atherogenic diet were protected by propranolol but not by hydralazine treatment [94]. The gravity of the atherosclerotic lesions correlated with the arterial flow disturbances induced by these drugs in hypertensive monkeys [95]. The occurrence of flow disturbances, estimated by the heart rate multiplied by the peak arterial velocity, was decreased by propranolol and increased by hydralazine. A membrane effect, independent of the beta-blocking properties, has also been proposed as an explanation of the protective effect of beta-blocking drugs.

As hypertension and atherosclerosis often develop simultaneously and exert reciprocal deleterious influences on arterial structure, preference will be given to antihypertensive agents with additional antiatherogenetic properties as soon as their efficacy is demonstrated in clinical trials. Prospective clinical studies are in progress to confirm the superiority of the calcium channel blockers preventing the cardiovascular complications of atherosclerosis [96].

Conclusions

(1) The obtention and maintenance of a normal blood pressure by anti-hypertensive therapy cannot guarantee the reversal or even the prevention of the cardiovascular structural changes. High blood pressure is a critical factor,

which has to be mastered (there are few examples of regression of hypertrophy without simultaneous correction of hypertension) but normotension is not the only criterium to fullfil. There are many situations, both clinical and experimental, in which a significant decrease in blood pressure is not associated with regression of the hypertensive structural changes. No inference should be made on the evolution of the structural changes from simple blood pressure data analysis.

(2) The earlier the treatment is started, the greater the chances to interfere with the development of cardiac and arterial hypertrophy. In this field, as in many others, preventive approach is more likely to be successful than late treatment. On the basis of this observation, the potential benefit of initiating a treatment at the earliest stage of hypertension in humans might deserve attention, as well as that of primary prevention programs at the general population level.

(3) Combinations of antihypertensive agents generally yield better results than monotherapy, probably because a greater number of trophic stimuli are inhibited by simultaneous administration of different antihypertensives.

(4) The different segments of the cardiovascular system, the heart, the large arteries, the arterioles, can evolve independently following antihypertensive therapy. There are many examples of dissociated responses of heart and microangiopathy, or heart and macroangiopathy. The structural changes in the large arteries seem the most resistant to treatment.

(5) Within one defined target, cell components also show differential responses to treatment. Usually, cardiac myocyte and smooth muscle cell hypertrophy are easily reversed. Connective tissue deposits appear considerably more difficult to control. There are, however, a number of circumstances where collagen excess was progressively resorbed or successfully prevented. Cell proliferation changes are the most resistant to treatment. In many instances, even a preventive treatment fails to inhibit smooth muscle cell hyperplasia, particularly in genetic hypertension.

(6) Among the different classes of antihypertensive agents currently available, diuretics and vasodilators *in monotherapy* often fail to induce reversion of the structural changes. The adrenergic drugs, and the more recently introduced converting enzyme inhibitors and calcium channel blockers, are more likely to act on cardiac and arterial hypertrophy.

References

1. Rose G (1987): Review of primary prevention trials. *Am Heart J* 114: 1013–1017.
2. Dahlof B (1987): The role of antihypertensive pharmacologic treatment in countering adverse pathophysiological profiles: influence on small arteries. *Am Heart J* 114: 984–991.

3. Lundgren Y, Hallback M, Weiss L, Folkow B (1974): Rate and extent of adaptative cardio-vascular changes in rats during experimental renal hypertension. *Acta Physiol Scand* 91: 103–115.

4. Lundin SA, Hallback-Nordlander MiL (1984): Regression of structural cardiovascular chan-ges by antihypertensive therapy in spontaneously hypertensive rats. *J Hypertension* 2: 11–18.

5. Sano T, Tarazi RC (1987): Differential structural responses of small resistance vessels to antihypertensive therapy. *Circulation* 75: 618–626.

6. Warshaw DM, Root DT, Halpern W (1980): Effect of antihypertensive drug therapy on the morphology and mechanisms of resistance arteries from spontaneously hypertensive rats. *Blood Vessels* 17: 257–270.

7. Freslon JL, Fiudicelli JF (1983): Compared myocardial and vascular effects of captopril and dihydralazine during hypertension development in spontaneously hypertensive rats. *Br J Pharmacol* 80: 533–543.

8. Sivertsson R, Hansson L (1976): Effects of blood pressure reduction on the structural vascular abnormality in skin and muscular beds in human essential hypertension. *Clin Sci Mol Med* 51 (suppl 3): 77s–79s.

9. Svensson A, Gudbransson T, Sivertsson R, Hansson L (1982): Haemodynamic effects of metoprolol and pindolol: a comparison in hypertensive patients. *Br J Clin Pharmacol* 13 (suppl 2): 259s–267s.

10. Jespersen LT, Nyborg NCB, Pedersen OL, Mikkelsen EO, Mulvany MJ (1985): Cardiac mass and peripheral vascular structure in hydralazine-treated spontaneously hypertensive rats. *Hypertension* 7: 734–741.

11. Hanson E, Eriksson BO, Sivertsson R (1981): Blood flow resistance in the hand after coartectomy. *Clin Physiol* 1: 257–262.

12. Sivertsson R, Andersson O, Hansson L (1979): Blood pressure reduction and vascular adaptation: a study on long-term effects of treatment with mefruside or atenolol. *Acta Med Scand* 205: 477–482.

13. Folkow B (1983): Neurotrophic effects on the vascular bed. *Acta Med Scand* suppl 672: 95–99.

14. O'Rourke MF (1985): Basic concepts for the understanding of large arteries in hypertension. *J Cardiovasc Pharmacol* 7 (suppl 2): S14–S21.

15. Wolinsky H (1971): Effects of hypertension and its reversal on the thoracic aorta of male and female rats. Morphological and chemical studies. *Circ Res* 28: 622–637.

16. Carlier PG, Rorive GL (1983): Evolution of aortic hyperplasia after reversal of renovascular hypertension in the rat. *Arch Intern Physiol Biochim* 96: 205–213.

17. Carlier PG, Rorive GL (1985): Pathogenesis and reversibility of aortic changes in experi-mental hypertension. *J Cardiovasc Pharmacol* 7 (suppl 2): S46–S51.

18. Carlier PG, Warling X, Rorive GL (1984): Prevention of the cardiovascular structural changes in the spontaneously hypertensive rat. *J Hypertension* 2: 429.

19. Owens GK (1987): Influence of blood pressure on development of aortic medial smooth muscle hypertrophy in spontaneously hypertensive rats. *Hypertension* 9: 178–187.

20. Sen S, Tarazi RC, Bumpus FM (1981): Reversal of cardiac hypertrophy in renal hypertensive rats: medical versus surgical therapy. *Am J Cardiol* 240: H 408–412.

21. Sen S, Tarazi RC, Bumpus FM (1976): Biochemical changes associated with development and reversal of cardiac hypertrophy in spontaneously hypertensive rats. *Cardiovasc Res* 10: 254–261.

22. Sen S, Tarazi RC, Bumpus FM (1977): Cardiac hypertrophy and antihypertensive therapy. *Cardiovasc Res* 11: 427–433.

23. Levenson JA, Simon AC, Bouthier JA, Maarek BC, Safar ME (1985): The effect of acute and chronic nicardipine therapy on forearm arterial haemodynamics in essential hypertension. *Br J Clin Pharmacol* 20: 107s–112s.

24. Safar ME, London GM, Safavian A, Laurent S, Pannier B (1987): Changes in arterial distensibility produced by converting enzyme inhibitors in hypertensive humans. *Clin Exper Hypertension-Theory Practice*, A9: 289–295.

25. Achimastos A, Girerd X, Simon AC, Pithois-Merli I, Levenson J (1987): The efficacy of a transdermal formulation of clonidine in mild to moderate hypertension and its effects on the arterial and venous vasculature of the forearm. *Eur J Clin Pharmacol* 33: 111–114.

26. Carlier PG, Rorive GL, Barbason H (1983): Kinetics of proliferation of rat aortic smooth muscle cells in Goldblatt one-kidney, one-clip hypertension. *Clin Sci* 65: 351–357.

27. Carlier PG, Radelet M, Montrieux C, Greimers R, Rorive G (1985): Réponse proliférative de la paroi artérielle dans l'HTA. Hyperplasie versus polyploïdie. *Arch Mal Cœur Vaisseaux* 78: 1710–1715.

28. Bevan RD, Eggena P, Hume WR, van Marthens E, Bevan JA (1980): Transient and persistent changes in rabbit blood vessels associated with maintained elevation in arterial pressure. *Hypertension* 2: 63–72.

29. Owens GK, Rabinovitch PS, Schwartz SM (1981): Smooth muscle cell hypertrophy versus hyperplasia in hypertension. *Proc Natl Acad Sci USA* 78: 7759–7763.

30. Wolinsky H (1971): Effects of hypertension on the rat aortic wall and their relation to concurrent aging changes. Morphological and chemical studies. *Circ Res* 30: 301–309.

31. Foidart JM, Rorive GL, Carlier PG, Nusgens B, Lapiere Ch, Lambotte R (1983): Hypertension expérimentale: modifications précoces du métabolisme du collagène. *Rev Méd Liège* 38: 537–59.

32. Foidart JM, Rorive GL, Nusgens BV, Lapiere CM (1978): The relationship between blood pressure and aortic collagen metabolism in renal hypertensive rats. *Clin Sci Mol Med* 55 (suppl IV): 27s–29s.

33. Rorive GL, Carlier PG, Foidart JM (1986): The structural responses of the vascular wall in experimental hypertension. In: Zanchetti A, Tarazi RC (eds), *Handbook of Hypertension*, vol 7: Pathophysiology of hypertension, pp 428–453.

34. Nakada T, Lovenberg W (1978): Lysine incorporation in vessels of spontaneously hypertensive rats: effect of adrenergic drugs. *Eur J Pharmacol* 48: 87–93.

35. Weiss L, Lundgren Y (1978): Chronic antihypertensive drug treatment in young spontaneously hypertensive rats: effects on arterial blood pressure, cardiovascular reactivity and vascular damages. *Cardiovasc Res* 12: 744–751.

36. Owens GK (1985): Differential effects of antihypertensive drug therapy on vascular smooth muscle cell hypertrophy, hyperploidy, and hyperplasia in the spontaneously hypertensive rat. *Circ Res* 56: 525–536.

37. Carlier PG (1987): Contribution expérimentale à la prévention des altératioons de structure cardiovasculaires associées à l'hypertension artérielle. Thèse de Doctorat en sciences biomédicales expérimentales, Université de Liège.

38. Ehrhart LA, Ferrario CM (191): Collagen metabolism of aortic medial hypertrophy in spontaneously hypertensive rats treated with methyldopa. *Hypertension* 3: 479–484.

39. Sen S, Bumpus FM (1979): Collagen synthesis in development and reversal of cardiac hypertrophy in spontaneously hypertensive rats. *Am J Cardiol* 44: 954–958.

40. Ruskoaho HJ, Savolainen ER (1985): Effects of long-term verapamil treatment on blood pressure, cardiac hypertrophy and collagen metabolism in spontaneously hypertensive rats. *Cardiovasc Res* 19: 355–362.

41. Udenfriend S, Cardinale G, Spector S (1981): Hypertension-induced fibrosis and its reversal by antihypertensive drugs, in: Laragh JH, Buhler FR, Seldin DW (eds), *Frontiers in Hypertension Research*, pp 404–411. New York: Springer-Verlag.

42. Oshima T, Matsushita Y, Miyamoto M, Koike H (1983): Effects on long-term blockade of

angiotension converting enzyme with captopril on blood pressure and aortic prolyl hydroxy-lase activity in spontaneously hypertensive rats. *Eur J Pharmacol* 91: 283–286.

43. Trimarco B, Wikstrand J (1984): Regression of cardiovascular structural changes by anti-hypertensive therapy. *Hypertension* 6 (suppl III): III 150–158.

44. Lundgren Y, Weiss L (1979): Cardiovascular design after 'reversal' of long-standing renal hypertension in rats. *Clin Sci* 57: 19–23.

45. Nordborg C (1987): The influence of antihypertensive treatment on the renal arterial struc-ture in spontaneously hypertensive rats. A morphometric study. *Clin Exper Hypertension-Theory and Pract* A9: 1567–1584.

46. Griffith R, Hummel R (1973): Prévention des lésions vasculaires du rat hypertendu. *Triangle* 12: 75–82.

47. Limas C, Westrum B, Limas CJ (1983): Effect of antihypertensive therapy on the vascular changes in the spontaneously hypertensive rat. *Am J Pathol* 111: 380–393.

48. Uhari M, Reinila A, Tarkka M (1983): Prevention of morpholigical changes in great arteries in coarctation of the aorta with antihypertensive therapy. *Br J Exp Pathol* 64: 191–197.

49. Laks MM, Morady F, Swan HJC (1973): Myocardial hypertrophy produced by chronic infusion of subhypertensive doses of norepinephrine in the dog. *Chest* 64: 75–78.

50. Blaes N, Boissel JP (1983): Growth stimulation effect of catecholamines on rat aortic smooth muscle cells in culture. *J Cell Physiol* 116: 167–172.

51. Bevan RD (1975): Effect of sympathetic denervation on smooth muscle cell proliferation in growing rabbit ear artery. *Circ Res* 37: 14–19.

52. Scott TM, Pang SC (1983): The correlation between the development of sympathetic inner-vation and the development of medial hypertrophy in normotensive and spontaneously hypertensive rats. *J Autonomic Nerv Syst* 8: 25–32.

53. Tomanek RJ, Davis JW, Anderson SC (1979): The effects of alpha-methyldopa on cardiac hypertrophy in SHR. *Cardiovasc Res* 13: 173–182.

54. Tomanek RJ (1982): Selective effects of alphamethyldopa on myocardial cell components independent of cell size in normotensive and genetically hypertensive rats. *Hypertension* 4: 499–506.

55. Yamori Y, Nakada T, Lovenberg W (1976): Effects of antihypertensive therapy and lysine incorporation into vascular proteins of the spontaneously hyperttensive rat. *Eur J Pharmacol* 38: 349–355.

56. Pegram BL, Ishise S, Frohlich ED (1982): Effect of methyldopa, clonidine and hydralazine on cardiac mass and hemodynamics in Wistar Kyoto and spontaneously hypertensive rats. *Cardiovasc Res* 16: 40–46.

57. Corea L, Bentivoglio M, Verdecchia P (1981): Reversal of left ventricular hypertrophy in essential ypertension by early and long-term treatment with methyldopa. *Clin Trials J* 18: 380–394.

58. Drayer JIM, Gardin JM, Weber MA, Aronow WS (1982): Changes in cardiac anatomy and function during therapy with alphamethyldopa: an echocardiographic study. *Curr Ther Res* 32: 856–865.

59. Greenberg S (1981): Effect of chronic administration of clonidine, propranolol and al-phamethyldopa on extensibility and biochemical properties of the veins in renal and sponta-neous hypertension. *J Pharmacol Exp Ther* 218: 779–790.

60. Greenberg S, Wilborn W (1982): Effect of clonidine and propranolol on venous smooth muscle from spontaneously hypertensive rats. *Arch Int Pharmacodyn* 258: 234–244.

61. Potter DD, Furshpan EJ, Landis SC (1983): Transmitter status in cultured rat sympathetic neurons: plasticity and multiple function. *Fed Proc* 42: 1626–1632.

62. Sen S, Tarazi RC, Bumpus FM (1980): Effect of converting enzyme inhibitor on cardiac hypertrophy in SHR. *Hypertension* 2: 169–176.

63. Kazda S, Stasch JP, Hirth C (1987): Nitrendipine in experimental hypertension: effects on cardiac hypertrophy, heart failure and atrial natriuretic peptides. *J Cardiovasc Pharmacol* 9 (suppl 4): S90–S95.

64. Prasquier R, Dufloux MA, Chatellier G, Plouin PF, Menard D, Corvol P, Menard J (1987): Comparaison de l'effet du captopril et du minoxidil sur la masse ventriculaire gauche. *Arch Mal Cœur Vaisseaux* 80: 911–918.

65. Kobrin I, Sesoko S, Pegram B, Frohlich ED (1984): Reduced cardiac mass by nitrendipine is dissociated from systemic or regional haemodynamic changes in rats. *Cardiovasc Res* 18: 158–162.

66. Antonaccio MJ, Kerwin L (1981): Pre- and postjunctional inhibition of vascular sympathetic function by captopril in SHR: implication of vascular angiotensin II in hypertension and antihypertensive actions of captopril. *Hypertension* 3 (suppl I): I 54–62.

67. Motz W, Strauer BE (1985): Regression of cardiac hypertrophy after therapy in animal hypertension. *J Cardiovasc Pharmacol* 7 (suppl 2): S56–S61.

68. Fenje P, Leenen FHH (1985): Effects of minoxidil on blood pressure and cardiac hypertrophy in two-kidney, one-clip hypertensive rats. *Can J Physiol Pharmacol* 63: 161–164.

69. Tomanek RJ, Wangler RD, Bauer CA (1985): Prevention of coronary vasodilator reserve decrement in spontaneously hypertensive rats. *Hypertension* 7: 533–540.

70. Drayer JIM, Gardin JM, Weber MA, Aronow WS (1983): Changes in cardiac muscle mass during vasodilation therapy of hypertension. *Clin Pharmacol Ther* 33: 727–732.

71. Drayer JIM, Gardin JM, Weber MA, Aronow WS (1983): Changes in ventricular septal thickness during diuretic therapy. *Clin Pharmacol Ther* 32: 283–288.

72. Sen S, Tarazi RC (1983): Regression of myocardial hypertrophy and influence of adrenergic system. *Am J Physiol* 244: H 97–101.

73. Schmitt G, Skrobek R, Hauss WK (1974): Uber die Wirkung von Cinnarizin (Stutgeron) auf die hochdrukbedingt Zell Proliferation in Herz und Aorta in Tierexperiment. *Med Welt* 25: 1096–1103.

74. Carlier PG, Rorive GL (1984): Pathogenesis of aortic hyperplasia in renovascular hypertensive rat: effect of chemical sympathectomy, platelet aggregation and renin-angiotensin blockade. *Mol Physiol* 6: 265–276.

75. Loeb AL, Mandel H, Straw JA, Bean BL (1986): Increased aortic DNA synthesis precedes renal hypertension in rats. An obligatory step? *Hypertension* 8: 754–761.

76. Mathy C, Carlier P, Yerna N, Rorive G (1987): Polyamines et hypertrophie cardiovasculaire dans l'hypertension expérimentale. *Arch Mal Cœur Vaisseaux* 80: 777–782.

77. Ruskoaho H, Raunio H (1987): Altered cardiac polyamine biosynthesis in spontaneously hypertensive rats. *Am J Physiol* 253: H262–269.

78. Carlier P, Smelten N, Yerna N, Rorive GL (1988): Can an 'anti-trophic' agent (DFMO) improve the control of the cardiovascular structural changes during antihypertensive therapy? *Clin Exper Hypertension* (in press).

79. Tytberg J, Fredholm B (1987): Induction of ornithine decarboxylase activity and putrscine synthesis in arterial smooth muscle cells stimulated with platelet-derived growth factor. *Exp Cell Res* 170: 160–169.

80. Kihara M, Utagawa N, Mano M, Nara Y, Horie R, Yamori Y (1985): Biochemical aspects of salt-induced, pressure-independent left ventricular hypertrophy in rats. *Heart and Vessels* 1: 212–215.

81. Lindpaintner K, Sen S (1985): Role of sodium in hypertensive cardiac hypertrophy. *Circ Res* 57: 610–617.

82. Yamori Y, Igawa T, Tagami M, Kanbe T, Nara Y, Kihara M, Horie R (1984): Humoral trophic influence on cardiovascular structural changes in hypertension. *Hypertension* 6 (suppl III): IIII 27–32.

83. Tobian L (1987): High-potassium diets prevent stroke death, brain hemorrhages and infarcts, artery hypertrophy, and renal disease in hypertensive rats, even though blood pressure is not lowered. *J Cardiovasc Pharmacol* 9 (suppl 4): S38–S48.

84. Henry PD, Bentley KI (1981): Suppression of atherogenesis in cholesterol-fed rabbits treated with nifedipine. *J Clin Invest* 68: 1366–1369.

85. Betz E, Hammerle H, Strohschneider T (1985): Inhibition of smooth muscle cell proliferation and endothelial permeability with flunarizine in vitro and in experimental atheromas. *Res Exp Med* 185: 325–340.

86. Blumlein SL, Sievers R, Kidd P, Parmley WW (1984): Mechanism of protection from atherosclerosis by verapamil in the cholesterol-fed rabbit. *Am J Cardiol* 54: 884–889.

87. Rouleau J, Parmley WW, Steven J, Wikman-Coffert J, Sievers R, Mahley RW, Havel RJ (1983): Verapamil suppresses atherosclerosis in cholesterol-fed rabbits. *J Am Coll Cardiol* 1: 1453–1466.

88. Willis AL, Nagel B, Churchill V, Whyte MA, Smith DL, Mahmud I, Puppione DL (1985): Antiatherosclerotic effects of nicardipine and nifedipine in cholesterol-fed rabbits. *Arteriosclerosis* 5: 250–255.

89. Ginsburg R, Davis K, Bristow M, McKennett K, Kodsi S, Billingham ME, Schroeder JS (1983): Calcium antagonists suppress atherogenesis in aorta but not in the intramural arteries of cholesterol-fed rabbits. *Lab Invest* 49: 154–158.

90. Tilton GD, Buja L, Bilheimer DW, Apprill P, Ashton J, MacNatt J, Kita T, Willerson JT (1985): Failure of a slow channel calcium antagonist, verapamil, to retard atherosclerosis in the Watanabe Heritable Hyperlipidemic Rabbit: an animal model of familial hypercholesterolemia. *J Am Coll Cardiol* 6: 141–144.

91. Van Niekerk JLM, Hendriks T, De Boer HHM, van 't Laar (1984): Does nifedipine suppress atherogenesis in WHHL rabbits? *Atherosclerosis* 53: 91–98.

92. Etingin OR, Hajjar DP (1985): Nifedipine increases cholesteryl hydrolytic activity in lipid-laden rabbit arterial smooth muscle cells. A possible mechanism for its antiatherogenic effect. *J Clin Invest* 75: 1554–1558.

93. Henry PD (1985): Atherosclerosis, calcium, and calcium antagonists. *Circulation* 72: 456–459.

94. Spence JD, Perkins DG, Kline RL, Adams MA, Haust MD (1983): Hemodynamic modification of aortic atherosclerosis: effects of propranolol vs hydralazine in hypertensive hyperlipemic rabbits. *Atherosclerosis* 50: 325–333.

95. Spence JD, Pesout J, Melmont KL (1977): Effects of antihypertensive drugs on blood velocity in Rhesus monkeys. *Stroke* 8: 589–594.

96. Hugenholtz PG, Lichtlen P, van der Giessen W, Becker AE, Nayler WG, Fleckenstein A, Hulsmann (1986): On a possible role for calcium antagonists in atherosclerosis. A personal view. *Eur Heart J* 7: 546–559.

CONCLUSION

36. The heart in hypertension: mechanical and humoral factors

J.I.S. ROBERTSON and W.H. BIRKENHÄGER

This chapter will focus on the interaction between mechanical and humoral factors in cardiac involvement in hypertension. Advances of knowledge in both of these areas have been spectacular in recent years, such progress resulting in large measure from the perceptive and imaginative research of the late Robert Tarazi. The momentum achieved will surely be sustained, indeed almost certainly increased, in the near future.

A most pressing need in the field of hypertension is an understanding of why, despite striking therapeutic success in treating or preventing many of the complications of hypertension, including hypertensive heart failure, we have made little impression on hypertension-related coronary artery disease and its consequences (Robertson 1987). We shall herein attempt, inter alia, to find some leads towards remedying this therapeutic deficiency.

The heart as a cause of hypertension

The notion that the heart could be the prime mover in the pathogenesis of essential hypertension has been extensively considered over the past 20 years (Birkenhäger, de Leeuw & Schalekamp 1982). Particularly attractive features in this connection have been the findings of increased heart rate with elevated cardiac output in young subjects with mild elevation of systemic arterial pressure. It has been speculated that these features could have their origin in heightened sympathetic nervous activity, possibly associated with systemic venous constriction leading to a relative increase in central blood volume. Enhanced tissue perfusion resulting from these causes might, by a process of autoregulation, proceed to increased peripheral resistance and more sustained blood pressure elevation, the characteristic features of established essential hypertension.

M.E. Safar & F. Fouad-Tarazi (eds.), The heart in hypertension.
© *1989 Kluwer Academic Publishers, Dordrecht –*

Despite the attractions, there are difficulties in the ready acceptance of these concepts. First, only a few studies have been performed in hypertensive subjects who were unaware of their diagnosis; in such cases cardiac output was not found to be increased. This raises the possibility that where cardiac output and heart rate were found to be elevated, these features may have resulted from introspection and anxiety rather than comprising intrinsic pathogenic mechanisms in the evolution of hypertensive disease. Second, subjects with a high cardiac output exhibit a proportional elevation of total oxygen consumption. Thus so-called 'luxury perfusion', a pre-condition for autoregulation, is lacking. Third, autoregulation is an almost instantaneous phenomenon; it provides an uncomfortable basis therefore for the supposedly gradual transition from high cardiac output to high peripheral resistance in the evolution of essential hypertension. Fourth, no evidence has been found of increased urinary excretion of adrenaline or noradrenaline, and thus of enhanced sympathetic activity, in untreated mildly hypertensive subjects (Brown et al. 1985).

Thus while the notion remains extent that a primary cardiac abnormality may initiate a series of events leading to established essential hypertension, the evidence at present is inconclusive and in many respects insecure.

Hypertension as a cause of cardiac hypertrophy

It has been remarkably difficult to establish whether the progressive ventricular hypertrophy which accompanies systemic hypertension is a straightforward result of the increased afterload, or whether, at least in part, both the hypertension and the myocardial hypertrophy are consequent upon neurohumoral influences (Östman-Smith 1981; Tarazi 1986; Fouad-Tarazi 1987).

The predominant involvement of the left ventricle in such hypertrophic changes, and their progression with advancing hypertension, point to a pre-eminent influence of mechanical factors. However, the presence often of distinct echocardiographic signs of left ventricular enlargement even in very mild hypertension has been taken by some workers to indicate that both phenomena drive from a common cause or causes, rather than that the hypertension leads simply to ventricular hypertrophy.

The argument has not been resolved by recourse to study in genetically hypertensive strains of rat. In newborn spontaneously hypertensive rats, left ventricular weight is often already increased, suggesting that hypertension and hypertrophy share a common pathogenetic pathway, rather than being linked in series. However, interpretation is not easy (Sokade 1979). Even though the arterial pressure of newborn spontaneously hypertensive rats may lie within the overall normal range, the average value is increased in comparison with control animals. Such minor elevation of blood pressure could have led to left ventricular hypertrophy in the rat, as indeed may also have been the case in mild hypertension in man.

Evidence on these tissues derived from intact animals is inevitably clouded because the effects of ventricular loading and other influences, such as autonomic activity, cannot be disentangled. Korner (Korner 1983) succeeded in standardizing external conditions in dogs with renovascular hypertension and a 50% increase in left ventricular weight together with matched control animals. Increasing the preload by elevating left atrial pressure, while maintaining heart rate and mean arterial pressure constant, resulted in a rise in intrinsic myocardial contractility ((dP/dt)max) in both groups, but more so in the hypertensive animals. When left atrial pressure was kept steady in the face of varying afterload, similar differences in myocardial contractility were observed. The ((dP/dt)max) on average was 28% higher in the hypertensive animals over a broad range of diastolic pressures (60–120 mmHg). Thus, in hypertensive dogs, studied under controlled conditions, myocardial hypertrophy went with an amplification of myocardial contractility in response to given pre- or afterloads. This amplifying factor was closely related to the degree of hypertrophy. Similar findings have been reported on pump function in that stroke volume increased more in hypertensive than in normotensive animals when filling pressure was increased, while mean arterial pressure and heart rate were kept constant (Korner 1983). These results suggest that hypertrophy is a straightforward response to the increase in 'true' afterload, i.e. the increase in isovolumetric wall stress in hypertension. The key observation is that the degree of left ventricular wall thickening almost exactly mirrors and offsets the increase in wall stress which would otherwise have occurred. This could be a strong point in favour of the basis for left ventricular hypertrophy in hypertension being purely mechanical.

Possible trophic factors other than systemic hypertension

Some of the arguments in favour of the left ventricular hypertrophy in hypertension being a consequence simply of an increased ventricular afterload have been set out in the preceding paragraph. The reasoning has appeared nevertheless inconclusive to some workers (Tarazi 1986; Fouad-Tarazi 1987). It has been argued for example that a neurohumoral factor could balance a given level of hypertension against a particular degree of hypertrophy because of an ancillary trophic property residing in that factor. Numerous putative trophins, demonstrable or speculative, have been considered in this context (Robertson and Ball 1989). Two avenues especially have been of interest: the possible role of the sympathetic nervous system and catecholamines; and the renin-angiotensin system. Re (1984), Dzau (1988), and Jin et al. (1988) amongst others have provided evidence that cardiac myocytes can synthesize renin, and that a paracrine or intracrine action of angiotensin II within the myocardium could be involved in ventricular hypertrophy. Any such trophins or their effects are not necessarily confined to the heart. Arterial myocytes might also synthesize and/or respond to these various agents. We shall discuss the vascular, as distinct from the cardiac, aspects, later.

Pursuing a related line, Skinner and colleagues (1986) showed that in man inactive renin underwent 58% extraction in one passage through the coronary circulation. They consider that circulating inactive renin could be a cardiotropic hormone.

One most fruitful approach in attempting to distinguish between mechanical and chemical trophic factors in left ventricular hypertrophy is to employ antihypertensive drugs which lower blood pressure to similar extents, but which have differential effects on the putative trophic factors. Tarazi and his colleagues, exploring this route produced much evidence in favour of the existence of chemical myocardial trophins (Tarazi 1986; Fouad-Tarazi 1987).

Histological and biochemical accompaniments of myocardial hypertrophy

The phenomena accompanying the cardiac adaptation to systemic hypertension have been studied at several levels, from muscle weight and bulk, through the size and composition of myocardial tissues, cells and organelles, down to molecular biochemistry. The myocardial hypertrophy is characterized by an enlargement of individual myocytes without an increase in their number. This is preceded by biochemical processes which occur very rapidly. There is an increase in ribonucleic acid and in mitochondrial proteins, shortly followed by increased myosin adenosine triphosphatase activity and myosin concentration (Wikman-Coffelt 1986; Sleight and Zanchetti 1988).

In experimental renal hypertension in various laboratory animals a rise in the ratio of left ventricular weight to body weight may be seen within days or weeks of an increase in systemic arterial pressure. A functionally critical feature of left ventricular hypertrophy in hypertension is a progressive loss of adrenoceptor numbers. Thus ventricular responses become increasingly dependent on the Frank-Starling mechanism rather than on neurohumoral factors (Fouad-Tarazi 1987).

Functional consequences of left ventricular hypertrophy in hypertension in man

In essential hypertension in man, (Tarazi 1986; Fouad-Tarazi 1987; Katz 1987,

1988; Laragh 1988) the morphological pattern of the cardiac accompaniments of the raised arterial pressure are initially harmonious and largely advantageous. There is a thickening of the left ventricular wall and septum, an unchanged or slightly diminished left ventricular volume, and elongation of the outflow tract.

The concentrically hypertrophied left ventricle goes on to manifest diminished compliance, and diastolic pressure is elevated even at a normal ventricular volume. Left ventricular filling is universally related to left ventricular bulk in hypertension. Because, as has been mentioned, the hypertensive heart is very dependent on the Frank-Starling mechanism, the diminished ventricular compliance ('negative lusitrophy') is a potent source of functional impairment (Katz 1987, 1988; Fouad-Tarazi 1987). Its correction should be a major aim of antihypertensive drug therapy.

Coronary artery filling is greatest during diastole; thus the diminished ventricular compliance, with its adverse effects on diastolic intramyocardial tension, will impede coronary blood flow. Consequently the subendocardial layers of the ventricle become chronically ischaemic (Katz 1987; Strauer 1988). Because the ability of the myocardium to extract oxygen from blood at diminished coronary blood flow is very limited (Strandgaard and Haunsoe 1987), myocardial ischaemia is compounded.

To these very prevalent developments in hypertension can be added often the problems accompanying atheromatous coronary artery stenosis.

Supervention of the malignant phase, with frequently high circulating concentrations of renin and hence angiotensin II, can additionally lead to angiotensin II induced multifocal myocardial necrosis. The malignant phase can further cause coronary arteriolar fibrinoid lesions (Gavras et al. 1975; Robertson and Ball 1989).

Given this pathophysiological sequence, it is hardly surprising that in the days before the availability of antihypertensive drugs, cardiac failure was one of the most frequent complications of hypertension. Even today, it remains clear that left ventricular hypertrophy in hypertension is associated with an increased prevalence of ventricular arrhythmias and carries a poor prognosis (Laragh 1988; Strauer 1988; Robertson and Ball 1989).

Structural vascular changes in hypertension

This paper has so far concentrated on the changes in cardiac, and mainly left ventricular, structure accompanying the progression of systemic hypertension. The cardiac changes proceed together with hypertrophy in the wall of both large and resistance arteries. Indeed, the cardiac and arterial changes may share both mechanical and chemical trophic stimuli.

The structural modifications in smaller resistance arteries and arterioles have long been recognized as contributing, through their geometrical consequences, to a disproportionate increase in peripheral vascular resistance, and thus as critically reinforcing the progression of hypertension (Falkow et al. 1983).

In the larger arteries, loss of compliance causes a diminution in their capability to dampen the pulsatile systolic blood flow impelled by the left ventricle (Safar et al. 1987). In the larger arteries also, hyper-responsiveness to vasoconstrictor stimuli can be demonstrated.

These several pathophysiological arterial changes clearly possess, as do those afflicting the heart, important implications for the progression and adverse consequences of hypertension, and for its therapy.

While the origins of the arterial and arteriolar changes in hypertension are close to those involving the heart, the vascular and cardiac changes, both before and during antihypertensive therapy, do not always proceed in close parallel. There are several possible explanations for the divergences. There are potentially important biochemical and morphological differences between cardiac myocytes and arteriolar smooth muscle; local growth factors may not be equally prominent or equally effective in the heart and peripheral vessels; while sympathetic nervous activity and hormonal systems such as atrial peptides and the renin-angiotensin axis are unlikely to be similarly active, at all levels (Tarazi 1986; Fouad-Tarazi 1987).

The renin and atrial peptide systems in hypertension

We shall be concerned here with the endocrine aspects of the renin and atrial natriuretic peptide systems in hypertension. The intracrine and paracrine functions of renin, and its possible trophic influence, have already been discussed.

The renin-angiotensin and atrial peptide systems can be regarded as counterpoised against each other, the former to protect the organism against salt and water depletion and hypotension; the latter to deal with fluid overload (Robertson and Richards 1987). In normal man, there is a clear inverse correlation between concurrent measurements of plasma active renin concentration and atrial natriuretic peptide (Richards et al. 1988). Plasma concentrations of renin have also been found to be inversely correlated with arterial pressure in untreated essential hypertension. Because body sodium content likewise rises with arterial pressure in essential hypertension, it might be supposed that such sodium retention would be the proximate cause of the fall in plasma renin (Beretta-Piccoli et al. 1982). However, this seems unlikely, because no correlation has been found between plasma renin and either total exchangeable or total body sodium in essential hypertension. A more likely explanation of the progressive fall in plasma renin is loss of compliance and hence of sensitivity to vascular stimuli in the wall of the afferent renal arterioles responsible for sensing and transmitting signals for renin release from the kidney (Swales 1975). If correct, this latter hypothesis would represent a special instance of the arterial involvement in hypertension already discussed. In untreated essential hypertension, it is usually only with the advent of certain complications, such as the malignant phase, or hypertensive heart failure, that plasma renin and angiotensin II are increased (Robertson and Ball 1989).

Plasma atrial natriuretic peptide, in contrast, is elevated, and significantly correlated positively with arterial pressure, in untreated essential hypertension (Montorsi et al. 1987). So far as we are aware, no mathematical exploration of the relationship between body sodium content and plasma atrial natriuretic peptide concentrations has yet been made in this condition, although, as both rise together, they could be correlated. Significantly higher values of atrial natriuretic peptide have been found in hypertensive patients with evidence of left ventricular hypertrophy than in those without (Montorsi et al. 1987).

Many patients with left ventricular hypertrophy and hypertension have moreover been seen to have plasma atrial natriuretic peptide levels above the normal range. Because atrial distention is the strongest candidate as the principal stimulus to atrial peptide secretion (Richards et al. 1986), it seems likely that the elevation of atrial natriuretic peptide in essential hypertension reflects the functional cardiac consequences of left ventricular hypertrophy which we have already discussed in some detail.

With the onset of cardiac failure, the inverse relationship between plasma concentrations of renin and of atrial natriuretic peptide which is characteristic of normal subjects and those with untreated and uncomplicated essential hypertension is lost. Renin and atrial natriuretic peptide are increased together in cardiac failure, and are then weakly, but significantly, positively correlated (Richards et al. 1988; Robertson and Richards 1988). The rise in plasma atrial peptide is almost certainly a consequence of an increase in atrial pressure, and is directed to protecting the organism against water and sodium overload. The increase in plasma renin is probably due mainly to circulatory changes within the kidney, which are an early feature of heart failure. A major, and crucially important effect of increased intrarenal renin, and hence of angiotensin II in heart failure, is a preservation of glomerular filtration rate and of urea excretion despite the fall in renal blood flow (Brown et al. 1970; Robertson and Richards 1988). That such intrarenal compensatory effects of the renin-angiotensin system are necessarily accompanied by less desirable features of elevated circulating angiotensin II, such as stimulation of secretion of aldosterone and vasopressin, and peripheral arteriolar constriction, are of secondary importance to the organism, but assume critical therapeutic consequences.

Cardiac and arterial structural changes in hypertension: therapeutic implications

One potentially powerful method of distinguishing between mechanical factors and other trophic influences on vascular and cardiac structural changes is the assessment of differential effects of various antihypertensive drugs. Tarazi and his colleagues have excelled in pursuing these aspects (Tarazi 1986; Fouad-Tarazi 1987). They showed that, in spontaneously hypertensive rats, methyldopa caused a substantial reduction in left ventricular weight, while hydralazine failed to do so, and minoxidil actually increased cardiac hypertrophy, despite similar reductions in blood pressure. A possible explanation offered was that these drugs, with widely differing effects on sympathetic drive, had unmasked a cardiotrophic effect of catecholamines. This notion was held to be further supported by the subsequent finding that propranolol diminished myocardial hypertrophy without measurably affecting blood pressure. These concepts have subsequently been widely explored both clinically and in the laboratory. Sympatholytics, including reserpine as well as methyldopa, have been confirmed as leading to regression of left ventricular hypertrophy. Similar reduction of left ventricular hypertrophy has been seen with converting enzyme inhibitors, calcium antagonists and the serotonin antagonist ketanserin (Fouad-Tarazi 1987; Meulemans et al. 1987).

Notwithstanding the studies with propranolol mentioned above, the effect of classical beta-adrenoceptor blockers on regression of clinical left ventricular hypertrophy remains controversial, as also is that of diuretics. Alpha-adrenoceptor blockers such as trimazosin seem not to be effective in this respect.

Attention has, rightly, not been confined simply to structural properties of the left ventricle. Ventricular lusitropy and filling rate, aspects of major importance for cardiac function, do not necessarily change in direct proportion to regression of ventricular hypertrophy (Katz 1987, 1988). Fouad-Tarazi (1987) has stated that consistent improvement in diastolic function could not be demonstrated in man during long-term treatment of hypertension with diuretics, classical beta-blockers, or calcium antagonists. Early evidence suggests that the new drug nebivolol may however possess the capacity to benefit diastolic function in hypertension (De Crée et al. 1988).

It has been repeatedly emphasized that hypertrophy in the wall of resistance arteries may both progress and, with treatment, regress, independently of left ventricular hypertrophy (Fouad-Tarazi 1987). Nevertheless, the outcome of therapy on such vascular hypertrophy has, for obvious reasons, been extensively examined. In this area also, hydralazine is largely ineffective, while, by contrast, diuretics and converting enzyme inhibitors do lead to regression of hypertrophic changes.

The potentially beneficial effects of antihypertensive drugs which enhance compliance in the walls of large arteries has, as has been discussed above, been increasingly recognised. There is evidence that cardiac hypertrophy is related to the decrease in aortic distensibility, independently of arterial vascular resistance. Thus, it is implied, improvement in arterial compliance is important in the reversion of left ventricular hypertrophy (Safar et al. 1987).

Hydralazine, and classical beta-blockers such as propranolol, have little effect in man in improving arterial compliance when employed in the treatment of hypertension. By contrast, converting enzyme inhibitors and the recently-introduced nebivolol increase arterial compliance (Safar et al. 1987; Van Merode et al. 1988). Almost certainly such improvement is not due simply to structural change; the speed with which compliance increases for example with nebivolol, clearly implies an important functional component.

The consequences of therapeutic remodelling and thus of both structural and functional improvements in the myocardium and arterial walls should include benefits in blood flow velocity and turbulence patterns (Spence 1982; 1986). Again, there should follow less tendency to atherogenesis and its consequences.

Conclusions

The undoubted success of antihypertensive drug therapy in preventing or controlling the malignant phase, hypertensive hart failure, stroke and renal failure, while creditable, leaves no room for complacency. Present treatment is obtrusively unsatisfactory in limiting hypertension-associated coronary artery disease and its consequences. In this brief article we have attempted to perceive some of the reasons for this therapeutic failure. We have directed attention to the myocardium, the coronary circulation, and to both large and small peripheral arteries. It is our view that the development and deployment of antihypertensive drugs with actions which also correct structural and functional abnormalities in these tissues offer a most fruitful therapeutic prospect.

References

Beretta-Piccoli C, Davies DL, Boddy K, Brown JJ, Cumming AMM, East BW, Fraser R, Lever AF, Padfield PL, Semple PF, Robertson JIS, Weidmann P, Williams ED (1982): Relation of arterial pressure with body sodium, body potassium and plasma potassium in essential hypertension. *Clinical Science* 63: 257–270.

Birkenhäger WH, de Leeuw PW, Schalekamp MADH (1982): *Control mechanisms in essential hypertension*. 2nd Edition Chapter 2, pp. 31–64. Elsevier Biomedical Press, Amsterdam, New York, Oxford.

Brown JJ, Davies DL, Johnson VW, Lever AF, Robertson JIS (1970): Renin relationship in congestive cardiac failure, treated and untreated. *Am Ht J* 80: 329–342.

Brown MJ, Causon RC, Barnes VF, Brennan GB, Greenberg G (1985): Urinary catecholamines in essential hypertension: results of 24-hour urine catecholamine analysis from patients in the Medical Research Council Trial for mild hypertension and matched controls. *Anart J Med* 57: 637–645.

De Crée J, Van Rooy P, Geukens H, Haeverans K, Verhaegen H (1988): Double-blind placebo controlled studies of nebivolol in patients with essential hypertension. *In: Proceedings, 'Cardiovascular Disease and β-Adrenoceptor Function'*. Antwerp, p. 20.

Dzau VJ (1988): Cardiac renin-angiotensin system: molecular and functional aspects. *Am J Med* 84 (3A): 22–27.

Folkow B, Hansson L, Sivertsson R (1983): Structural vascular factors in the pathogenesis of hypertension. In: JIS Robertson (ed), *Handbook of Hypertension, Volume I: Clinical Aspects of Essential Hypertension*. Elsevier, Amsterdam pp. 133–150.

Fouad-Tarazi FM (1987): Structural cardiac and vascular changes in hypertension: Response to treatment. *Current Opinion in Cardiology* 2: 782–786.

Gavras HP, Kremer D, Brown JJ, Gray B, MacAdam RE, Medina A, Morton JJ, Robertson JIS (1975): Angiotensin- and norepinephrine-induced myocardial lesions: experimental and clinical studies in rabbits and man. *Am Ht J*.

Jin M, Wilhelm MJ, Lang RE, Unger T, Lindpaintner K, Ganten D (1988): Endogenous tissue renin-angiotensin system: From molecular biology to therapy. *Am J Med* 84 (3A): 28–36.

Katz AM (1987): A physiologic approach to the treatment of heart failure. *Hospital Practice* 22: 117–148.

Katz AM (1988): Influence of altered inotropy and lusitropy on ventricular pressure-volume loops. *J Amer Coll Cardiol* 11: 438–445.

Korner PI (1983): The role of the heart in hypertension. In: JIS Robertson (ed), *Handbook of Hypertension, Volume I: Clinical Aspects of Essential Hypertension*. Elsevier, Amsterdam, pp. 97–132.

Laragh JH (1988): Cardiac pathophysiology and its heterogenecity in patients with established hypertensive disease: the first Robert C Tarazi Lecture. *Am J Med* 84 (suppl 3A): 3–11.

Meulemans AL, De Clerck NM, Brutsaert DL (1987): Effects of ketanserin, captopril and alinidine on cellular cardiac hypertrophy in spontaneously hypertensive rats. *Acta Cardiol* 42: 365–366.

Montorsi P, Tonolo G, Polonia G, Hepburn D, Richards AM (1987): Correlates of plasma arterial natriuretic peptide in health and hypertension. *Hypertension* 10: 570–576.

Östman-Smith I (1981): Cardiac sympathetic nerves as the final common pathway in the induction of adaptive cardiac hypertrophy. *Clinical Science* 61: 265.

Re RN (1984): Cellular biology of the renin-angiotensin systems. *Arch Int Med* 144: 2037–2041.

Richards AM, Cleland JGF, Tonolo G, McIntyre GD, Leckie BJ, Dargie HJ, Ball SG, Robertson JIS (1986): Plasma α-natriuretic peptide in cardiac impairment. *Brit Med J* 293: 409–412.

Richards AM, Tonolo G, Tree M, Robertson JIS, Montorsi P, Leckie BJ, Polonia J (1988): Atrial natriuretic peptides and renin release. *Am J Med* 84 (3A): 112–118.

Robertson JIS (1987): Hypertension and coronary risk: possible adverse effects of antihypertensive drugs. *Am Ht J* 114: S1051–1054.

Robertson JIS, Ball SG (1989): In: Julian DG, Camm J, Poole-Wilson PW, Fox K (eds), *Hypertension in Diseases of the Heart.* Butterworths, London (in press).

Robertson JIS, Richards AM (1988): Cardiac failure, the kidney, renin and atrial peptides. *Europ Ht J* 9 (suppl H): 11–14.

Robertson JIS, Richards AM (1987): Converting enzyme inhibitors and renal function in cardiac failure. *Kidney Int* 31 (suppl 2): 216–219.

Safar ME, Pannier BM, Soubies PL, Laurent S, Safavian A, London GM (1987): Intrinsic alterations of the arterial wall in hypertension and the effect of antihypertensive therapy. *Current Opinion in Cardiology* 2 (suppl 1): 26–32.

Skinner SL, Thatcher RL, Whitworth JA, Horowitz JD (1986): Extraction of plasma protein by human heart. *Lancet* 1986/1: 995–997.

Sleight P, Zanchetti A (eds) (1988): The renin-angiotensin system and the heart. *Am J Med* 84 (3A): 1–162.

Sokade H (1979): Proceedings, III International Symposium on the spontaneously hypertensive rat and related studies. *Japanese Heart Journal* 20 (suppl 1).

Spence JD (1986): Antihypertensive therapy and atherosclerosis. In: Rapaport E (ed), *Cardiology Update.* Elsevier, New York, pp. 137–155.

Spence JD (1984): Hemodynamic effects of anti-hypertensive drugs: possible implications for the prevention of atherosclerosis. *Hypertension* 6 (suppl III): 163–168.

Strandgaard S, Haunso S (1987): Why does antihypertensive treatment prevent stroke but not myocardial infarction? *Lancet* 1987/2: 658–660.

Strauer BE (1988): Coronary hemodynamics in hypertensive heart disease: basic concepts, clinical consequences, and experimental analysis of regression of hypertensive microantiopathy. *Am J Med* 84 (3A): 45–54.

Swales JD (1975): Low-renin hypertension: nephrosclerosis? *Lancet* 1975/1: 75–77.

Tarazi RC (1986): Cardiovascular hypertrophy in hypertension. *Hypertension* 8 (suppl 2): 187–190.

Van Merode T, Van Bortel L, Smeets F, Reneman R (1988): Effect of nebivolol on the vessel wall properties of the carotid artery in hypertensive patients. In: *Proceedings, 'Cardiovascular Disease and β-Adrenoceptor Function'.* Antwerp, p. 24.

Wikman-Coffelt J (1986): Biochemical regulation of myocardial hypertrophy. In: A. Zanchetti, RC Tarazi (eds), *Handbook of Hypertension.* Pathophysiology of hypertension; Cardiovascular aspects. Elsevier Amsterdam 7: 25–52.

Developments in Cardiovascular Medicine

1. Ch.T. Lancée (ed.): *Echocardiology*. 1979   ISBN 90–247–2209–8
2. J. Baan, A.C. Arntzenius and E.L. Yellin (eds.): *Cardiac Dynamics*. 1980
           ISBN 90–247–2212–8
3. H.J.Th. Thalen and C.C. Meere (eds.): *Fundamentals of Cardiac Pacing*. 1979
           ISBN 90–247–2245–4
4. H.E. Kulbertus and H.J.J. Wellens (eds.): *Sudden Death*. 1980   ISBN 90–247–2290–X
5. L.S. Dreifus and A.N. Brest (eds.): *Clinical Applications of Cardiovascular Drugs*.
    1980   ISBN 90–247–2295–0
6. M.P. Spencer and J.M. Reid: *Cerebrovascular Evaluation with Doppler Ultrasound*.
    With contributions by E.C. Brockenbrough, R.S. Reneman, G.I. Thomas and D.L.
    Davis. 1981   ISBN 90–247–2384–1
7. D.P. Zipes, J.C. Bailey and V. Elharrar (eds.): *The Slow Inward Current and Cardiac
    Arrhythmias*. 1980   ISBN 90–247–2380–9
8. H. Kesteloot and J.V. Joossens (eds.): *Epidemiology of Arterial Blood Pressure*. 1980
           ISBN 90–247–2386–8
9. F.J.Th. Wackers (ed.): *Thallium-201 and Technetium-99m-Pyrophosphate. Myocar-
    dial Imaging in the Coronary Care Unit*. 1980   ISBN 90–247–2396–5
10. A. Maseri, C. Marchesi, S. Chierchia and M.G. Trivella (eds.): *Coronary Care Units*.
    Proceedings of a European Seminar, held in Pisa, Italy (1978). 1981
           ISBN 90–247–2456–2
11. J. Morganroth, E.N. Moore, L.S. Dreifus and E.L. Michelson (eds.): *The Evaluation of
    New Antiarrhythmic Drugs*. Proceedings of the First Symposium on New Drugs and
    Devices, held in Philadelphia, Pa., U.S.A. (1980). 1981   ISBN 90–247–2474–0
12. P. Alboni: *Intraventricular Conduction Disturbances*. 1981   ISBN 90–247–2483–X
13. H. Rijsterborgh (ed.): *Echocardiology*. 1981   ISBN 90–247–2491–0
14. G.S. Wagner (ed.): *Myocardial Infarction*. Measurement and Intervention. 1982
           ISBN 90–247–2513–5
15. R.S. Meltzer and J. Roelandt (eds.): *Contrast Echocardiography*. 1982
           ISBN 90–247–2531–3
16. A. Amery, R. Fagard, P. Lijnen and J. Staessen (eds.): *Hypertensive Cardiovascular
    Disease*. Pathophysiology and Treatment. 1982   IBSN 90–247–2534–8
17. L.N. Bouman and H.J. Jongsma (eds.): *Cardiac Rate and Rhythm*. Physiological,
    Morphological and Developmental Aspects. 1982   ISBN 90–247–2626–3
18. J. Morganroth and E.N. Moore (eds.): *The Evaluation of Beta Blocker and Calcium
    Antagonist Drugs*. Proceedings of the 2nd Symposium on New Drugs and Devices,
    held in Philadelphia, Pa., U.S.A. (1981). 1982   ISBN 90–247–2642–5
19. M.B. Rosenbaum and M.V. Elizari (eds.): *Frontiers of Cardiac Electrophysiology*.
    1983   ISBN 90–247–2663–8
20. J. Roelandt and P.G. Hugenholtz (eds.): *Long-term Ambulatory Electrocardiography*.
    1982   ISBN 90–247–2664–6
21. A.A.J. Adgey (ed.): *Acute Phase of Ischemic Heart Disease and Myocardial
    Infarction*. 1982   ISBN 90–247–2675–1
22. P. Hanrath, W. Bleifeld and J. Souquet (eds.): *Cardiovascular Diagnosis by
    Ultrasound*. Transesophageal, Computerized, Contrast, Doppler Echocardiography.
    1982   ISBN 90–247–2692–1

Developments in Cardiovascular Medicine

Developments in Cardiovascular Medicine

43. S. Sideman and R. Beyar (eds.): [3-D] *Simulation and Imaging of the Cardiac System.* State of the Heart. Proceedings of the International Henry Goldberg Workshop, held in Haifa, Israel (1984). 1985   ISBN 0–89838–687–X
44. E. van der Wall and K.I. Lie (eds.): *Recent Views on Hypertrophic Cardiomyopathy.* Proceedings of a Symposium, held in Groningen, The Netherlands (1984). 1985
ISBN 0–89838–694–2
45. R.E. Beamish, P.K. Singal and N.S. Dhalla (eds.), *Stress and Heart Disease.* Proceedings of a International Symposium, held in Winnipeg, Canada, 1984 (Vol. 1). 1985   ISBN 0–89838–709–4
46. R.E. Beamish, V. Panagia and N.S. Dhalla (eds.): *Pathogenesis of Stress-induced Heart Disease.* Proceedings of a International Symposium, held in Winnipeg, Canada, 1984 (Vol. 2). 1985   ISBN 0–89838–710–8
47. J. Morganroth and E.N. Moore (eds.): *Cardiac Arrhythmias.* New Therapeutic Drugs and Devices. Proceedings of the 5th Symposium on New Drugs and Devices, held in Philadelphia, Pa., U.S.A. (1984). 1985   ISBN 0–89838–716–7
48. P. Mathes (ed.): *Secondary Prevention in Coronary Artery Disease and Myocardial Infarction.* 1985   ISBN 0–89838–736–1
49. H.L. Stone and W.B. Weglicki (eds.): *Pathobiology of Cardiovascular Injury.* Proceedings of the 6th Annual Meeting of the American Section of the I.S.H.R., held in Oklahoma City, Okla., U.S.A. (1984). 1985   ISBN 0–89838–743–4
50. J. Meyer, R. Erbel and H.J. Rupprecht (eds.): *Improvement of Myocardial Perfusion.* Thrombolysis, Angioplasty, Bypass Surgery. Proceedings of a Symposium, held in Mainz, F.R.G. (1984). 1985   ISBN 0–89838–748–5
51. J.H.C. Reiber, P.W. Serruys and C.J. Slager (eds.): *Quantitative Coronary and Left Ventricular Cineangiography.* Methodology and Clinical Applications. 1986
ISBN 0–89838–760–4
52. R.H. Fagard and I.E. Bekaert (eds.): *Sports Cardiology.* Exercise in Health and Cardiovascular Disease. Proceedings from an International Conference, held in Knokke, Belgium (1985). 1986   ISBN 0–89838–782–5
53. J.H.C. Reiber and P.W. Serruys (eds.): *State of the Art in Quantitative Cornary Arteriography.* 1986   ISBN 0–89838–804–X
54. J. Roelandt (ed.): *Color Doppler Flow Imaging and Other Advances in Doppler Echocardiography.* 1986   ISBN 0–89838–806–6
55. E.E. van der Wall (ed.): *Noninvasive Imaging of Cardiac Metabolism.* Single Photon Scintigraphy, Positron Emission Tomography and Nuclear Magnetic Resonance. 1987
ISBN 0–89838–812–0
56. J. Liebman, R. Plonsey and Y. Rudy (eds.): *Pediatric and Fundamental Electrocardiography.* 1987   ISBN 0–89838–815–5
57. H.H. Hilger, V. Hombach and W.J. Rashkind (eds.), *Invasive Cardiovascular Therapy.* Proceedings of an International Symposium, held in Cologne, F.R.G. (1985). 1987   ISBN 0–89838–818–X
58. P.W. Serruys and G.T. Meester (eds.): *Coronary Angioplasty.* A Controlled Model for Ischemia. 1986   ISBN 0–89838–819–8
59. J.E. Tooke and L.H. Smaje (eds.): *Clinical Investigation of the Microcirculation.* Proceedings of an International Meeting, held in London, U.K. (1985). 1987
ISBN 0–89838–833–3

Developments in Cardiovascular Medicine

Developments in Cardiovascular Medicine

Developments in Cardiovascular Medicine

100. J. Morganroth and E.N. Moore (eds.): *Risk/Benefit Analysis for the Use and Approval of Thrombolytic, Antiarrhythmic, and Hypolipidemic Agents.* Proceedings of the 9th Annual Symposium on New Drugs and Devices (1988). (forthcoming)
ISBN 0–7923–0294–X

101. P.W. Serruys, R. Simon and K.J. Beatt (eds.): *PCTA – An Investigation Tool and a Non-operative Treatment of Acute Ischemia.* 1990   ISBN 0–7923–0346–6

102. I.S. Anand, P.I. Wahi and N.S. Dhalla (eds.): *Pathophysiology and Pharmacology of Heart Disease.* 1990 (forthcoming)   ISBN 0–7923–0367–9

103. G.S. Abela (ed.): *Lasers in Cardiovascular Medicine and Surgery.* Fundamentals and Technique. 1990 (forthcoming)   ISBN 0–7923–0440–3

104. H.M. Piper (ed.): *Pathology of Severe Ischemic Myocardial Injury.* 1990 (forthcoming)   ISBN 0–7923–0459–4

105. S.M. Teague (ed.): *Stress Doppler Echocardiography.* 1990 (forthcoming)
ISBN 0–7923–0499–3

106. P.R. Saxena, D.I. Wallis, W. Wouters and P. Bevan (eds.): *Cardiovascular Pharmacology of 5-Hydroxytryptamine.* Prospective Therapeutic Applications. 1990 (forthcoming)   ISBN 0–7923–0502–7

107. A.P. Shepherd and P.A. Öberg (eds.): *Laser-Doppler Blood Flowmetry.* 1990 (forthcoming)   ISBN 0–7923–0508–6